Women, violence and social change

Women, Violence and Social Change demonstrates how refuges and shelters stand as the core of the battered women's movement, providing a basis for pragmatic support, political action and radical renewal. From this base, movements in Britain and the United States have challenged the police, courts and social services to provide greater assistance to women.

Well-known for their research on violence against women and as the authors of the acclaimed book *Violence against Wives*, Rebecca and Russell Dobash provide important evidence on the way social movements can successfully challenge institutions of the state, as well as salutary lessons on the nature of diverted and thwarted struggles. The Dobashes analyse the development of new therapeutic approaches aimed at abused women and violent men, and show how these have detracted from efforts to assist women and end violence. They show how differing national research agendas have affected the identification and definition of the problem of violence against women and, in some cases, have actually hampered efforts to assist abused women and challenge male violence.

Women, Violence and Social Change is unique among books about violence against women. By focusing on the dynamic relationship between the battered women's movement and the state, the Dobashes highlight the complexity and contradictions of efforts to achieve social change. This scholarly and timely book provides revealing insights into the process of achieving positive changes for women.

R. Emerson Dobash and Russell P. Dobash teach in the School of Social and Administrative Studies, University of Wales College of Cardiff and are Co-Directors of the Institute for the Study of Violence.

Women, violence and social change

R. Emerson Dobash
and Russell P. Dobash

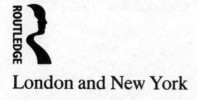

London and New York

First published in 1992
by Routledge
11 New Fetter Lane, London EC4P 4EE

Simultaneously published in the USA and Canada
by Routledge
a division of Routledge, Chapman and Hall Inc.
29 West 35th Street, New York, NY 10001

Typeset from authors' disk by Leaper & Gard Ltd, Bristol, England
Printed and bound in Great Britain by
Mackays of Chatham plc, Chatham, Kent

British Library Cataloguing in Publication Data
Dobash, R. Emerson (Rebecca Emerson) *1943-*
   Women, violence and social change.
   1. Families. Violence
   I. Title
   362.8292

Library of Congress Cataloging in Publication Data
Dobash, R. Emerson.
   Women, violence and social change / R. Emerson Dobash and Russell
   P. Dobash.
   p.   cm.
   Includes bibliographical references and index.
   1. Abused women – Services for – Great Britain. 2. Abused women –
   Services for – United States. 3. Abused women – Government policy –
   Great Britain. 4. Abused women – Government policy – United States.
   5. Women's shelters – Great Britain. 6. Women's shelters – United
   States. I. Dobash, Russell. II. Title.
   HV1448.G7D63   1992   91-14397
   362.82'928'0941–dc20   CIP

ISBN 0–415–02921–X (hbk)
ISBN 0–415–03610–0 (pbk)

HV
1448.G7
D632
1992

For our parents

Helen and Ike
Helen and Paul

Contents

Acknowledgements

In many ways this book began several years ago when we first started researching violence against women. In working with activists from Britain and the United States, we have been impressed by their dedication, commitment and skills, and by the movements they have created in order to deal with this problem. In *Women, Violence and Social Change* we have focused on the battered-women's movements in Britain and the United States and the innovations that have resulted from their struggles for change. As activist researchers, we support the goals of providing safety, shelter and autonomy for abused women, and of working to eliminate violence against women, yet we have attempted to conduct a critical evaluation of these developments in both countries.

We owe an inestimable debt to people in both countries. In compiling information for this book we benefited from discussions and interviews with activists, advocates, academics and representatives of various agencies. We would like to thank: Susan Schechter, Sharon Vaughan, Fran Wasoff, Alison Mackay, Ellen Pence, Michael Paymar, Hamish Sinclair, Donna Garske, Mary Pat Brygger, Barbara Hart, Laurie Woods, David Adams, Esta Solar, Sue Martin, Del Martin, Gail Sullivan, Mary Jane Cronin, Cheryl Howard, Annette Van Dyck, Margo Wilson and Martin Daly. For commenting on various chapters, we are grateful to Susan Schechter, Sharon Vaughan, Donna Garske, Ellen Pence, Michael Paymar, Jeff Edelson and David Adams. We are particularly grateful to Marjorie Fields who read and commented on the entire manuscript and provided invaluable reference materials.

Newsletters of Scottish Women's Aid, Welsh Women's Aid, National Women's Aid England, the National Center of Women and Family Law in New York City and the Center for Women Policy Studies in Washington DC have provided an invaluable source of information about developments in Britain and the USA.

We began working on this book while we were visiting scholars at the Rockefeller Center, Belliago, Italy. A period of research at the Institute for the Study of Social Change at the University of California, Berkeley, enabled us to gather materials on developments in the United States. The Carnegie Trust for Scotland provided partial support for travel in the United States in order to interview activists and government officials.

Abbreviations

ART	Activist Research Task Force
CEASE	Community Effort for Abused Spouses
CETA	Concentrated Employment and Training Act
CJ (S)	criminal justice (system)
CTS	Conflict Tactics Scale
DAIP	Domestic Abuse Intervention Project
DSS	Department of Social Services
FV	Family Violence
FVP	Family Violence Project (San Francisco)
HEW	Department of Health, Education and Welfare
HHS	Health and Human Services
HUD	Housing and Urban Development
LEAA	Law Enforcement and Assistance Administration
NCADV	National Coalition Against Domestic Violence
NIMH	National Institute of Mental Health
NOW	National Organization of Women
NWAF	National Women's Aid Federation
R and D	research and demonstration
USCCR	United States Commission on Civil Rights
VAW	violence against women
VOCA	Victims of Crime Act
WAFE	Women's Aid Federation England

1 Violence against women

For the women who have been physically abused in the home by the men with whom they live, the past two decades have seen both radical change and no change at all. The lives of some have been touched by an ever expanding, worldwide movement to support women who have been battered and to challenge male violence. Some legal and social institutions have begun to respond, while others remain in a nexus of traditional tolerance of male violence and indifference to those who suffer from such violence. This is a time marked by social change and resistance to change, by innovation and reassertion of tradition. Both the new and the old responses are used, challenged and defended by those with differing views about the nature of this problem and how best to confront it. The arena of change and challenge is alive with ideas and activity.

Increasingly, women who have been abused come forward for support in directly challenging the violence or organizing their escape from it. Although relatively few violent men are being confronted with the unacceptability of their violence and their responsibility for its elimination, the numbers are growing. The fact that this occurs at all is due almost solely to the efforts of the battered-women's movement in bringing the issue to public attention and organizing a pragmatic response to assisting women based on a wider philosophy of feminist inspired change. The story of the development of these innovative changes covers individual terror and personal triumph as well as institutional action and reaction. It is a story of one of the important social movements of our time. It is about deeply held cultural beliefs, entrenched patterns of response and the struggle to move away from supporting male violence and towards its rejection. It is a story that is at once personal and institutional, local and international, depressing and inspirational.

In many countries it is now well known that violence in the home is commonplace, that women are its usual victims and men its usual perpetrators.[1] It is also known that the family is filled with many different forms of violence and oppression, including physical, sexual and emotional, and that violence is perpetrated on young and old alike. It is the battered-women's movement, with the support of the media, who have put the issues of the physical and sexual abuse of women and girls firmly on the social agenda. The now familiar stories of personal pain and degradation fill out the statistics with human dimensions and make the social facts comprehensible. For some, familiarity with accounts of violence breeds indifference and inaction; for others they bring indignation and a call for action.

Although the stories may now be familiar, they still remain both painful and powerful. For women who have been attacked, there is a litany of abuses from repeated assaults to rape and murder. In the 1970s the stories at once described what were then unfamiliar accounts of abuse, and informed a disbelieving public of its wide-spread nature. Women's accounts revealed the nature of men's violence and the sources of conflict leading to attacks. They also described women's emotions and reactions as well as the inaction of social and legal institutions. The words of only a few of the millions of women who have been abused describe the nature of the violence ranging from slapping and shoving to brutal assaults and sometimes murder:

> I have had glasses thrown at me. I have been kicked in the abdomen when I was visibly pregnant. I have been kicked off the bed and hit while lying on the floor – again, while I was pregnant. I have been whipped, kicked and thrown, picked up again and thrown down again. I have been punched and kicked in the head, chest, face, and abdomen more times than I can count.[2] (American woman)

> It was punching, banging my head on walls. Kicking everything.[3] (Northern Irish woman)

> He tried to strangle me last night. I was terrified. I did manage to get out of the house but I had to go back the next morning. You see it was Easter weekend and my two children were afraid the Easter Bunny wouldn't come if mummy and daddy were fighting.[4] (Canadian woman)

> He once used a stick, he hit me once with a big fibreglass fishing pole, six foot long. And he just went woosh, he gave me such a

wallop with that. I had a mark ... right down my back. I thought
my back had broke.[5] (Scottish woman)

He'd kick me or hit me on the back of the head (so it wouldn't
show). He raped me once, then smashed me in the face.[6]
(Northern Irish woman)

He used to bang my head against the wall or the floor. I finally left
him when I thought he was trying to kill me.[7] (English woman)

The injuries inflicted during these attacks range from cuts and bruises
to broken bones, miscarriages and permanent damage. Again, women
from numerous countries recount similar incidents and report a full
range of injuries:

I wasn't badly hurt. My ear was bruised and my hair was pulled
out.[8]

Punching, I had my nose broken, ribs broken, two black eyes – he
dragged me out of bed by the hair and pulled me along the ground.
He smashed the door of my parent's house down when I was there.[9]

Each one got harder and harder ... one time he hit me so hard on
the back of the head he broke his own hand.[10]

The elbow was all lying open, the top of my legs was lying open ...
gashes all over.[11]

I had treatment for a fractured skull and I lost a child in a mis-
carriage due to violence.[12]

The effect upon women's physical and emotional state is frequently
recorded:

[The worst aspects of the experience of battering are]: Feeling so
ill and tired after the beatings, and so useless, I couldn't face
people with the marks on my body.[13]

I was always terrified. My nerves were getting the better of me....
He knew this and I think he loved this.[14]

The fear of not knowing what he would do – I feared for my life.[15]

I remember the tension of becoming aware that I had to notice
what I was saying all the time, to make sure I didn't offend him. I
had become afraid of him.[16]

Was he going to scare me all my life? Was he going to punch me in
the head and knock me out and I'd die?[17]

The sources of conflict leading to violent events reveal a great deal about the nature of relations between men and women, demands and expectations of wives, the prerogatives and power of husbands, and cultural beliefs that support individual attitudes of marital inequality:

> I realized I was under terrible strain the whole time ... I'd go into a blind panic about what side the spoon had to be on. It was that sort of detail everyday.[18]

> There was too much grease on his breakfast plate and he threw his plate at me.[19]

> I had a poker thrown at me – just because his tea was too weak – he just takes it for granted, if you're married you'll have to accept it. It's part of being a wife.[20]

> And then he had his belt and I was whipped over the shoulders everywhere, on my face and everything. And this was to teach me not to argue with him.[21]

> He would stay out all night and become violent when questioned.[22]

The four main sources of conflict leading to violent attacks are men's possessiveness and jealousy, men's expectations concerning women's domestic work, men's sense of the right to punish 'their' women for perceived wrongdoing, and the importance to men of maintaining or exercising their position of authority.[23] For many women, a sense of shame and responsibility, along with fear of reprisals, keeps them silent, sometimes for years. The US National Crime survey of domestic violence cases from 1978 to 1982 found that 48 per cent were not reported to the police (because it was viewed as a private matter or because of fear of reprisal).[24] An Irish woman who went to a refuge after twenty years of violence, explains her silence:

> I hid what was happening to me from everyone. I made excuses for my bruises and marks. I thought I should put up with it ... accept my lot as being part of marriage ... I wanted to keep it hidden.[25]

It should be noted that in the same US survey 52 per cent of women did report the violence to the police because they hoped this would prevent further incidents.[26] The problem of women's reluctance to report men's violence is often exacerbated by social, medical and legal institutions whose actions reveal a powerful legacy of policies and practices that explicitly or implicitly accept or ignore male violence and/or blame the victim and make her responsible for its solution and elimination.[27]

By the late 1980s, public accounts had chipped away at persistent images of the violence as a problem confined to the working class, ethnic groups or the poor. The United States was rocked by revelations that John Fedders, one of President Reagan's high ranking legal officials, had beaten his wife for eighteen years.[28] The image of the perfect marriage of a member of the Washington establishment was crushed in the account of a daily life of repeated attacks. Insult and further injustice were added to injury when the courts awarded him a percentage of the royalties from the book she wrote about the relationship on the grounds that she could not have written the book had he not made it possible by abusing her.[29]

Equally as sensational and as destructive of myths of middle-class immunity was the trial of a wealthy, Jewish, New York lawyer for the murder of his adopted daughter in what has been described as a vast inventory of abuse and intimidation also directed at his female partner, a well educated, Jewish editor of children's books:

> The 6th Precinct officers were so shocked by Hedda's condition that they videotaped her, lumps of hair missing, clusters of small scabs on the bare scalp – were they cigarette burns? Deep ulcers on gangrenous legs. A bruise on the buttock the size of a football. Bruises on her back. A pulverised nose. Jaw broken in two places. Nine broken ribs, a cauliflower ear, a split lip ... a ruptured spleen, removed in hospital, a broken knee, a bruised neck and innumerable black eyes – 10 in one year – and after her arrest doctors discovered minor brain damage.[30]

The case became sensational not so much because of the violence itself but because it took place in an affluent home. Controversy increased when he was found guilty of manslaughter rather than murder because the use of cocaine may have meant he was not completely aware of his actions. There was even more controversy about the responsibility of a seriously abused woman for stopping her abuser from also abusing their child.[31] The case fuelled a new wave of interest in domestic violence in the United States, added some new dilemmas and brought a new twist to victim blaming.

With repeated male violence, death sometimes occurs. In one case, a retired vicar from the affluent south of England 'bludgeoned his wife to death' over two hours when he had trouble with radio reception. At the end, his son, who lived in an adjoining house, heard him shout 'Are you dead yet?'. It was reported that the 74 year old vicar 'was "arrogant and self-centred with an explosive temper" and had previously beaten his 85 year old wife during their forty-six year marriage'.[32] The claim of diminished responsibility was used to reduce the charge from murder to manslaughter and the judge initially stated he intended to put the Reverend on three years probation to be spent in a Benedictine Abbey. The Abbot later decided the Vicar was medically unsuited for their facility.[33]

Stories of death are more sensational and therefore more likely to be reported in the press, but they often reflect the final event following a history of male violence not deemed sufficiently important or dramatic to appear in print or in police statistics. The ultimate victim of domestic homicide may, of course, be either the woman or the man. When the woman dies, it is usually the final and most extreme form of violence at the hands of her male partner. When the man dies, it is rarely the final act in a relationship in which she has repeatedly beaten him. Instead, it is often an act of self-defence or a reaction to a history of the man's repeated attacks.[34] No matter who dies, the antecedent is often a history of repeated male violence, not of repeated female violence. This is a common pattern known in the United States at least since the 1950s,[35] and one that continues today. The following Scottish case illustrates many features common to cases in which men kill wives and female partners:

> Mary Khelifati was murdered ... by her violent husband. She had been rehoused [after a stay in a refuge] ..., but her husband had traced her to her new address. By this stage, Mary was convinced that the end was near. Her solicitor had achieved everything possible on her behalf [an exclusion order and an interdict (injunction)] but the danger had not lessened. Khelifati stabbed Mary to death in front of their six year old daughter. At his trial ..., the jury unanimously found him guilty of murder, and he was sentenced to life imprisonment. Press coverage of the trial focused on Khelifati's defence claim that Mary had said she would take the child abroad and he would never see her again.... No mention was made of his continual violence and threats towards Mary, nor of her attempts to escape from him. Even after her brutal death, Mary's life of hell was being trivialized and her suffering negated.[36]

Some abused women think about escaping violence by killing their male abuser or themselves, and some actually do so:

> And we had this great big carving knife downstairs and I used to go upstairs and stand there with it and think 'If I stick it in him – will I get done for murder?' And sometimes if he threw me out I used to go and get three or four bottles of aspirins and go into a cafe and think 'Get myself a couple of cups of tea – take all these

and the problem's solved – all this will be finished with'. But there was always [my son] to consider, I used to think if I leave [my son] with him what's he going to grow up like – twisted – like his dad.[37]

In their comprehensive and scholarly examination of homicide in many countries, Daly and Wilson strongly support the idea that it is men's sexual jealousy and possessiveness, or proprietary rights, that lead to spousal homicide, be it committed by the man or the woman. They conclude that:

> In every society for which we have been able to find a sample of spousal homicides, the story is basically the same: Most cases arise out of the husband's jealous, proprietary, violent responses to his wife's (real or imagined) infidelity or desertion.[38]

They cite evidence from industrial and primitive societies. In spousal homicides, sexual proprietariness (jealousy and attempts to stop a wife's desertion) was cited in 81 per cent of cases in a 1955 study in Baltimore, Maryland,[39] while a 1980 study in Virginia noted this factor in nearly every case excluding those with diagnosed psychiatric disorders.[40] Peter Chimbos found a similar pattern in his 1978 Canadian study of convicted men and women.[41] Daly and Wilson note that:

> Men ... strive to control women, albeit with variable success; women struggle to resist coercion and to maintain their choices. There is brinksmanship and risk of disaster in any such contest, and homicides by spouses of either sex may be considered the slips in this dangerous game.[42]

Chimbos notes that one of the most important single findings from his Canadian study is that spousal homicide 'is rarely a sudden explosion in a blissful marriage' but is based on the situation at the time and on a history of quarrels, usually about sexual jealousy and possessiveness.[43] It was the 'endpoint' in a series of conflicts, and 70 per cent reported prior assaults.[44] He also found that apart from stabbing (38 per cent) and firearms (30 per cent), 32 per cent of the killings he studied were the result of beating, always by men, who can use their body and strength as tools for killing.[45] In another study of spousal homicide in Florida, it was found that 73 per cent of the women who killed reported that they had previously been beaten by their partner,[46] while in Totman's the rate was 93 per cent.[47] Zimring and his colleagues have referred to this as the 'female use of lethal counterforce'.[48]

As stated earlier, the dynamics are usually very different when women kill their husband or male partner. It is usually a response to years of male violence and not a culmination of years of female violence. The following letter from a battered woman who killed her husband reveals some of these dynamics.

I was used and abused, battered stupid and nearly strangled. I passed out, had hair torn out of my head. I was actually pulled along the street by my hair. I've had my ear stitched, my cheek bones fractured, my nose fractured, my jaw fractured. I still remember the doctor saying you must have a jaw like [a professional boxer].

It was pure agony, life was hell. I often thought of taking the easy way out but I had a young son to consider and it was always him I thought about. I tried pills once and I actually had a knife on my hand to cut my wrists but I kept thinking about my son, he kept me sane....

I could write a book about my fifteen years of anguish because you see I killed my husband, not deliberately, it was an accident, but as the doctors said it was like the straw on the camel's back. I snapped. I took it until I could take no more and for that I got three years imprisonment.[49]

In every country where the issue of battering has now been recognized there are well-known cases of women in prison who have killed their male partners after years of his violent abuse. Some have become '*causes célèbres*' and are subsequently released. Others remain unknown and serve out sentences because they were first abused by their male partners and then failed by a society unwilling or unable to provide the necessary means of protection or escape.[50] In her historical and contemporary study of *Women Who Kill*, Ann Jones cites numerous such cases:

Katherine Rohrich shot her husband four times as he slept, but only after she and her eleven children had endured years of battering, and only after she had been denied the help of local law-enforcement personnel several times.... [The judge] described [her] as a woman 'pushed to the wall'.[51]

New Orleans district attorney's office in July 1978 dropped charges against Viola Williams, who shot her common-law husband, Harold Randolph, twice in the head and neck and eleven times in the back. Pretrial investigation determined that Randolph had beaten her for ten years, shoved her face into an anthill, and once pled guilty to a simple battery charge after clubbing her with a baseball bat; at the time she shot him, he was attacking her with a knife. She shot twice in self-defence, she said, and then eleven times more for what he had done to her. [The District Attorney acknowledged she had a] 'a valid self-defence claim.... I'm sorry the system didn't help her sooner.... We have evidence that she sought help many times.'[52]

For Jones, 'Homicide is a last resort, and it most often occurs when men simply will not quit'.[53] Examples include:

[She] left her husband, but he kept tracking her down, raping and beating her; finally when he attacked her with a screwdriver, she shot him.[54]

[She] filed for divorce, but her husband kept coming back to beat her with a dog chain, pistol-whip her, and shoot at her. At last, after she had been hospitalized seven times, she shot him.[55]

... teaching submission, [he] made her watch him dig her grave, kill the family cat, and decapitate a pet horse. When she fled he brought her back with a gun held to her child's head.[56]

Angela Browne's study of battered women who kill is filled with similar accounts of women repeatedly beaten, abused, raped and terrorized before killing their abuser.[57] Jones notes that many case records show men following, harassing and beating their wives for years before they are themselves killed by the woman who had for so long been their victim. For Jones, it is misdirected to ask 'why women stay' and more telling to address 'Why don't men let them go?'.[58]

With expanding awareness of the problem, thousands of accounts from across the world can be added to the British and North American voices above. The accounts reveal patterns strikingly similar across countries even as they reflect important and distinct cultural differences. In India and Bangladesh, for example, women are beaten and killed because of men's possessiveness and demands about women's domestic work, but also because of the price of a wife and the bereavement of a widow. Dowry deaths are common and sati, the burning of a widow upon the death of her husband, has been the subject of a vigorous, though not completely successful, women's campaign for abolition.[59] In urban Maharashtra and Greater Bombay, nearly a quarter of deaths among women between 15 and 44 years of age are due to 'accidents' caused by burns.[60] The pattern is worst among the youngest women and reflects the problem of dowry deaths. Although the Dowry Prohibition Acts have been passed in both countries, the social custom of dowry is still practised.[61] Women are frequently beaten or killed when her family fails to meet payments or the husband or his family decide they want more than originally agreed.[62] Doused with cooking oil and set alight they become the victim of an 'accident' in the kitchen. In Bangladesh they have also had to legislate against the practice known as acid throwing.[63] In both countries, women are often harassed and abused until they commit suicide.

In Papua, New Guinea, the Constitution guarantees equality for women and prohibits punishment that is cruel or violates human dignity. Many government officials strongly resisted these new laws and men still beat and kill their wives, sometimes in unfamiliar ways but usually for familiar reasons:[64]

> A man in Gulf Province has been arrested for shooting his wife in the ribs with an arrow and inflicting a severe axe wound to her head....[65]

> A blind man was charged with murder for beating his wife to death with his cane on Independence Day.... He is alleged to have beaten up his wife after hearing stories that she was being unfaithful to him.[66]

In many African countries, women are triply abused within the family, the economy and the state: by husbands who beat them, by the ravages of war and as exploited workers who make up most of the farm labourers in agricultural economies.[67] Genital mutilation of women and girls in order to control their sexuality is also widely practised in many African countries.[68] In Latin American countries the image of the macho man continues and violence against women is perpetuated within that cultural context. For example, in Quito, Ecuador, over 80 per cent of women interviewed in one study had been beaten by their partners, and such incidents make up 70 per cent of all crimes reported to the police in Peru.[69] In the two years between 1986–7, 18,000 cases of woman abuse were reported to the police in Sao Paulo, Brazil,[70] and a Women's Police Station was established in 1986 as part of an effort to combat violence against women.[71]

In Israel, with its emphasis on the importance of the family and the belief that violence has no place in Jewish society, wives are still beaten by husbands.[72] The fashion for stress reducing 'toys' in Japan in the late 1980s included an 'I am sorry doll' who speaks only when spoken to, and begs 'Please forgive me' and 'Please don't hit me'. There are three types: the company boss, the female police officer and the wife.[73] In Malaya, the stereotypes and myths about the abuse of wives are all too familiar:

- Only poor and uneducated men batter their wives
- No one should interfere in the domestic affairs of man and wife
- Unhappy families are better than no families
- Alcohol causes battering
- She must have enjoyed it. Otherwise she'd leave.
- Husbands have every right to do what they want with their wives
- Women who are beaten obviously deserve it
- Its just the odd domestic tiff [74]

In response to this violence and to the unwillingness or inability of social, legal and medical agencies to act effectively to assist women after abuse, refuges and shelters have now been established throughout much of the world by activists who provide an immediate, pragmatic response to the problem. Usually against great odds, and often resourced primarily by women volunteers, refuges and shelters have opened in country after country forming a watershed in the response to this social problem. Countless women from all over the world speak of the importance of the refuge in their lives: the value of escaping from violence, the importance of mutual support and solidarity; the end of isolation; and support for self-reliance rather than continued dependence. An Israeli woman tells of the relief after thirty years of marital violence:

> I had no family who could help me and I suffered great fear. He said he would kill me, and I believed him. I stayed to take care of the children and when the last one left home, somehow I got up the courage to come here.... I'm afraid to go out in the street. Every night I dream that he is coming to kill me. My daughter tells me she has the same dreams. If I hadn't had the centre to come to, I don't know what I would have done.[75]

From New Zealand, a 52 year old woman tells of the return to normal life after twenty years of violence:

> At long last we were able to be normal loving human beings. My children and I could laugh and joke with one another out in the open.... Friends could visit me without me worrying about him coming in and being so rude and aggressive that they wouldn't come back again.[76]

Their British and North American counterparts also emphasize the importance of the refuge in changing their lives:

> You weren't there eight years ago when I needed a place to go with my baby. Thank God you're there now for those in need![77] (American woman)

> I used to be ashamed to talk about battering to people. I can really talk openly here because they've all been through the same thing.[78] (English woman)

> We all run it as a group, so we all take decisions. It's like a small community – we all help each other.[79] (English woman)

> A lot of women here give you courage. At first I asked, 'Did I do the right thing? Is it me?' Now I say, 'I don't have to take this. We, women, are in this together.'[80] (American woman)

The beginning of the social movement dealing with violence against women, like most beginnings, was rather unspectacular and went without too much notice. But this changed quickly as refuge provision grew from local groups to national organization, and recognition of the problem became international. In 1972, the first refuge for battered women opened in Britain. Others were soon to follow throughout Britain[81] as well as in Europe, the United States, Canada and Australia[82] as activists travelled within and between countries, sharing ideas and providing support for opening new refuges.

The battered-women's movement has now extended throughout much of the world, providing shelter and working for social change. For example, in 1988 Welsh Women's Aid sponsored an international conference with delegates representing over forty countries.[83] The process of innovation and change evident in this worldwide movement is the focus of this book. While examples of the old ways, the old attitudes and beliefs and the old responses of agencies and social policies abound and indicate continued support for the abuse of wives and female partners, they offer no hope or useful direction for action. Hope and inspiration for positive action lay in the innovations, the breaks with the legacy of violence. It is here that present and future changes are being formed and reformed; here, that the nature of women's lives may be freed from the constant possibility that force might be unleashed against them as they conduct the business of daily life; here, that attention might productively turn in pursuit of an end to the centuries of protection and support for male violence and a beginning of the era of its rejection.

In this book we shall concentrate on the process of change, including innovations at local, institutional and national levels, and upon the actions of a social movement attempting to move ideas and practices from the status quo to a new and fundamentally different level. The focus is on the battered-women's movements in Britain and the United States. While much narrower than the world stage upon which these changes are actually being played, this is, nonetheless, a sizeable arena in which many important innovations have emerged. Britain and the United States lend themselves to comparison because of shared legal and cultural traditions and a similar language. Differences, however, are often great, and the 'common language' sometimes causes more confusion than clarity.

We are not primarily concerned with exploring the nature of the violence itself, since we and others have done that elsewhere,[84] but it is crucial that the violence not be forgotten as we examine the responses to it. Nor is it our intention to produce a comprehensive history of the movements as such. This has been written for the United States by Susan Schechter and awaits writing in Britain.[85] The present work concentrates on the efforts of a new social movement to change cultural and institutional patterns, and on the responses to those efforts. In order to do this, we have interviewed activists and officials in Britain and the United States, used the published works of others and compiled information from countless documents, pamphlets and newsletters produced by the movement and both governments.

In pursuing this analysis of change, we shall inevitably concentrate on innovations that reject violence and its foundations rather than on established patterns that support them. The intention is to examine change in progress and consider models for development that are challenging and innovative. But this should not be taken as an indication that innovations are the norm or that resistance to change is not strong. We shall also examine how innovations have been blocked and sometimes diverted as they have been implemented in a wider, less supportive social context. That is, how challenging ideals have sometimes been subverted, undermined and reshaped by legislation and institutional response.

This involves consideration of the internal dynamics of the movement: its resources and organization; the diversity of goals and tactics; and negotiations with the community, institutions of the state, policy makers, researchers, violent men and others. None of these facets are ossified but are themselves changing with time and circumstances. Thus, the task of characterizing a living movement while still in the process of development is inevitably more complex than charting one that has become a memory. The battered-women's movement has negotiated for social change within the wider context of the existing economic, political and social position of women in society, and the established philosophies, priorities and practices of existing institutions and agencies of the state. Negotiations with institutions of the state shall be examined particularly in terms of proposals for innovative change and the responses to them. Notions about the nature of the problem, the most effective strategies and solutions, and who or what is in need of change vary and are themselves the subject of debate, and these will also be considered. These differences shall be examined and some of their consequences considered. The nature of social change, the dynamics of a social movement and the ideas and practices of feminism are all at work as the process of change stops and starts, moves forward and backward, and occasionally takes a step sideways.

2 The rise of the movement
Orientations and issues

The great mobilization of women began with a vision supported by action. The vision was of a world transformed, of a society in which women occupied a place no longer subordinated and participated fully in all facets of society. A world in which women were revalorized, fully integrated and set free from male domination was a bold notion. This transformative vision could not be achieved without major social changes in all facets of cultural, political and economic life. Such an expansive vision was suggestive of limitless arenas for action.

In charting the discovery of the problem, the building of a movement and the formulation of responses to women who have been abused, it is only possible to touch on some of the most important events and issues within this larger struggle for social change. This characterization of the movement can, nonetheless, provide a foundation for examining its relationship with agencies of the state: agencies with whom activists have alternately worked with and against in their efforts to seek change. We shall consider the wider context in which the battered-women's movement arose, including the legacy of the women's liberation movement, and explore various approaches to understanding social movements and social change. We shall then focus more closely on the movement for battered women including: the initial recognition of the problem and attempts to raise public awareness; the vision or goals of the movement's action, tactics and achievements; the building of national organizations; and internal issues confronted by the movement. A closer examination of refuges/shelters and of the relationship between the movement and external organizations, including government, legislators, the justice system, professionals and research, shall be covered later.

In both Britain and the United States, the women's movement of the late 1960s and 1970s provided the base of membership and the overall perspective from which numerous issues could be addressed and actions organized. Wage work and the economy, domestic work and the family, reproduction and medicine, mental health and psychiatry, knowledge and the university, sex and the double standard, violence against women and many others became the sites of protest against disadvantages historically constructed and maintained through economic segmentation, cultural beliefs and institutional practices. Male domination and power were fundamental to all. The task of transformation was enormous, but the spirit and energy of the time was of equal measure, and so began the struggle for change.

Women were not alone in their attempts to build a better world, nor were they alone on the building site. Other new social movements – peace, civil rights, students and the New Left – were also there, and they, in turn, had followed the older labour movement for the working class. The modern site was being built on still older foundations of early feminism, socialism and utopian communities. A mixture of both old and new fused in the emerging analysis of contemporary conditions giving impetus to the efforts to shape a better society for all. The women's movement of the 1960s and 1970s drew from all these sources, although some more so than others. It also had a legacy of its own, although this had to be rediscovered in the rubble of historical neglect. Once rediscovered, the change efforts of earlier generations of women, and some men, left powerful and compelling ideas that could be made new in the modern world. They provided inspirational stories of struggles against great odds and victories. They also provided salutory lessons of defeats, diversions and periods of indifference and neglect.

ISSUES – OLD AND NEW

In creating their present, the new women's movement was innovative. Everything was up for consideration. Debates about the nature of the problem and possible solutions ranged widely.[1] There was a legacy of ideas and action from earlier periods of struggle and change, such as the mid-nineteenth and the early twentieth centuries.[2] Based on personal experience, and sometimes using the new scholarship, they engaged anew the debates about women's nature, the importance of citizenship and political representation, higher education, wage work, the state, independence, autonomy and freedom, motherhood, the 'moral superiority' of women, the family, patriarchy, power, domination, oppression and many, many others. Some ideas date back to the Enlightenment of the late seventeenth century, others to the French and American revolutions, the Industrial revolution, Evangelicalism and the religious revivalism of the late eighteenth and early nineteenth centuries and early anti-slavery movements of mid-nineteenth century Britain and America.[3] The knowledge that women are in a secondary position to men both in society and in the family, and that this results in numerous problems for women, including economic disadvantage and the use of violence against them, was becoming common currency in the women's movement. The new issue of the physical abuse of women in the home simply extended this knowledge of women's oppression beyond the more public spheres of wage work, safety in public places and the like and into the very heartland of private life, the family. Thus, the fact that women were beaten by husbands and cohabitants was a logical extension of earlier discoveries.

SOCIAL MOVEMENTS IN CHANGING TIMES

The context of emerging movements

Social movements tend to come in waves, with numerous groups such as women, ethnic and religious minorities and workers all seeking to change their social, political and economic circumstances. The times that foster such development are often more open and visionary, giving hopeful glimpses of better conditions for all. In their two volume history of women in Europe, Anderson and Zinsser note that feminist movements flourish during liberal revolutions and decline during conservative periods. They cite the flourishing of feminism at the time of the French revolutions of 1789, 1848 and 1871, the German revolution of 1848 and the liberal movement in Russia of the 1850s. They also note its decline during the conservative or repressive periods thereafter, such as during the first and second Napoleonic empires.[4] In Haug's study of the current women's movement in fifteen European countries, she found fairly similar conditions in each country as the movement emerged in the late 1960s and early 1970s.[5] The movements followed a phase of economic growth, the extension of welfare-state provision and, for most, a social-democratic government. Reform, greater opportunities, more security, higher standards of living and more state regulation of the private spheres, usually occupied by women, formed the general backcloth to the emergence of the new women's movement.[6] Apart from the wider structural conditions, Jo Freeman views three factors, mostly relating to the potential membership of a new movement, as essential for their emergence, and Dahlerup adds a fourth:

1 a pre-existing communication network or infrastructure within the base of the movement;
2 susceptibility of the network to new ideas;
3 a situation of strain or crisis that actually triggers off the movement;[7]
4 international diffusion of ideas.[8]

The nature of social movements

Since neither social movements nor the times in which they exist remain static, any description of goals, strategies and membership is always a tentative, rather than a definitive, characterization. However, theories about social movements can help conceptualize their nature, goals and consequences. While social movements may effect changes in political, economic and social conditions, they also arise out of and are themselves affected by changes in these external contexts, as well as by changes within their own membership or organization.

The development of social movements has been characterized in diverse ways. The early work of Blumer defined the collective behaviour associated with social movements as a usual process in society which emerged out of 'social unrest' and developed and changed through various forms of interaction and communication.[9] He thought it important to study the forms of such behaviour, the situational contexts in which they occur, relationships between those situations and the broader sociocultural frameworks, and the short- and long-term impact of collective behaviour on previously established sociocultural frameworks.[10] Another traditional model focuses on the membership as the key to success and survival in responding to strategic and doctrinal challenges.[11] Accordingly, as new movements challenge older movements or events challenge group ideology, the internal responses of movement members are viewed as crucial to the eventual outcome.

More recently, particularly in the USA, resource mobilization theory has focused on the type of resources mobilized for action. They may be material (money, labour, land,[12] facilities[13]), or the human and social resources necessary for collective action (authority, moral commitment, trust, friendship, skills and habits of industry).[14]

The theory also focuses on external factors, emphasizing either resources of political influence in the management of the movement[15] or economic rationality (especially funding) and the role of professional leaders.[16] External factors and the upper tier of the movement, rather than the membership, are sometimes viewed as crucial in effectively responding to changing times and circumstances in order to ensure growth or, in some cases, survival itself.[17] Still others see social movements as maintaining continuity during periods of less activity and thereby avoiding their own demise through 'abeyance structures' which allow challenging groups to continue in 'non-receptive political climates'.[18]

Piven and Cloward focus on the goal of radical change rather than on interaction, membership or resources.[19] They maintain that once grass roots movements shift from direct action and support by members to building an organization and dependence on third parties for support, the potential for radical change is lost. Based on their study of poor people's movements in the USA, they maintain that truly radical change movements are by their very nature ephemeral. They burst on the scene and make an impact using mass support and direct action. They then cease to exist or are utterly transformed through organization, bureaucratization and external pressure. For Cloward and Piven, institutionalized tactics, dependence on external funding and established political influence, may sustain the existence of a movement but, in the process, destroy its goals of sustained social change.

Other writers focus on the importance of radical factions within social movements, not because they represent the original or most important goals or identity of the movement, but because they serve as a subgroup that presses for the greatest change and uses the most extreme forms of action. The radical faction not only makes the claims and actions of other subgroups look more moderate, both inside and outside the movement, but also mean that any backlash will likely result in purging of the radical faction rather than crushing the entire movement.[20]

Others argue that social change can only be sustained by penetrating deeply into the institutional and ideological structures of society so that the ideals and restructuring associated with bursts of political action can become firmly established after the period of most visible direct action has passed. The Greens of West Germany and Poland's Solidarity provide examples of such shifts from trade union and social movement to political party.[21] The more disillusioned, or some might say realistic, contend that the established order cannot be changed fundamentally, and the only possible approach to social change is to establish a separate culture apart from the mainstream.[22] The dilemma of participating in the political process is one of holding on to the goal of change while trying to influence organizations which, by their very nature, would be expected to resist or subvert such goals. Whatever the orientation, all social movements must find solutions to the dilemma of maintaining their goals of social change while finding the means of support necessary for survival.

While emphasis upon resource mobilizaton theory is a more familiar approach to studying social movements in the USA, recent literature from Europe focuses on what are called the new social movements. Ecology, peace, anti-nuclear and the women's movements are distinguished from older movements (especially the working-class labour movement) in terms of values, issues, forms of action and constituencies.[23] The new social movements stress cultural rather than economic issues, and focus on quality of life, equality, individual autonomy, participation, democracy and human rights.[24] Conflicts are about what Habermas calls the 'grammar of forms of life'.[25] The new movements aim to recover personal identity, create 'new public spaces' free of administrative control using decentralized forms of participation and organization rather than representative forms of democracy.[26] Membership has been defined as the 'new middle class', or a reworked definition of the American term 'new class', particularly specialists in social and cultural services.[27]

Alain Touraine analyses social movements as central to how people create the world in which they live.[28] They are not simply attempts to seek the assistance of the state in creating a more modern and advanced version of the society we now have, but are a class or group 'searching for an alternative', 'defending another society' or way of life.[29] Social movements are composed of the collective action of those seeking control of 'the great cultural orientations by which a society's ... relationships are normatively organized', what he calls 'historicity'.[30] 'The social movement is the organized collective behaviour of a class actor [in this case women] struggling against his [her] adversary for the social control of historicity in a concrete community.'[31]

Touraine's image is of collective action guided by an idea, an orientation or a plan. Social movements are not striving to become political parties or to transform state power. Their action is fundamentally directed towards social change and not towards a conquest of state power. There may, nonetheless, be some alliances with state power in seeking social change.[32] Touraine analyses social movements in terms of three interrelated components which constantly affect one another. They are identity, the totality and opposition:[33] that is, how the movement identifies itself, who or what is in opposition to the desired change, and what is at stake or being sought (goals, the totality). 'If one is to fight ... should one not know in whose name one is fighting, against whom, and on what grounds.'[34] Touraine depicts these three as a triangle and analyses the relationships between each combination of facets as the social movement works for change.[35] The nature of the movement thus includes its goals and the forces which must be overcome in order to achieve change. This does not exhaust the coverage of the phenomenon of new social movements. While still other thinkers would alert us to still other issues, it is not possible to cover all of this work here.[36]

It is not always easy to define what goals might constitute social change or how they might be sustained against external pressure.[37] Mathiesen's idea of 'the unfinished' is useful in thinking about the ability of the new alternative to be expansive in nature and have longevity. At the point at which any new way of thinking or acting emerges, it is 'unfinished'; there is no closure. Almost everything can be considered, the widest possible changes are imagined and discussed. This is especially embodied in the women's movement's ideal of changing the status of women in all spheres of society. Closure begins by settling on specific tasks as necessary for achieving the ultimate goal, such as when the Suffragettes concentrated solely on the vote rather than also upon the wider vision of change in women's status throughout society. Such closure can signal the end of the new alternative but only if the wider, long-term goal is completely supplanted by the narrower, short-term task. Alternatives such as changing the status of women or ending male violence have an open, expanding nature allowing for many specific tasks to be achieved along the way. It is only when a specific task, such as achieving the vote or opening a certain number of refuges, becomes the ultimate goal *per se*, rather than one of the necessary tasks for achieving the wider goal, that the alternative is finished.

Mathiesen's model considers the potential for change embodied in the goals of any social policy, public demand or piece of social research.[38] In order to stand as a true alternative to the status quo, a change proposal must both *contradict* the existing order, that is represent a real alternative, and, at the same time, seriously *compete* for adoption or acceptance. In this case, it must *contradict* the established acceptance of men's violence against women and the general failure to respond concertedly or effectively to end such violence. In order to have a chance at becoming a reality, this goal must also *compete* for serious attention on the agenda of social change. The pressures pulling away from the goal of social change include varied attempts to encourage or coerce activists in the name of reason, co-operation or clarity to redefine the goal in terms that no longer contradict the existing order. Also included are pressures either to return to the fold or risk being defined as too extreme for serious consideration, and thus cease to compete for attention. Both eliminate the challenge. Both ensure that the 'unfinished' is finished.

The analysis of social movements portrays a complex interplay of issues, values, goals, organizational forms, internal dynamics and external relations which continue to shape and reshape the organic development of a movement as it emerges, expands and wins and loses struggles in its attempt to bring about social change. Although the dynamic nature of social movements is subject to debate, and the ideas presented here do not exhaust the field, many are resonant with debates and dilemnas facing the women's movement and its offspring, the battered-women's movement. Focusing on values and goals, internal developments and external relations with the public and institutions of the state we shall explore the efforts of this new social movement to transform the daily lives of women and men, cultural beliefs and institutions of the state. Of particular relevance to our analysis are Touraine's ideas about the nature and importance of the identity of the movement and its membership, and the relationship between the movement and its adversaries. Also of importance are Mathiesen's ideas about constructing and maintaining a goal of change which has the possibility of being realized.

EMERGENCE OF THE WOMEN'S MOVEMENT AND SOME FIRST PRINCIPLES

In the USA, the new women's movement developed from three general groupings: previously politicized women from the New Left who became oriented to issues affecting women's social, political and especially their economic life; those from civil rights activism; and women who had little or no experience of political thinking or action but were drawn to issues affecting their everyday life. For the most part, they may be defined as members of what has been called the new class, that is members of the middle classes drawn mostly from education and the social and human services.[39] In 1968, the first meeting of twenty-two women in Sandy Springs, Maryland debated whether the movement should become an independent, autonomous women's movement or remain a branch of the radical left.[40] A national meeting held in Chicago in November of the same year and attended by 200 women from twenty states and Canada debated whether the issue was capitalism or male-dominated institutions and values, and the divide between the 'politicos' (New Left) and the 'feminists' (civil rights and others) was articulated and became the source of a bitter divide outside the movement and, to a lesser extent, within it. The balance towards an autonomous women's movement was soon tipped by the rapid increase of previously apolitical women. Nevertheless, the principles of the women's liberation movement reflected an agenda of radical social change, even if one outside the tradition of the New Left with its focus on class and economic change.[41] Radical feminism and Liberal feminism were to take the centre ground in the USA, and socialist feminism, particularly in the context of a weak socialist tradition throughout the country, became a small minority within the movement.

The women's movement in Britain had an independent beginning, although it was also influenced by radical feminism from the USA.[42] The emphasis on political analysis, the importance of class, the traditions of trade union organization, and Labour and left party politics were much stronger and more respected in Britain, and attempts to insert women into the agendas of the radical left gave impetus to socialist feminism and provided a platform for early, influential works such as Juliet Mitchell's 'The longest revolution' (1966) and Sheila Rowbotham's 'Women's liberation and the new politics' (1969).[43] Although radical feminism also became the mainstay in Britain, the influence of socialist-feminist thought and the general environment of Labour and left politics have been more influential in the overall nature of the movement than in the USA.

Goal: equal rights or liberation

Of particular importance within past and present women's movements has been the different orientations to rights or to liberation. They represent differences in ideology, strategies, issues to be addressed and approaches to be taken. Fundamentally, they form differences in the definition of the nature of the problem and the solutions to be sought, and these strands of feminism were later to be represented in the battered-women's movement in the two countries.

The section of the women's movement oriented to women's rights is known as liberal, equal rights or reform feminists. It usually works on civil and political equality or political reforms within the context of the existing social order and uses traditional pressure group tactics.[44] NOW, The National Organization for Women, created in 1966, is the main exemplar in the USA, and the struggle for ERA, The Equal Rights Amendment to the US Constitution, is a recent example of this approach.[45] For such women's rights activists, legislation is the main approach to reforms which are sought within the context of the present society with its established hierarchies. Equal rights ideas are usually set within a Liberal political discourse. In examining the Liberal political discourse on equality used in two US campaigns of the 1980s (women's poverty and equal wages), Brenner discusses how the Liberal discourse of reform accepts hierarchy and inequality within the overall society and attempts simply to allow each group to compete 'equally' for the unequal distribution of resources, power and rewards.[46]

Women's liberation or emancipation is a broader approach than civil or political equality, striving instead for 'freedom from oppressive restrictions imposed by sex, for self-determination and for autonomy'[47] or 'advocating the liberation of all oppressed people'.[48] The term 'liberation' is used in quite distinct ways by socialist-feminists, emphasizing class relations and a socialist society, and radical feminists emphasizing gender and cultural transformation. The radical feminists of New York City wrote the first policy statement for the women's liberation movement. The sex–class analysis viewing women as an oppressed class was a bold and dynamic theory of power, rather than one simply of unequal relations arising out of a fixed distinction of gender. It made an important contribution to feminist thinking about male domination and power, and to the development of the 'pro-woman line'.[49] With women as the primary focus, emphasis was placed on culture, changing consciousness and lifestyles.

The different types of feminism, liberal/reform/equal rights feminists, radical feminists and socialist-feminist, all influenced the new women's movement, and, in turn, the battered-women's movement. The groupings have sometimes formed coalitions and at other times created divisions within the movements.[50] Within each country, the differences in these political positions have helped shape the movement and the different approaches to the question of change.[51] Developments in the two nations are similar and mutually influencing in many ways, and hold in common the rapid development and powerful influence of radical feminism. However, the greater influence of Liberal or equal rights feminism in the USA and the more established position of Labour and left politics along with socialist-feminism in Britain help explain some of the differences in the respective battered-women's movements. Similarly, Myra Marx Ferree's analysis of the women's movement in West Germany and the USA notes the influence of the different national contexts on the movement, its issues and strategies, with ideas of equality and the issue of race shaping thinking and action in the USA and ideas of autonomy and the issue of class as more central in West Germany.[52]

In Britain, National Women's Liberation Conferences were held from 1970 to 1978, and seven demands were worked out at successive conferences. They focused on equal pay, education and job opportunities, reproductive freedom, child care, financial and legal independence, sexual preference and, most important for our present concern, violence against women. The seventh demand, adopted in 1978, reads:

> freedom from intimidation by threat or use of violence or sexual coercion, regardless of marital status; and an end to all laws, assumptions and institutions which perpetuate male dominance and men's aggression towards women.[53]

The demand for an end to male violence merely confirmed in principle within the women's movement what had already begun in practice with the establishment of refuges for women fleeing from violent partners.

THE BATTERED-WOMEN'S MOVEMENT – VISION AND ACTION

The recognition of wife abuse and collective action

The battered-women's movement (shelter or refuge movement) is a direct product of the women's movement in both countries, and most of the early shelter groups arose out of women's liberation consciousness raising groups which had decided it was time to move from thought to action. In Britain, founding the first refuge was the result of pioneering efforts of the group of women who opened Chiswick Women's Aid.[54] It emerged in a rather unexpected manner, beginning with a campaign to protest against the elimination of free school milk and ending with a refuge for battered women. The story is now well known. Five hundred women and children and one cow marched through an English town in support of their claim. The cow aptly served as a symbol of their cause and the amiable spectacle brought considerable attention.

While not a direct success, the march did bring solidarity among the women and initiated a successful attempt to set up a community meeting place for local women. It was here that women began to tell one another horrific stories of the violence they had received at the hands of their male partners. Here, that the doors were first opened for them to find refuge. Here, that violence against women began to be defined as a problem of epic proportions. Here, that publicity was, and continues to be drawn. Here, that the inspiration for a social movement began.[55] Erin Pizzey soon emerged from the original group as the powerful, indomitable figurehead of Chiswick Women's Aid. She was able to capture public attention and define the problem as a crisis requiring action. She became the visible, moral entrepreneur launching the issue as an emerging social problem, developing and controlling her refuge, and proffering strong personal ideas about possible causes and solutions.[56]

In the United States, the battered-women's movement began a few years after its birth in Britain. Its initial character, while informed by the British experience, was affected most specifically by the preceding women's liberation and anti-rape movements in the USA. In many ways, the 'discovery' of wife abuse was not the surprise that it had been in Britain, partly because of some early contact with British groups, particularly Chiswick, but also because of the base of knowledge and experience gained by American activists who had already worked on the issue of rape.

The battered-women's movement in the USA had its first real beginnings in 1973 and 1974 with the opening of Women's Advocates in Minnesota and Transition House in Boston, but wider public recognition and widespread activity similar to that in Britain did not come until somewhat later.[57] Although the Salvation Army and a few other organizations had provided accommodation for women who were homeless or had been beaten by alcoholic partners, their primary focus was on alcohol and not on violent abuse or its social supports. As such, this activity cannot be seen as the beginning of the movement in the United States as Chiswick's is in Great Britain.

Women's Advocates and Transition House in the USA, like Chiswick in Britain, began from the foundations of women's liberation, particularly through consciousness-raising groups that provided an early network of communication for beginning the process of turning from thought to action. Beginning with a focus on the status of women and women's issues made it possible to turn their attention to the issue of battering as a social problem and to move from consciousness raising to social action. Focusing on the wider context allowed them to seek explanations, causes and effective responses not in terms of individual deviance, such as alcohol abuse, but in terms of power relations between the sexes, from the most personal level to the wider social and cultural spheres. This included a consideration of the criminal justice system, social services, medicine, legislation, the economy and deeply held and highly revered beliefs about male domination and female subordination which underpinned, supported and maintained systems of male control.

Both within and across the two countries, Women's Advocates, Transition House and Chiswick Women's Aid initially served as models for the expanding movement. Also important in the early recognition of wife abuse as a social problem were early articles by Lisa Leghorn and Betsy Warrior.[58] In 1976, Betsy Warrior also published a directory, *Working on Wife Abuse*, which provided a unique, international resource of information about new groups opening throughout the world, practical information and 'think pieces' about central issues.[59] The Directory was invaluable in establishing a network of early contacts between shelters and building coalitions across vast geographical distances, and it remains a unique and important source to date. From these early beginnings, although not always as a direct consequence of them, shelters began opening all over the USA, and from the mid-1970s, public attention was increasingly turned to exposing the existence of wife, or woman, abuse.

As awareness spread in both countries, women activists began to respond in increasing numbers either by forming new groups or by taking on this new issue as a part of the agenda of an existing group. There was an explosion of activity which is typically associated with the early stages of the recognition of a social problem.[60] Efforts to raise public awareness about the very existence of this abuse and its severity required extensive mobilization of material and social resources including an active involvement with the media and the public. Attempts to set up refuges in Britain and safehouses, hotlines and shelters in the USA were monumental tasks requiring hours of work, usually with little or no pay, to raise funds, find accommodation, answer telephones and deal with the details of providing assistance for women fleeing from violence.

Most of the time and energy focused on meeting the immediate needs of the women seeking support and assistance. This involved a host of activities dealing with: the physical injuries of women still suffering the aftermath of an attack; the emotional aspects of experiencing violence and of leaving a relationship; the problems of escaping violence and living in a new and unfamiliar environment; the children who had witnessed or even experienced violence and were also now living in a new and unfamiliar setting; and, finally, the numerous legal, social and medical agencies often approached for help.

There were no set ways of doing things nor any textbook theories or professional philosophies to be adhered to in formulating responses to this plethora of issues. Responses were developed through direct contact with the women in terms of their own needs. New issues arose constantly. New solutions were created daily. New issues necessitated the development of a variety of innovative responses subject to fairly quick adoption, modification or rejection depending upon how useful or successful they were in practice. This time of innovative development and expansion was open, rather than rigid, and, like in Mathiesen's early stage of 'becoming', anything was possible. Since no narrow or specific definition of the task had been set, the whole problem could be addressed. Establishing refuges/ shelters and hot-lines, educating the public, pressing for changes in public agencies as well as attempting to reorder the wider social conditions that underpinned the continued use of male violence, were all on the agenda.

The vision: goals of the movement

There is considerable diversity in the specific programmes and immediate goals within and between local shelter groups and, at a wider level, in the more general, ideological perspectives within the movement itself. Although philosophy and pragmatics, ideology and action can be diverse, there are also commonalities. Stripped to the barest level, central issues may be considered in terms of the orientation to long-term change. The central goals concern the protection of abused women and change for all women: that is, to provide assistance to abused women and their children and to change gender inequalities in the domestic, economic and political arenas that form the foundation of and provide the support for male violence. Related foci concern reducing the frequency and/or severity of the violence of individual men or, more expansively, completely eliminating male violence and domination. It should be stressed that the focus has not usually been on violent men as such, but on the assistance and protection for women that can be obtained by seeking from agencies such as the justice system an effective response to violent men. Thus, there are three general goals: assisting victims, challenging male violence and changing women's position in society. All three are not adopted equally or in the same fashion throughout the movement.

Providing assistance for the victims of violence is, however, universally endorsed within the movement. This is the symbol of the movement's identity and provides the impetus for development and expansion. The initial and primary response has been the provision of refuges and shelters. The other aims reflect differing positions within the movement. Protecting abused women and addressing male violence often involves efforts directed at the criminal justice system. Programmes for violent men remain controversial. Both shall be discussed in later chapters. The general aim of changing the position of women in society is also fairly universal, although somewhat stronger in Britain than in some segments of the movement in the United States. For some groups in the USA, the provision of services has either voluntarily become the final goal or been pressed upon the movement in religiously and socially conservative communities which view the wider goal of social change as socially unacceptable and/or politically unobtainable. In such communities, activists oriented to social change dare not speak about egalitarian principles and must alter their message or risk being purged by funding agencies in favour of groups who will not challenge the status quo. There are varying degrees of pressure to conspire in continuing the traditional responses, which make it difficult to hold on to the vision of change. This focuses our attention on the most innovative approaches brought to the three goals of assisting victims, responding to male violence and changing women's position in society. Innovative responses that reflect these three changes most closely are of particular interest since they provide inspiration, possible models for adoption and modification, and insight into the means of achieving effective change.

In order to work towards achieving their goals, a variety of tactics have been adopted. In the beginning, public marches and rallies were more common. In Britain, there were also a few instances of squatting houses for use as refuges. Then, as now, tactics include lobbying legislators and negotiating with local agencies such as the police and social work departments, and, in Britain, the housing department. Thousands of documents have been written by activists for public education and for disseminating information within the movement itself. The media have also been used as an important tool in conveying to a wider public the message of women in need of assistance, agencies in need of change and a general public in need of enlightenment.

Division of labour and styles of working

The style of working towards these goals has become a goal in itself. Within the recent tradition of the women's movement, as in historical groups such as the St Simonians, the notion of group participation, consensus decision making, non-hierarchical structures and divisions of labour are seen as important, living examples of social relations based on equality and achieved through merit rather than based on domination and status acquired through race or sex. When the movement first began, it emerged out of women's groups that had adopted flexible, participatory and collective forms of structure and divisions of labour. Tasks were to be universally allocated rather than specialized, and authority was to be democratic rather than rigid and hierarchical. With little experience of how to make such a form of organization work or existing models to follow, implementation of this new style was as difficult to implement as other new forms had been for other innovative groups such as the early utopians of the Oneida colony in the USA, New Lanark in Scotland or the Communes of Paris during the French revolution.

Being 'new' within one's own historical period may mean a freedom to work out how to reconstruct social life in an alternative fashion, but it also means that activists have to continue to work to develop the model while at the same time finding little or no support, and possibly a great deal of external opposition, from other organizations with whom it is in constant contact and upon whom it might actually depend for existence. In the USA, funding bodies often demanded a hierarchy of officials seen as responsible for decision making and implementation, usually in the form of Boards of Directors and Executive Committees. The pressure was less in Britain, but so was the funding. Outside organizations do not know how to work with personnel who are constantly changing, and, indeed, this was later found to be an organizational problem in terms of completing tasks as well as negotiating with others. Representatives from the media wanted to know who was in charge as they gathered material for stories and/or wished continuity of spokeswomen as they built a story. Funders wanted to know who was in charge of spending their money. In the beginning, the response to this pressure varied within local groups, some creating hierarchical leadership, others creating informal leaders or task leaders. Some established a hierarchical structure and rotated individuals into the positions in order to continue to operate a collective style internally. It should be noted, however, that some groups created hierarchical forms of organization on their own initiative.

In some ways the non-hierarchical, or 'flat' structure of authority is one way in which the form of organization is meant to ensure that no individual or group gains through more decision making power than any other. This, of course, ignores informal or personal forms of power. This was once referred to in America as town hall democracy in which each person had the same right as any other person to speak and vote on every issue. By comparison, within representative democracy such tasks are delegated to a few who are meant to represent the interests of the many, and are retained as long as they do so. With executive authority, a single person or a few individuals have the authority given to them, either by the membership or by some external or higher body. They may make decisions with little or no consultation with the membership and with less chance of removal should they deviate from the general wishes of the membership. Each style has its advantages and disadvantages, and may be more or less applicable to different settings, and each may be used for 'good' or 'ill'. It is generally believed, particularly in America, that more democratic structures of authority will lead to more benevolent or better outcomes because of the necessity to be more sensitive to issues among the broadest membership or citizenry. As such, one might expect wide support for the notion of collective authority emanating from a broad base of women representing many different groups and interests. This was not generally the case. As we shall see, there were numerous external pressures pulling away from a flat structure of authority and a diffuse division of labour. In addition, there were also internal pressures created by the rapidly increasing size of the organization and the growing number of tasks to be undertaken.

Much of the pressure pulling away from collective and towards more structured or hierarchical forms of authority comes from a perceived conflation of forms of authority with types of division of labour. The lack of hierarchy in the former is often perceived to mean a lack of differentiation in the latter, and it is here that the nub of the criticism of non-hierarchical forms of authority and perceptions of its failure seems to lie. Some degree of specialization does seem to be useful in completing tasks and doing them well. It is clear, both inside and outside the organization, who is ultimately responsible for the work, and such individuals have an opportunity to develop skills and expertise in a given area. While it is theoretically possible to have undifferentiated forms of decision making and authority combined with a specialized division of labour, there is a danger that certain tasks will become more highly valued and may be translated into vehicles of authority and control.[61] Extreme specialization may also result in the formation of subgroups who develop and reflect different interests and become factionalized within the organization. Like it or not, the movement has had the thorny questions of power, authority and divisions of labour thrust upon them simply because they seem, inevitably, to form constituent parts of action and of organizations.

Recognition of the problem by activists was followed by massive efforts to develop awareness and gain support in the community and within the agencies of the state. Media campaigns help to inform the community further about the issue and of the need to support the pragmatic efforts of activists. Time spent making contacts, informing them about the issue and the movement, and contributing to programmes and articles was and still is seen as beneficial. Journalists generally support the efforts of the refuge/shelter groups and are often oriented to the development of positive responses to abused women. From the beginning, articles have appeared in major newspapers, women's magazines and news magazines. Local and national television programmes have been numerous, and major programmes depicting the experiences of abused woman include The Phil Donahue Show and 60 Minutes in the USA and Panorama in Britain as well as a major television film, 'The Burning Bed'.

Although the media continue to be of great importance in sustaining public interest and education, it can also have its drawbacks. Some coverage is sensationalist and journalists may assert unsubstantiated yet damaging 'theories' about the problem, its victims, perpetrators and solutions, such as those of the provocative masochistic woman, the alcoholic or inadequate man (and sometimes woman), and the notion of husband beating which has taken a particularly strong form in the USA. Such notions implicitly assume that this is strictly an individual problem suffered by deviants needing psychiatric care rather than a social problem in need of wider remedies.

The usual practice of seeking experts both to inform journalists about the subject and to quote in giving authority to their articles or programmes has also had some negative effects on the social movement. While those with the most direct experience of the problem are women living and working in refuges, they are often overlooked by the media in favour of others, often with much less experience or knowledge but with the academic or professional credentials thought necessary to give more authority and accuracy to the coverage. In short, the advantages of good media coverage are at times contradicted by the disadvantages of coverage which may convey a narrow

and erroneous definition of the problem and its causes, asserts the
authority of the professional as the expert with superior knowledge to
that of battered women themselves and/or experienced activists, and
may deny or ignore wider feminist approaches and interpretations.
This has sometimes been exacerbated, particularly in Britain, by a
form of isolation of some groups. At times this has been in response
to previous programmes thought to be damaging to abused women or to
the movement itself. At other times it appears to reflect the reluctance of particular groups to provide continuity of spokeswomen or
those deemed by the media to be likely to be effective on radio or
television. Freeman comments on the history of media hostility to the
women's movement in the USA and also notes how structurelessness
and the lack of spokespersons selected by the movement means that
the media choose those individuals with whom they will work and
only the press, not the movement, can remove or change the person
to whom they will listen.[62] Thus, failing to select spokeswomen within
the movement or choosing those deemed unsuitable by the media
leave the movement either without a voice or with one selected by the
media itself. This is an issue both of organization and of personalities.

BUILDING FROM THE BOTTOM UP: SHAPING THE NATIONAL ORGANIZATIONS

Britain

Although the first British refuge began at Chiswick Women's Aid, the
national movement grew out of a split over philosophy and approach
that quickly separated Chiswick from the other Women's Aid groups
who became the National Women's Aid Federation (NWAF). The
Federation began in 1974 at the first national gathering of the newly
formed Women's Aid groups from England, Scotland and Wales.
The occasion was marked by a split over principle, with the majority
wishing to form a democratic, egalitarian organization (NWAF) and
Chiswick, in the person of Erin Pizzey, wishing to maintain central
control, power, publicity and exclusive access to funds donated by the
public.[63] The National Federation began without the group that had
started it all, and the one that had so thoroughly captured media
attention that, for years to come, it was often believed to be the only
refuge in Britain. In writing the following letter to social work and
housing departments throughout the country, Pizzey responded to the
split by attempting to ensure that no other refuge would receive
funding without her personal approval:

We are particularly worried and unhappy that there are groups who seem to be trying to use Women's Aid as a platform for Women's Liberation and Gay Women's Liberation.

We would strongly advise Social Services and Housing Departments to look very carefully at the groups in their areas who are offering to set up refuge before giving them your support. If in doubt please feel free to contact us at Chiswick for any information.[64]

The split was fraught with conflict between the two factions, and there was considerable fear in the Federation that it would damage the new social movement. For their part, much of the media never quite forgave the tarnishing of an idol nor forgot the sole and privileged position once occupied by Chiswick. In the United States, the split over principle came much later in its development. Splits are, of course, common in all social movements, including labour, anti-nuclear, civil rights, ecology and Solidarity. The participatory and decentralist nature of the new movements make them particularly prone to such factions.[65]

The Federation began with thirty-five founding groups. The five aims adopted in 1974 were retained with some modifications when adopted as constitutional objectives in 1987. They currently read as follows:

1 Promoting the development of a network of autonomous locally based groups to provide temporary refuge on request, for women and their children who have suffered mental, emotional or physical harassment in their relationships, or rape or sexual harassment or abuse.
2 Encouraging the development of facilities which offer advice, support and practical help to any woman who seeks it, whether or not she is resident of a refuge, and which gives continuing support and after-care to women and children after they have left the refuge.
3 Researching into and campaigning for the provision of facilities which meet the emotional and educational needs of the children of women who seek refuge.
4 Providing information and assistance to local groups who are members of the Federation and to create a forum for the exchange of information and ideas on all aspects of the objects of the Federation.
5 Educating and informing the public, the media, the police, the courts, the social services and other authorities with respect to the

violence women suffer, mindful of the fact that this is a result of the *general position of women in our society* [our emphasis].[66]

The only original aim not reformulated in this new statement is, 'To encourage women to determine their own futures and to help them achieve them, whether this involves returning home or starting a new life elsewhere.[67] The reason for its exclusion is not stated. The fifth principle immediately presented a dilemma. In attempting to obtain charitable status, important for reasons of funding and taxation, the reference to the cause of the problem as 'relating to the status of women in society' was deemed a political aim, thus disqualifying them from charitable status. Principles and funding, both necessary for change and survival, were poised against one another by external forces. Either solution would in some way be problematic.

The National Women's Aid Federation initially covered all of Britain. Soon distinct national organizations were established in England, Scotland, Wales, Northern Ireland and the Republic of Ireland, each administering their own local groups. The National Women's Aid Federation, now renamed Women's Aid Federation England (WAFE), is composed of a National Office, a National Co-ordinating Group, an Employment Group and a Finance Group as well as several special interest groups. The National Office, based in Bristol, is strictly a co-ordinating body. It is meant to assist new groups with policy development, campaigning, fund-raising, research, public education, internal and external training, and to organize the annual general meetings (AGMs) and national conferences The Federation has no economic or managerial power over local refuge groups. There are twelve regions, each with an elected representative, who meet quarterly. The twelve regional representatives forming the National Co-ordinating Group are meant to transmit information between their local refuges and the National Office in Bristol. Decisions are made by the membership at the annual general meeting. Between AGMs, the twelve member National Co-ordinating Group serve as the decision-making body of WAFE. In addition to the National Co-ordinating Group, others include Employment, Finance and special interest groups.[68] The national organizations of Scotland, Wales and Northern Ireland differ some-what from England, but not in ways that represent a significant departure from these overall aims and approach.

The United States

Discussions about forming a national organization began among activists attending several different conferences: the Wisconsin Conference on Battered Women (October, 1976); the White House meeting about battering (July, 1977); and the International Women's Year Conference in Houston, Texas (November, 1977). They culminated at the United States Civil Rights Commission Consultation on Battered Women held in Washington DC (January, 1978) where The National Coalition Against Domestic Violence (NCADV) was formed.[69] Previous discussions were translated into action over the few days of the Washington meeting as sixty women worked to create regional caucuses, an interim structure and a statement of purpose.[70] Ten federal regions elected two-woman steering committees and nine task forces were formed until a national meeting could be held. The initial goals emphasized gaining financial aid for shelters and grassroots services, sharing information and supporting research beneficial to the movement. The style of working emphasized consensus, and representation was to include those of all ages, races, classes and sexual preferences. The three initial goals of the steering committee were to set up a structure, hold a national conference and influence national legislation.[71]

The simple fact of American geography served as a major impediment to forming a national organization, particularly for groups without sufficient funding to run their local shelter, much less travel the vast distances necessary to meet even on an infrequent basis, making the telephone essential in bridging the gap created by hundreds or even thousands of miles between locations. Work continued, but the first national conference was not held until two years later, in 1980. Meanwhile, the steering committee decided on the goals:

1 To monitor and impact legislation relating to domestic violence and family policy.
2 To aid in the develoment of state and regional coalitions.
3 To develop a national network of shelters.
4 To educate the public to a non-acceptance of violence and to strive towards the complete elimination of violence in our society.
5 To support and initiate change in traditional sex-role expectations for women and men.[72]

These principles established the basic orientation to the issue of battering and the task forces and committees formed the basic structure for carrying out responsibilities and managing relationships between the different subgroups within the Coalition, as well as with outside agencies.

State coalitions began to form in the USA after the formation of the National Coalition. Combining shelter groups into larger state-wide organizations required local groups, already greatly overworked opening and running shelters, to take on yet another task of developing a state-wide organization. Many, however, saw this as crucial in gaining greater political influence, particularly in working for legislation and funding, and in solidifying the grassroots, feminist base of the movement. With the pressing demands of local work, the importance of developing some overarching organization for the purpose of extending political influence may have seemed like an unnecessary luxury. Some, no doubt, felt less need to form larger groups oriented to wider social change than to expand the number of smaller groups working directly on the issue at the local level. In such an atmosphere, there is a tendency to see national organizations as large bureaucracies administering over local groups than as a vehicle undertaking other facets of wider social and political change.

Diversity and identity

If the sheer volume of accomplishments is one of the most obvious characteristics of the movement in America, diversity is the other. Although there are differences between the British and American movements, diversity within the movement itself is more pronounced in the USA. It is evident in everything from stated ideals to programme development and organizational structure, and reflects the broader base of membership. Ideology, tactics and short- and long-term goals for change continue to be worked through local decision making, programme development, forms of organization and resolution of conflicts. The diversity of membership within the American move-ment brings a broad base of support to the movement, thus ex-panding the range of those seeking change. This strength also has its limitations. The broader base of membership may offer such a breadth of ideas and orientations that, at a certain point, they cease to enhance the original vision and goals and begin to fragment or dilute them. The enhanced need for compromise in order to retain the group as a whole may similarly reach a point where the movement departs from an agenda of social change, away from 'the alternative'. The outcome may lead to greater conservatism, a more restricted approach to change and a dilution of the 'the contradiction'. These issues remain problematic in a movement seeking growth and expansion and, at the same time, retention of the original goals of the earlier, more circumscribed membership.

As social movements emerge and expand, a variety of issues must be addressed. Pressing questions include: Who are we? What are we seeking? Who is the opposition? For Touraine, they involve issues concerning the fundamental nature of the social movement and its relationship with others. They include the identity and nature of the movement itself; what is being sought;[73] and who or what is in opposition to the changes. The identity of the movement itself raises issues about who they are and how they are formed as a movement, including internal dynamics, organization and relationships between differing subgroups. The focus upon what is being sought of necessity includes a definition of the nature of the problem being addressed by the movement and the consequent solutions to be sought. Identification of who or what constitutes the opposition may sometimes be as problematic as defining the nature of the movement's relationship with the opposition, be they violent men, the government, agencies of the state or the community at large. The practical solutions to these issues help form the dynamic nature of the movement.

The identity of the battered-women's movement contains some elements that are adopted throughout the movement and others characterizing only smaller segments. The movement is most specifically oriented to providing protection and support for battered women and is against male violence. For the most part, the members are women working on an issue of violence against women. There are differences, however, concerning whether the movement is also in the name of change for all women within the social order. The question of who or what constitutes the opposition has been variously answered in terms of batterers, men in general, agencies of the state, especially the criminal justice system, and/or the social and economic supports for violence against women.

The nature of the new, alternative world being sought also varies within the movement. For some, it is a vision of expanding and changing the nature of services available to the individuals currently experiencing violence, especially shelter accommodation and support or advocacy in dealing with social agencies. For others, the vision includes such services but is also oriented to transformations in the general social and material conditions of all women that, in turn, support the abuse of women, i.e. male domination and women's subordinated place in society. What is being sought is either restricted solely to a variety of individual services for those already experiencing violence, or is expanded to include such services as well as wider changes in the social and material status of women and men.

Issues internal to the movement reflect various facets of the problem (women, children, employment), forms of organizational structure, especially hierarchy and collective styles; the nature of shelters and other programmes; concerns about interests/problems of subgroups within the movement and the relationships between them; and, of course, the problem of funding which embodies issues of co-optation, expansion and survival. Fundamental to all the specific issues addressed by groups is, however, the general question of whether they are more narrowly oriented solely to the delivery of individual services or are also working for wider social changes to deal with the conditions that support and continue this form of violence.

INTERNAL ISSUES

In addition to the vision, the action and the forms of organization, a variety of issues continue to be of importance within the movement itself. These include language, funding, style of working, divisions of labour, men, professionals and grassroots activists, class, race, homophobia and research. Of course, not all of these issues have the same importance in each country. Orientations and emphasis vary locally and nationally. Some of the solutions are very similar across countries while others are quite different, reflecting the context in which they have been developed and must operate.

Language: for battered women and against male violence

In both countries, the movements continue to debate and refine the terms used to define the problem, the organizations and the individuals involved. Is the problem wife abuse or woman abuse? Wife abuse implies that the social institution of marriage as well as gender is central, but has the drawback that it may also imply that violence is only directed at women living in the legal, rather than the social state of marriage. Woman abuse focuses on gender and avoids the problem of assuming legal marriage but, in so doing, loses emphasis upon the analytical insight that the social institution of marriage as traditionally constructed forms much of the foundation of the problem. The nature of abuse itself: does it include physical as well as other forms of violence? Beating and battering may be more descriptive, but are they too literal and emotive? As descriptive terms, domestic, spousal and family violence obscure the gendered nature of the problem and ignore the nature of the relationship involved.

Similar difficulties arise in terms used to describe the women subjected to violence. Battered wives, battered women, abused women and victims of violence have all been used. All have the problem of implying a permanent status, a master identity that can never be escaped. The terms used to try to overcome this problem ('formerly battered/abused woman', 'women who have been abused' and 'survivors of spouse abuse') are helpful but cumbersome. They also imply a permanent, albeit transformed, status. The term 'victim' has been used in two ways: implying a master status of the individual woman (i.e. she is a victim), and as a description of the experience itself (i.e. she was the victim of a violent attack). The first has recently come in for strong criticism and is often replaced by the term 'survivor'.[74] The second remains important for describing the act and women's role within it.

It is not difficult to imagine the problems facing activists as they tried to name their national and local organizations, those affected by the problem, and even the movement itself. Some groups simply inherited a name from a previous group or retained one for reasons of continuity and external recognition even though the political implications of such a name may be unclear or even misleading. Nonetheless, names are the purveyors of identity and meaning, and language continues to be debated and reworked within the movement. For Touraine, the identity of any social movement, both for itself and for others, is crucial in relation to what is at stake and what or who is defined as the opposition. In Britain, the national organizations are named in terms of aiding women (Scottish Women's Aid, etc.). In the United States, the national identity stands against the violence (National Coalition Against Domestic Violence). The term 'domestic' leaves unarticulated the fact that the focus is upon violence against women within the domestic arena. Without crediting too much to the name alone, one may, nonetheless, ponder possible implications of the different foci for the projected image of the problem as well as for the activities of providing refuge, tackling the criminal justice system, and the like.

Funding: the dilemmas of free vs. paid labour and co-optation vs. survival

Early funding through jumble and garage sales, community donations and free labour in redecorating and running shelters has been largely replaced by funding from local and national government in Britain, and local and state government, as well as charitable and corporate funds in the USA. Whether the source of funding comes from the community, individual philanthropy, corporations or the state, it is rarely given without conditions, in some cases involving an attempt to alter the principles of the movement. Initial debates about funding focused on two major facets of the interface between social change and money: free vs. paid labour, and co-optation of principles vs. survival of the movement.

Work, principles and goals all intertwine in dilemmas about funding. Questions concern why those oriented to assistance, caring or social change should be expected to work extraordinarily long and hard hours for little or no pay. Why should women work for little or less than men or professionals? Is this the price necessary to maintain principles and goals? Can an organization be built and survive with little funding? Does expansion, or even survival, require funding that would undermine or destroy the original principles and goals of the movement? More explicitly, will funding necessarily bring co-optation of the original principles of service to individuals and social change, and ultimately restrict the movement solely to the provision of service? Does changing from volunteer labour to paid labour, or from under-paid to well paid labour, bring a transformation in the type of person involved, from grassroots worker or philanthropists to professional? Is it possible to accept funding, thus ensuring survival of the movement and acceptable wages for work, and, at the same time, negotiate successfully with funding agencies to maintain the basic principles necessary for working towards 'the alternative'? – that is, working within the system while at the same time contradicting the status quo.

Before grassroots groups in the USA truly had a chance to get their feet on the ground, build their organizations and firmly establish their explanations and solutions, there was, by British standards, an explosion of State and Federal funding for more development. While the existence of this new funding was due largely to activists' own successes, the new funding was by no means theirs simply for the asking. The search for funding was intense and the demands of the search itself, as well as the conditions attached to accepting funds, often brought as many problems as it solved. Problems of new personnel, new programmes and new demands for compromise were met in a variety of ways, some expanding the efforts towards assistance and wider social change while others narrowed the focus more closely on the provision of services.[75]

Some examples illustrate different outcomes of this process. In Austin, Texas, a radical grassroots group with limited financial support and principles of wider social change was completely transformed by funding as people and principles were replaced in order to make way for massive funding and building of one of the few purpose-built shelters in the world.[76] In Minneapolis, Women's Advocates obtained both financial, corporate and community support while also retaining grassroots activists and original principles of social change. Transition House in Boston maintained its grassroots principles, gained little funding and eventually closed.

A recent study of 111 shelters in the USA found that funding was given the 'highest possible priority'.[77] This reflects an orientation to ever expanding programmes and diversification of activities. The pressure for funding on a large scale in the USA is also related to the need to purchase shelters and take on large mortgages, a problem which does not exist to the same extent in Britain because of the availability of public housing which is often provided by local government at a reasonable rent. However, recent changes by the Conservative government have drastically reduced the stock of public housing, and legislation concerning board and lodging for those in need has begun to plague groups in Britain. It must also be stressed that wealth is always relative as US shelters also feel the strain of financing, and, as in Britain, some have had to close because of lack of funding.

In Britain, funding has been mostly limited to local government and some local fund raising, and has been much more modest than in the USA. This means that the movement is much poorer in financial terms than their American cousins, but lack of funds to pay professional salaries has also meant the retention of activists, albeit underpaid, and volunteers committeed to the original principles and vision. Lack of corporate funds may mean a loss of material wealth but also avoids a powerful source of external pressure on principles and practice. The fact that the British movement was more firmly established in their principles and practices, and more firmly identified with the issue before even this limited funding became available, reduced some of the external pressure pulling away from their original ideas and practices and helped them resist some of the more traditional responses and forms of organization. In some ways, Women's Aid has become a part of the established landscape without becoming a part of traditional modes of practice. In others, it has been excluded by other organizations or excluded itself because of an inability to find a way of communicating and/or a fear of compromise should they do so. By comparison with groups in the USA, they have generally remained more 'pure' or unreconstructed in ideas and principles but much poorer in material resources. In both countries, tremendous efforts and energy continue to be spent trying to obtain the funds necessary for survival without too much compromise.

Men

The question of men raises several different issues within the movements. It is generally agreed that men, and not women, are responsible for spousal violence, and that this is structured within a context of male power and domination and supported through cultural beliefs and institutional organization and practice. While this forms an overall perspective upon the problem itself, it leaves open questions of the place of men in trying to eliminate this problem. Two main issues have arisen: (1) the place of men in local shelter/refuge programmes, the national organization and the movement itself; and (2) the development, nature and funding of programmes for batterers.

The question of the participation of men in shelters, the national organization and the movement arose at the very beginning of both movements. In Britain, Women's Aid initially decided to prohibit men from obtaining any positions of power and decision making throughout the organization, but local groups could decide whether to allow their participation in specific programmes such as children's play groups and periodic maintenance of refuges. The decision remains to date. Some early, negative experiences with men doing volunteer work within a few local refuges meant that even this activity has been very circumscribed or completely eliminated in Britain. As such, Women's Aid remains exclusively an organization of women. This has the effect of making it easier to maintain feminist principles and practice within an all woman group. On the other hand, it reduces the experience of taking those ideas into mixed groups and learning the techniques of negotiation, deciding on the acceptable levels of compromise and co-operative working between women and men.

In the USA, early debates were similar, and men were similarly excluded from the national organization and the movement itself. Although men have not been so clearly excluded from involvement in the activities of local groups, they are generally not present in large numbers. Men have generally excluded themselves from involvement, seeing this as a women's issue and one in which few have any interest. A few men work as volunteers or support staff in shelters. Some local groups have men in positions of power and status, as members of Boards of Directors and serving as public figures. In some cases the participation of men is chosen by local groups and actively used in support of feminist goals. In others, it is imposed or strongly influenced by funding bodies or as a condition of community support. While in still others, the presence of men, particularly in positions of power and status, signifies a group which departs from feminist goals, usually in preference for a narrow, individual focus on therapy and social service.

Both countries focus on the need for social and legal agencies to respond swiftly and effectively to men who use violence against women. This involves pressing legislators to pass new laws against men's violence and justice personnel to enforce them. Particular emphasis has been placed on the justice system and equitable treatment of this kind of violence, like other forms of violence, as a crime punishable by arrest and vigorous prosecution. Here, the involvement with men is twofold, indirectly with male batterers and directly with the criminal justice system with its overwhelming numbers of male personnel and its legacy of principles and forms of organization that are male dominated.[78] This does not involve the movement in direct contact with batterers. It is not, therefore, seen as the responsibility of the movement actually to do anything about batterers themselves, but, rather, to ensure that the criminal justice system protects women from male violence by taking up its responsibility to uphold the law and thereby control violent men.

While obtaining passage of legislation is itself difficult, ensuring enforcement from police, prosecutors and judges is even more problematic,[79] particularly in light of the traditional preference for ignoring or minimizing this kind of violence. The difference between the movement and the justice system in aims and orientations to violent men has meant protracted struggles for change and limited compliance with hard won reforms.[80] For some activists, the experience has lead to disillusionment, or at least a less optimistic view about using a reluctant justice system as a component of social change. This illustrates the complexity of the problem and highlights the fact that solutions include both the men who batter and the man-made institutions that allow it to continue. If institutions form part of the problem (and also involve the interests of men), how can they be changed by women who are largely outside the power structure? In the campaigns for legislative reform directed at arrest of batterers and enforcement of the law against assault, both the institutional orientation to male power and individual responsibility for the use of power in this form of violence are tackled at once. This shall be covered in some detail in the chapters on criminal justice. What is important here is that activists have been left with the dilemma that leaving the concerns about violent men to the criminal justice system alone has not been effective in meeting the movement goals of protecting women from male violence.

Programmes for violent men are another way of attempting to eliminate male violence, yet they present the movement with another set of issues. The first programme for batterers, EMERGE, began in Boston in 1977. It was started by a group of men who were informally linked to the movement. Using a feminist analysis of male domination and control, they adopted the principles of focusing on the violence and rejecting it unequivocally. The story of these programmes shall be told later, but it is important to state here that they remain an issue for the movement. Pro-feminist groups with a perspective sensitive to the issues concerning battered women and positive ties with the local women's shelters are seen by some activists as a necessary departure from the usual responses to battering, while for others they are to be avoided if possible. For all, there is concern about competition for scarce funding as well as wider issues about the content and orientation of batterers' programmes and whether they will individualize the wider social problem.[81]

The overall dilemma for the movement is one of maintaining their general goals and vision, what Mathiesen refers to as the *contradiction*, while at the same time being taken sufficiently seriously to be able to *compete* with other groups for adoption of these changes. It is obviously easier to maintain new or alternative goals and visions, i.e. contradictions of the status quo, in groups where the membership is sufficiently circumscribed that those basic ideas are not challenged, but confinement within a circumscribed group does not easily allow the message of change to compete for adoption in wider arenas of more diverse groups. On the other hand, competing for the adoption of new ideas always means negotiating, developing tactics and finding the acceptable limits of compromise that allow the movement to participate in the process of social change while at the same time holding on to proposals that constitute real change. The dilemmas of working for this '*competing contradiction*'[82] are revealed yet again as the movement continues to respond to the issue raised by batterers' groups. Ignoring such groups may help retain the vision (the *contradiction*) untouched but offers little or no possibility of having an impact upon the goals or practice of men's groups, that is, to *compete*. Directly attacking men's groups retains the feminist vision but also allows for the possibility of having no impact on men's programmes. Trying to work co-operatively with men's groups allows for the possibility of having an impact upon their practice (*competing*), but, at the same time, runs the risk of losing the feminist goals and vision because of the inevitable need to negotiate and compromise within any such working relationships and thus providing an agreement with rather than a *contradiction* of the status quo. There is no obvious position to be taken. The outcome of this will depend on the skill and tactics of the movement as well as the impact of wider issues such as government support, public opinion and the like. This could be an opportunity for expansion of the original vision of the movement and for inclusion of a much wider section of the community in these efforts. It could develop into two separate and unrelated movements against male violence, or it could signal an eclipse of either one.

Activists and professionals

The concern about the balance between social change and social service, political work and service provision has been expressed most persuasively by Schechter,[83] who notes that the possible shift and its fundamental transformation of the movement could occur and might reach advance stages before it is even noticed. She anticipated the possible loss of the new way, 'the alternative', and has tried to retain within the movement the process of working more self-consciously and concertedly towards those activities, tasks and types of relationships that form the conditions of social change.

The possible shift from social change to social service is embodied in the debate about professionals and their place in the movement. This is particularly relevant to the USA, although it might become more important in Britain with the emergence of psy-professionals, particularly in the new programmes for violent men. The question of the role of professionals involves the very identity of the movement and the goals to be sought. At stake is whether it continues as a social movement seeking social change for all women and improved conditions for those who are abused, or becomes a social service providing individual assistance and/or therapy for a few. That is, whether they remain activists and advocates *contradicting* the status quo and *competing* for adoption of their vision of social change or are transformed into or replaced by hostel managers and therapists supporting the status quo.

At its base, the issue of grass roots and professionals may not be so much a question of the exclusive presence of one group or the other, but, rather, of how they combine and what they strive to achieve. The membership of most new social movements is composed of community activists and those from the 'welfare and creative professions', what has sometimes been called the 'new class'. For example, the membership of British CND, the Campaign for Nuclear Disarmament, during one of its most active phases, contained members from social work, medical services, teaching, the Church, journalism, art, architecture and scientific research.[84]

From the beginning, there has always been some combination of grass roots and professionals in the movement in both countries. It has remained at a fairly constant, low level in Britain while the number of professionals has increased in the USA. A characterization of the changing combination reveals that the initial discovery of the problem, the establishment of the primary response of shelters, the pressure for changes in legislation and the explanation of the problem came from activists. While some lawyers, social workers and researchers were involved, it was usually as participants using their respective skills, and not as wage earning employees engaged in their occupational work. As participants in a social movement, they used their particular skills to assist in the process of change, including shaping reforms and mounting criticisms within their own professions. This process involved using what they have gained from their profession to help create new forms of responses and relationships within it, instead of adopting the traditional stance and status of their professions to colonize the new social problem for the purpose of expanding the profession itself.

In addition to what might be called these 'visionary' or 'activist' professionals are their colleagues who might be called the 'occupational' professionals. While the former seek meaningful change in society using their field of work, the latter simply seek work. The latter do not provide critiques or call for change. Instead, they attempt to establish the relevance of their profession in responding to the new problem and to establish the necessity of having their members built into required staffing for shelter programmes. This sometimes requires minor modification or expansion of professional concepts, terminology or techniques, which then have a new sound to accompany the new problem, but nothing fundamentally different is actually proposed.[85] The relationship between the occupational professional and the individual, now redefined as the 'client', is usually a hierarchical, one-way line of communication, with the professional as a knowing, acting 'subject' and the individual/client as the passive, receiving 'object'.[86] The explanation of problems becomes individualistic in nature and the solution becomes individual legal actions or personal therapy. By its very nature, this moves away from wider social explanations and issues of social change. This approach not only retreats from the vision of social movements seeking change but is positively disdainful of, or at least fearful of, such activity. Accordingly, social change efforts are defined by occupational professionals as outside the 'proper' professional role. In failing to see the place of their own activities in the reproduction of the existing social order, they falsely view activist professionals' attempts to change to a new order as 'ideological, political or subjective' while viewing their own attempts to retain the traditional order as 'neutral' and 'non-political'.

The appearance of occupational professionals did not occur until the problem had been established and sufficient funding obtained to make it possible to carve out a place for employment. Then there appeared to be some attempts in the USA to try to establish the pre-eminence of their respective occupations as the experts who should fill such jobs. Within the movement in the USA, articles appeared about the grassroots and the professionals, asking: Who are the experts?[87] Who speaks for battered women? Who has legitimacy with the public, the state, legislators and policy makers? The answers could be posed in terms of those with credentials or those with vast experience of the problem, that is, abused women and activists. Commenting on the problems of a division between battered women and professional staff in shelters, Schechter states that 'hiring more professionals only increases these tendencies. In fact, professionalization of services is a dangerous goal for any movement that hopes to organize and liberate women.'[88]

At times, alliances between grassroots groups and professionals have been both useful and sought after by shelter groups. External requests for the voice or skill of an 'expert' or professional are often ably met and benefit both the movement and abused women. However, this sometimes has the unfortunate effect of giving the impression that only experts know such things or are able to articulate them. This further enhances the usual hierarchies of knowledge and worth. This is not to say that the particular vantage point of each does not result in differences in knowledges and skill, but, rather, to note that experience, and all it teaches, and theory and professional skills are not such that one is always better, or truer or more relevant than the other. Ultimately, there is a delicate yet important relationship between activists and visionary professionals, and a territorial one between activists and organizational professionals. At stake for the movement is its identity, membership and purpose: whether it is a charity helping the poor, a professional service providing therapy for the sick and deviant, or a modernizing, democratic, participatory social movement seeking change for all.

A broad based movement: pluralism and sectionalism

'Never trust anyone over thirty.' 'The only place for women in the movement is prone.' These infamous statements from leaders of the student and black activist movements of the 1960s illustrate how divisions can be used to identify which groups may belong to a social movement and to specify their place or function within it. They also illustrate the external contexts of social division and discrimination in which all social movements exist, and are reminders of internal issues to be addressed. Divisions around gender, race, ethnicity, sexual preference and social class are endemic in most western societies, and liberating social movements are not free from these problems even as they work to eliminate them. While it would be comforting to think that by opting to eliminate one area of subordination or discrimination all of the others will simultaneously be eliminated, this is patently not true. The well-worked debates about class and gender illustrate how social changes for white working-class men have not automatically brought changes for members of ethnic minorities and women.[89] It would also be comforting to think that by declaring a movement to be in support of liberating and emancipating principles that they will be adopted by members and put into practice with a minimum of effort, leaving the real work to that of changing the rest of society. This is also untrue. Since social movements emerge within the context of a divided society, they inherit this legacy and must explicitly deal with its manifestations within their movement. It is neither realistic nor fair harshly to judge a movement working to eliminate discrimination because the goal is not instantly achieved. Nor is it productive to ignore or excuse discrimination within a movement as the inevitable product of the wider, divided world in which the movement exists. Somewhere in between lies the struggle to put non-discriminatory principles into practice. In her call for sensitivity training for staff and residents, a black shelter director in the USA clearly articulated the immediate problem and its wider context:

> Everyone is racist within this society; it's inevitable. We can't help each other by pointing fingers and confronting each other hostilely.

We need to create a safe space to talk about our feelings, fears, and attitudes. We must start from, 'we all have negative attitudes'.[90]

It is this middle area between absolute bigotry and complete enlightened emancipation that characterizes the movement. The treatment of each of these issues could and should fill volumes in their own right, and some have done so. By comparison our treatment shall be brief. Each issue encompases its own questions about the wider social and institutional contexts of discrimination and poses dilemmas within the movement itself concerning differences among and between women who live and work in refuges and form the decision-making structure of the movement.

In order to encompass a substantial section of society, a social movement must have a broad base and appeal to a variety of groups within society. This has the benefit of expanding a popular movement and bringing a variety of perspectives to bear upon formulating new directions and structures. It also poses the dilemma of how to deal constructively with the interests of the various groups within the movement so that they strengthen the movement rather than become crystallized and result in internal struggles that become the primary focus of the movement. The battered-women's movement, particularly in the United States, is one of the very few examples of an organization actually crossing over the lines of race, class and sexual preference among its members. This is by no means universal or unproblematic, but where women of different races, classes and sexual preference work together and find some way of managing the obvious differences between them, even with strife and difficulty, this is a major step forward. This involves a combination of both pluralism and sectionalism built into the organizational structure.

Race

In the United States, the issues of race and ethnicity were raised very early. With the background of a strong civil rights movement and a society composed of almost every racial and ethnic group in the world, this is to be expected. As early as 1978, the issues of race and grassroots involvement brought strong debate at a conference in Denver, Colorado sponsored by the Department of Health, Education and Welfare (HEW) to consider findings of their sponsored research and demonstration project on various models of shelter provision. Concern was expressed about the failure to deal with race in shelter programmes and research. From the outset, the Coalition developed regional caucuses and task forces within the organizational structure in order to reflect the interests and concerns of women of colour, feminist socialists, rural women, handicapped women and different geographic regions.[91]

At the first national conference in 1980, the feminist-socialist caucus put forward a seven-point plan of action to form priorities and shape the work plan of the leadership. They included: concrete anti-racist work at all levels; development and participation of leadership of former battered, third world, rural, handicapped and low-income women at every level of the organization; recognition of lesbian women and a public stance against homophobia; an analysis of the dangers of co-optation in all facets of the work; ongoing discussion among the membership addressing issues of gender, race and class in the operation of daily work; a plan to share community organizing skills throughout the membership in order to build and mobilize at grassroots level; and giving priority to building alliances with other struggles in the women's movement and other progressive forces in housing, day care, civil rights, welfare rights and labour organizing in order to create a mass movement working to end violence against women.[92] The First National Conference on Third World Women and Violence was sponsored by the Washington DC Rape Crisis Center in August 1980, focused on the issue of race, and in December 1981, a national network of 100 women of colour was formed through the efforts of the Coalition's Women of Color Task Force.[93] The questions of race, as well as class and sexual preference, were addressed explicitly when they formed the central theme of the NCADV national conference in Wisconsin in 1982.[94] They were tackled head on and viewed both as elements providing a broad base of membership and diversity of experience and perspective, and confronted as elements with considerable potential to divide and factionalize the movement.

In Britain, the issue of race was not originally recognized nor built into the early organizational structure. Somewhat later, a separate group was formed within WAFE for a brief period. A group for Asian and Afro-Caribbean women has recently been reconvened in response to a desire for a black woman-only workshop at the national conference.[95] For the most part, Asian women became active before Afro-Caribbean women, and then primarily to set up separate refuges in order to deal with very distinctive cultural differences surrounding language, food and religion, as well as racial prejudice.[96] There are now separate refuges, particularly for Asian women in England and

Scotland. Amina Mama's book *The Hidden Struggle* provides an account of violence against black women, the responses of voluntary and statutory agencies, and their place in the movement in Britain.[97] It illustrates how the movement is actively working to find responses to very real problems created to a large extent by a racialist society.

Questions of race and ethnicity raise several important issues within the movement and pose some problems concerning the nature of the problem of violence against women. These include: (1) the economic, social and familial position of the woman of colour who is subjected to violence and of the man who abuses her; (2) the nature of ethnic communities and the special importance attached to the traditional family and kinship ties; (3) provisions in shelter for accommodating different languages, customs, food and/or the development of refuges specifically for women from different racial and ethnic groups; (4) inclusion of women of colour in the organizational structure of shelters and on committees dealing with proposed policies, legislation and funding. At the core is the fact that women of colour, both those living and working in refuges, experience a double oppression based both on gender and on race. This, combined with different cultural heritages and family and community cohesions, means that they have additional problems and priorities. Many feel that racial oppression is a more pervasive and serious problem than sexual/gender oppression, and many align first by race and only second by gender.

The additional factor of racial oppression means that movement ideas about male domination may be less clear, or contradictory. At least three ideas articulate various standpoints. First, that men of colour use violence against their partners because of the stresses and frustrations they experience because of white racial oppression and not so much as a form of male domination and control over women. That is, race is a stronger explanatory factor than gender. Second, that women of colour are bound by a greater cultural allegiance to the family and their community, and thus to leave a violent man presents greater difficulties for them. This is further exacerbated by their poor position in the economic market where they experience the double discrimination against women and against people of colour. Third, while it is both difficult and relatively unacceptable to leave a violent man, it is also unacceptable to seek assistance from the authorities, especially the police, since their response, particularly arrest, may be interpreted less as a support for women, as it might be for her white counterpart, and more as a further act of racial oppression against men of colour. These throw up a whole series of double binds for women of colour who are beaten, and for all activists within the movement as well as for social agencies responding to male violence.

The woman of colour who lives in a racialist society and is also beaten by her partner faces impossible choices: she may escape her man's violence but at the cost of family and community membership and solidarity, or she may remain ensconced within family and community but at the cost of her personal safety and well-being. Unless the ethnic community actively rejects male violence among its members and polices it themselves or allows others to do so, women of colour are, in fact, being expected to bear the brunt of gender violence within a racial or ethnic group in order that the group itself or its violent members not be exposed to further racial oppression. This stance is not completely unique and bears some resemblence to issues of class oppression and gender violence. For example, some commentators have excused the violence working-class men have used against their partners because of their oppression within the capitalist system. In so doing, white women have also been asked, particularly in the past, to remain silent, excuse the violence used against them and cope in the name of respectability for themselves, their man, their family and their community.

While the focus on race raises legitimate concerns about discrimination against men of colour, and fears of stigmatizing the family and community, a failure also to consider gender oppression leaves women of colour in much the same position as before the movement. It tends towards adopting a position that, quite unwittingly, excuses the violence of men of colour by placing its cause beyond his control, outside his sphere of motivations and, therefore, not truly his responsibility, like that of the white working-class man excused because of his oppressed place in the capitalist system. This denies the illegality of assaulting a woman of colour and the legitimacy of intervening on her behalf and/or at her request.

To address the question of the man's use of violence as a purposeful and useful act for which he is responsible is one which is obviously very difficult since it turns the object of racial oppression, the man of colour, into the subject of gender oppression, an abuser of women. If the victim of one form of oppression acts as an oppressor, albeit in another arena, then activists fear that public sympathy and understanding of racism will diminish. Indeed, this is not uncommon as the public often adopt spurious rationales for justifying violence as a convenient means of allowing it to continue rather than facing the difficulties and complexities of seeking its elimination. At the base of this lies a notion that victims of oppression must themselves be perfect, or at least not the oppressors of others. Only such 'worthy victims' warrant concern and deserve to be free from oppression. Based on the behaviour of some of its members, whole groups can be classified as 'worthy' and deserving freedom from oppression or as 'unworthy' and thereby justifying indifference or inaction. If some men of colour, no matter how many or how few, are violent to women of colour, then the entire group ceases to be 'worthy victims' of racial violence and oppression, and whites need not trouble themselves about eliminating this problem from the social landscape. Instead of delineating the extent and the severity of each of these problems, placing them in perspective and addressing them accordingly, the mere existence of one form of violence is simply used to offset and justify that of another. If some men of colour abuse their 'own' women, then, the thinking goes, why should whites worry about how they discriminate against all people of colour?[98]

To a large extent, the strength of the movement lies in its broad base of support and its potential for meaningful social change lies in this coming together of racial groups to work on a common task (itself a major accomplishment), while at the same time addressing the question of racism itself. The efforts of the battered-women's movement in dealing with racism are certainly not complete nor without problems and difficulties. Nonetheless, these efforts, particularly the scope of those in the USA, stand as something of a landmark among social movements and as an example to others who would seek to struggle for racial equality and harmony within and outside their organization.

Sexual preference

The issue of sexual preference and public intolerance of a variety of sexual and family lifestyles has always been a part of the women's movement with its orientation towards free choice of partners in developing non-hierarchical relationships. It has sometimes become an issue in its own right, usually to assert the right of lesbians openly to live a lifestyle other than the idealized monogamous nuclear family – working husband, dependent wife and 2.2 children – which, at present, composes only 5 per cent of British society.[99] Within the movement, it has also been important to acknowledge the right of lesbian women to live the private life they choose and to combat homophobia within the movement and thus decrease the possibility that the dominant group of heterosexual women will not exclude or purge lesbians in order to satisfy external or, sometimes, internal demands that the legitimacy of the movement be signified by the real or perceived conformity of all activists to an idealized family lifestyle.

While one's personal, sexual preference may have little direct connection to the issue, the provision of shelters, funding, legislation, running a national organization or public speaking, it remains an issue because of public pressure to deny the existence of lesbians and gay men and to deny their achievements and contributions to community life. The justification for exclusion is often expressed in the homophobic fear that lesbian women will sexually seduce women who live in shelters and/or 'convert' them, and that they have a particular interest in breaking up families and, thus, will not encourage women to go back to violent men. The fact that no woman should be encouraged to return to further abuse, and that seductions in shelters, in the few cases that have occurred, are, as elsewhere, usually done by men, seem to be forgotten or ignored by those inside or outside the movement who would construct this thin veil of legitimacy for intolerance.[100]

In order to prevent what could become a creeping form of self-censorship and increasing external demands for suppression, particularly in times of economic stringency when questions of survival of shelters become even more pressing, the national level of the movement in the USA responded by reaffirming the right of all women to choose their own private sex lives, acknowledging the important work done by lesbian women within the movement and directly tackling homophobia as a possible means of external discrediting and/or a source of internal disunity. This was done by directly acknowledging the issues of race, class and homophobia as factors that could lead to disunity and making them the theme of the 1982 national conference of NCADV.

Retaining a broad based and diverse membership cannot be done without achieving at least a minimum level of internal unity and solidarity, and diversity cannot be retained without respecting heterogenity. In a sense, this is perhaps like a latterday form of integration in which the mixed membership of a group is made clear and visible both to itself and to the outside world. All groups must thus acknowledge, rather than dispute or deny, the diverse nature of the organization itself as they conduct the business at hand which is addressing the issue common to all, that of working to eliminate the abuse of women.

Social class

The social class of women within the movement also provides diversity of membership and raises several important issues. There is widespread and persistent belief among the public and the media that this is a working-class problem that does not affect the rest of society. Studies which include the middle classes, famous cases that cannot be kept out of the media and the many middle-class women now willing to admit to their partner's use of violence against them dispute the popular myth and strengthen the notion that violence against women is a universal rather than a class-specific problem. This also helps provide a bridge within the movement across the traditional social divide between middle- and working-class women.

Given the nature of shelters and refuges as crisis accommodation usually crowded and with sparse provisions, it is most likely that the residents will be those working-class and poor women who cannot afford alternative accommodation and/or whose friends and relatives do not have sufficient space to house them and their children. Residents sometimes become volunteer or paid workers in shelters and some obtain positions in the local or national organization. Some also become spokeswomen in public meetings, on television and at national conferences. However, like most new social movements, the membership is mostly middle class. As Olive Banks notes, they have the 'education and political skills' necessary for rebellion and the 'free time' that makes 'it possible to translate rebellious ideas into political action'.[101] While the political acumen of many working-class struggles may challenge middle-class exclusivity in such areas,[102] it is, nonetheless, true that members of the middle classes and the intelligentsia have almost always been a part of struggles for major social changes even when their own class stood to be disadvantaged by it.

Within the battered-women's movement, as with many of the other new social movements, the middle classes, particularly those in the social and educational professions, form a substantial proportion of the membership. The fact that middle-class women predominate among activists and organizers and working-class women among residents has had an affect on the movement and highlights important issues. As with race, it is relevant to consider the cross-cutting allegiances between social classes, the difficulties of communication and the positions of decision making and power within the organization of local groups and the movement itself. The social and cultural divides in the wider society may not be as extreme as those concerning race and more blending may occur, but these social conditions do exist and need to be considered by the movement if they are not to be recreated therein.

As the movement has matured it is noticeable that the voice of abused women, once a requisite feature of speaking in any public forum, is less frequently heard. Perhaps this reflects a desire not to use the pain of women in order to educate the public and policy makers, a laudable desire. It may also be that activists have come to value their own skill and experience to such an extent that they alone represent abused women without considering the importance, both to the women themselves and to the public at large, of hearing women's stories over and over again until they are truly understood.[103]

Coalitions

Building coalitions with other groups and social movements can serve two important purposes. Temporary coalitions may be effectively formed in order to address a specific issue, such as pressing for or objecting to a piece of legislation or a public policy. Temporary coalitions are very task oriented and may even involve groups not completely in sympathy with one another. More permanent coalitions may expand still further the base of participation and of issues while creating an even larger mass movement. In Britain, traditional alliances exist between the women's movement and the Labour party, trade unions and some sections of local government, particularly the recently established Women's Committees. Voluntary organizations for single parents, housing and homelessness, anti-rape and others form natural and sympathetic partners on many issues. The practice, however, is usually one of operating separately and only combining on rare occasions. By contrast, coalition building was stated as one of the initial aims of the movement in the USA, and it has been used quite frequently to amass support for various issues, as shall be illustrated in Chapter 4 on the state and public policy. Schechter makes repeated reference to coalitions of women's groups used to pressure for specific gains within the movement and to resist detrimental developments. Progressive alliances are viewed as an important means of resisting government cuts and regressive steps, particularly in the current political and economic climate which is not favourable to progressive social movements and their proposed changes.[104] She warns, however, of entering into alliances of temporary expedience with right-wing groups whose principles are, in fact, at variance with the movement as this will ultimately undermine the movement itself. She also notes that this does not mean merging with other groups, losing movement goals or membership. Particular importance is given to retention of the autonomy of women's organizations, noting that 'the women's movement is too young and sexism too old for women to give up their own base of support'.[105]

Any comment concerning the sheer volume of achievements of the movement since its inception would, of necessity, be an understatement. Providing shelters where once there were none and establishing public recognition of the problem where it did not exist stand as monumental achievements on their own, but there is more. In both countries, innovations at the local level are countless, including successful efforts to obtain funding, public education, conferences and workshops, children's programmes, community outreach, and, specific to the USA, advocacy, counselling and telephone networks.[106] At the national level, the grassroots movements have also managed to initiate an impressive list of action, including: public hearings held by Parliament (GB) and the Senate and Civil Rights Commission (USA); National/Federal legislation (GB/USA), reforms in the social services and the justice systems; housing reform (GB); and civil actions against the police for failure to protect abused women (USA). In the USA, legislative reforms alone represent a massive effort primarily because of the necessity to pass laws in each of the fifty states rather than at the national level as in Britain. Finally, building national organizations for each movement and influencing similar actions internationally have taken both movements on to a world stage.

The identity of the movement is to a large extent revealed in its goals, styles of working, forms of organization and the internal issues it addresses and how it addresses them. In forging its identity the movement constitutes a new way of thinking and working that contradicts the status quo and competes for adoption of its proposals for social change. Creating a new alternative also requires negotiating with the opposition in order to establish these goals. It is in this process that the movement risks the transformation of its wider vision of social change to one that does not contradict the status quo or to one that does not compete on the field of change. Such negotiations necessitate raids and reconstructions within the camp of the opposition, sometimes winning, sometimes compromising and sometimes experiencing setback or defeat. In this process, the central task of the movement is to hold on to its alternative message, to resist the external pressures to transform it into some form that reproduces the status quo, albeit it with a new sounding name, but also to compete for acceptance where it is unlikely to be given easily or without compromise. It is a process of walking on the edge, sometimes inside, sometimes outside, sometimes progressing towards the goal of change, sometimes maintaining a steady state and sometimes losing. Walking on the edge does not demand that every struggle for change be won if the alternative is ultimately to be achieved, but that 'the alternative' not be lost in the ongoing struggle over specific issues, and, of course, that the ultimate goal is eventually achieved.

3 Refuges and housing

The refuge stands at the heart of the battered-women's movement and is important for a variety of reasons. For the woman, it serves as a physical place where she can temporarily escape from violence, find safety and make decisions about her own life. Contact with other women helps overcome isolation and a sense of being the only one with a violent partner. For the movement, it provides the physical location from which to organize, and serves as a base for practical and political thought and action. Refuges vividly illustrate women's continued dependence in marriage and economic disadvantage whereby they must rely on a man for the basic necessity of accommodation. It raises most powerfully the issue of women's autonomy by illustrating so clearly their present state of dependence upon others: husband, family, the state or charity for the material basis of daily existence. Thus, the refuge itself becomes a fundamental means by which feminist politics is developed, sustained and rekindled within the context of the problem itself and in close contact with the daily lives of its sufferers. The refuge provides an almost unique opportunity for creating a change for women that not only assists women who have been battered but also stretches beyond those who seek refuge. The provision of a physical space so thoroughly enmeshed in the problem itself and in the lives of the women and refuge workers is unique for most social movements, and it is doubtful that a movement, rather than just a provision of service, could have developed or been sustained without it.

Historically, the refuge has often served as a haven for women in distress, those escaping cruel fathers or husbands or those without means of support.[1] Housing has also been a rallying point for women's popular protest such as in the Highland Clearances of the late nineteenth and early twentieth centuries where Scottish women fought bailiffs seeking to remove them from their homes in order to use the land to graze sheep and in the nineteenth century Glasgow rent strikes organized because of high prices and poor conditions.[2] More recently, in the 1980s the women of the barrios in Mexico City have organized a tenants' union after the devastation of an earthquake in order to protect their families from eviction by unscrupulous landlords, negotiate with the government about the size and design of rebuilding, and to keep watch over construction workers and their managers. Shelter has often been provided for dependent or disadvantaged groups including women, children, the poor, the sick and the elderly; and sometimes for entire communities or whole societies as refugee camps develop to support victims of war, civil strife, racial violence and economic disaster.

The concept of the refuge represents a haven, a place of respite or a last chance to escape oppressive or dangerous circumstances. Indeed, the metaphor of the refuge was used in the fourteenth century by one of the first feminist writers, Christine de Pizan, in *The Book of the City of Ladies* (1405).[3] The image was of a medieval, walled city constructed by women to serve as a protection against the slander of influential men of letters in their assertions about the innate inferiority of women. As a writer in the French court, she was the first woman known to enter into the literary and philosophical debate about the value of women relative to men, *querelles des femmes*, in which learned men debated whether women were human, their basic nature, if they could be educated and whether they were good for men. Noting the almost universal assertion of women's inferiority among men of learning, she maintained that women were left defeated, either to accept these views and join an inferior cast, or to try to identify with men and become false and inauthentic.[4] She distinguishes herself as a feminist thinker, a term unknown until much later, by rejecting both and constructing a response asserting the intellectual and moral equality of women and men. She asserted women's basic humanity and called for better education and kinder treatment in marriage, accusing men of cruelty to wives and beatings:

> How many harsh beatings – without cause and without reason – how many injuries, how many cruelties, insults, humiliations, and outrages have so many upright women suffered, none of whom cried for help?[5]

Pizan used the walled city as a metaphor for rejecting men's false assertions of women's inferiority. For her, she

must shovel away the 'dirt' of men's false views of women before

she can build the city on a firm foundation [on a 'field of letters'].
The 'stones' forming the city's walls are the lives of exemplary
women, which provide a refuge to protect other women from male
slander.[6]

Three ladies, Reason, Rectitude and Justice, reviewed and rebutted
male disparagements of women and used examplars from the lives of
virtuous women to show women equal or superior to men. In
'building' for women this refuge from the cultural traditions that
subordinated them to men, Pizan constructed an ideology which
united women with similar beliefs over subsequent centuries.[7] She
also provided an early, compelling imagery of the importance of
refuge not only in individual attempts to escape male abuse but also
as a location for action directed at building a different environment
for all women.

For battered women, the provision of refuge first began in Britain
in the early 1970s and quickly spread nationally and internationally.
Refuge is, of course, a sensible, practical first step in assisting women
to leave violent men, but its general function may be viewed more
widely as a crucial, material means of responding to one of the fundamental aspects of men's control over women. To the extent that
women are solely or primarily dependent on a husband or male
partner for basic human needs such as food and shelter, they may
have to endure any number of abuses simply to maintain these basic
necessities of life itself. Women who challenge the abuses and the
abuser face the bleak prospect of losing the material requirements of
existence provided by their abuser. Thus, a woman's challenge to
violence must always be undertaken in the hope that she alone will be
able to provide decent housing for herself and her children, and in the
certain knowledge that this must be done in a world where women as
a group are economically disadvantaged. Housing for displaced
women is often undertaken by relatives or a new partner, and sometimes by philanthropists, the Church or the state. Even then, women
must expend great effort to secure this accommodation and, for the
most part, it usually means a drop in their standard of living. Historically, it has also meant that women must adhere to the rigid religious
and disciplinary regimes of the convent, magdalen house, the poor
house and, in this century, hostels for the homeless. The ability of
women to escape from male violence has always involved this most
basic of human requirements.[8] Thus, if women are to become free of
male domination or abuse, they must first find a means of securing
the basic human needs of food and shelter.

The economic dependence of women upon men is a crucial part of patriarchal control. As such, the refuge stands simultaneously as an essential aspect of supporting women subjected to male violence and of rejecting patriarchal control of women. In both symbolic and material terms, the refuge stands at the heart of attempts to eliminate men's abuse of wives and female partners. It can readily be seen that the obverse, men needing accommodation in order to escape abusive women upon whom they are economically dependent for the daily necessities of life, is rarely, if ever, true. While this may seem an obvious point to most observers, it must, nonetheless, be made because some American researchers believe they have found symmetry of violence among women and men in the United States, thus making the US a curiosity in international terms.[9] We shall return to this puzzle in the chapter on the research, but here we wish to stress the importance of the refuge in seeking positive social changes directed at protecting women and eliminating male violence.

THE FIRST REFUGES AND EARLY EXPANSION

The first refuge, and probably the most famous, Chiswick Women's Aid, opened in Britain in 1972. It was started by a consciousness-raising group who established a community centre to be used as a meeting place for women. Hounslow Council (London) provided a small terraced house with two rooms downstairs, two upstairs, a kitchen and outside lavatory. It had been derelict for six years and, like others nearby, was due for demolition.[10] When a woman arrived who had escaped from her husband because of years of violence she was taken in despite the licence limiting use to office hours only. Soon more women came, some for several days, others for months. Within a year there were over thirty women and children in residence. By April, 1973 there was an average daily population of twenty-five women and children. All four rooms were filled with mattresses on the floor, and a room of 12ft by 10ft slept three women and four children.[11] Thirty enquiries were received each day and 'overcrowding and uncomfortable conditions' were the norm.[12] No one was turned away, the refuge was literally bursting at the seams with 'women and children sleeping head to tail, like sardines in a can'.[13] The media were actively covering the new problem and helping to put pressure on existing agencies to respond to the plight of the women and their need for refuge.

The refuge was financed in a haphazard fashion, with the house and rates (local property taxes) paid by the Council (local government), social security payments covered the living expenses of women and children, with other necessities provided by proceeds from jumble sales and donations of furniture and clothes from the community. A large number of volunteers provided help and legal aid.[14] This refuge was soon replaced by a very large, Victorian mansion with ten large rooms and three inside lavatories donated by a socialist millionaire. On the first day, fifty-four women and children were in residence.[15] Despite its size, it, too, was soon overcrowded as more and more women heard of the refuge and sought relief from violence. The policy of overcrowding was viewed by Erin Pizzey, the charismatic leader, as important because women simply could not be turned away. It also made a strong point about the large number of women needing refuge. Overcrowding was viewed with alarm by health and safety officials and became the source of disputes with local authorities. It was difficult for residents, but made a strong point and created considerable media interest. To the visitor, the atmosphere in the refuge was chaotic, with bunk beds everywhere, children overflowing the back garden and the kitchen and bathrooms stretched beyond even the gracious proportions of a Victorian mansion.

In the United States, there is some debate about which refuge was first, but the one most closely identified with the battered-women's movement was Women's Advocates in St Paul, Minnesota. It began as a consciousness-raising group which became interested in action and social change. In 1972, the collective began a telephone service for women in the county Legal Aid office and soon found that the majority of calls were from women being assaulted by their husbands. Little help was provided by local services and so women and children were taken into the homes of volunteers.[16] In February, 1973, a one-bedroom apartment was obtained to provide more permanent shelter, but after six months the group was evicted by a disgruntled landlord. After a great deal of effort and serious financial difficulties, a mortgage was secured and Women's House opened in October, 1974. The house had five bedrooms, two and a half bathrooms, a large living and dining space, a basement and an attic on the third floor. Like all new shelters, it was the subject of considerable media attention and was immediately filled to capacity, taking in twenty-two women and fifteen children during the first months.[17]

Also in 1974, the first refuges were opened by Women's Aid in Scotland. The houses in Glasgow and Edinburgh were provided by local Housing Authorities (government-owned housing). In 1972, six women from the Edinburgh Women's Liberation Workshop began Edinburgh Women's Aid. After a workshop in Chiswick, they were inspired to open their own refuge and obtained a three bedroom flat from the Town Council with the proviso that it had to get off the ground within six months or close.[18] After two weeks, they had thirty-five women and children. The rent for the house was divided by the number of families in the refuge, all work was by volunteers and the group begged and borrowed equipment: '... there was plenty of spirit and enthusiasm'. 'We were very, very green....'[19]

In spring 1973, sixteen women from Glasgow Women's Liberation workshops and consciousness-raising groups formed Glasgow Women's Aid and began the one year battle to obtain a refuge. They had to prove there was a need for a refuge, that women did not deserve or like violence and that Women's Aid was not simply breaking up families. 'I must admit, in those early days, we were very naive and very indignant.'[20] Interval House opened in February, 1974.

> After campaigning for over one year, we were given this horrendous first-floor flat in the Gorbals [one of the most notorious slums in Glasgow]. It had a big kitchen where women cooked and ate, four bedrooms, a communal living room and one horrible toilet. The building was located underneath a railway line and on top of a haulage contractor. It had rats. It wasn't just a hard-to-let flat, it was due for demolition, except there were two other families who were still living there!.... It was very difficult to keep it looking welcoming. It was terribly depressing for any woman walking into that flat. It was dark. It was dingy. And we didn't have the money to carry out repairs.[21]

At first they also had an 'open door' policy and were overcrowded almost from the day of opening. At one point during the first year they had ten women and twenty-nine children sharing. 'They were sleeping everywhere except in the bath.'[22] This caused friction between the women about housekeeping, and wear and tear made the flat even less inviting. Women were leaving because of the conditions so the group established a basic housekeeping procedure and set a limit on numbers. Women kept coming, sixty-two during the first year alone. Both Glasgow and Edinburgh Women's Aid operated with the feminist principles of self-help and non-hierarchical organization. They were funded by volunteer assistance from members, fund raising, donations of money and furniture, social security payments to women for rent and food, and small grants from local government.[23] The first refuge soon opened in Wales followed by Northern Ireland and the Republic of Ireland.

Early expansion

Soon there was a flurry of activity as more groups began to form, more refuges opened, and more women sought shelter in more and more countries. In 1977, both the British and the US governments responded to activists pressure and, in co-ordination with activists, commissioned research on provisions for battered women. The results show the expansion of shelters and refuge, some aspects of life within them and, particularly in the USA, diversity of types of shelters. *Leaving Violent Men* tells the story for England and Wales and *A Monograph on Services to Battered Women* for the USA. These two studies of refuges, while not directly comparable, provide numerous points of comparison between the two countries. It is fortunate that they were conducted almost co-terminously, although it should be noted that the British movement was more advanced in refuge provision at that time because it had mushroomed a few years earlier.

The rationale for the British study was that alternative housing is a basic need expressed by battered women when seeking help and its absence a chief obstacle to escaping violence. Thus, its provision is essential if battered women are to have any real choice of leaving a violent man.[24] The British study was conducted against a backdrop of recently passed legislation meant to assist women in obtaining permanent accommodation, Parliamentary recommendations for refuge provision throughout the country and a welfare state with a large stock of council housing and an established commitment to the homeless. While the theory is always better than the practice, there was, nonetheless, significant commitment to housing provision.

This first and only large-scale study of refuge and permanent housing for battered women in England and Wales included a national, postal survey of 114 refuges and in-depth interviews with 656 women living in refuges, of whom eighty-four were interviewed in a follow-up eighteen months after the survey.[25] The findings show the extent of expansion within five years of the opening of the first refuge. During the one year period of the research, between September 1977 and 1978, 11,400 women and 20,850 children were housed, and many more were turned away because of lack of space.[26] Yet by 1978, only one-sixth of the one thousand refuges recommended by the Select Committee were available.[27] Refuges were found to have only basic amenities, usually only one kitchen and cooker, one bathroom and no dining room or laundry. Most were overcrowded. The women were critical of these conditions and the researchers recommended refuges with separate bedrooms, a kitchen and bathroom shared with only one or two families and communal living and play areas.[28] Women were allowed to stay as long as they needed in order to make decisions and, if required, to find permanent accommodation. Residents thought a stay of two months was ideal and six months a maximum. In reality, the average stay was five and a half months, and sometimes over a year, primarily due to difficulties in finding permanent accommodation.[29]

British refuges had very little money. They were funded primarily through the rent of residents, usually from social security benefits. Some groups received temporary government funds, such as Manpower Services Commission (now defunct) and Urban Aid available only for cities or regions of special need. At the time of the research, half the groups had less than five thousand pounds per year to cover all running costs.[30] They were grossly underfunded, and temporary sources of government funding were being cut and local authorities (local government), seen as the only realistic source of permanent funding, were not taking over as Women's Aid had hoped.[31] Despite all this, the women interviewed while they were in refuge and in the follow-up eighteen months later highly valued the refuge for offering a respite from violence, an end to isolation and an atmosphere of mutual support, sharing and assisted self-help.

By contrast, the USA had little of this infrastructure. The back-drop to the US study was one of providing welfare and public housing only for the poorest women, and a more restricted approach to material provision for those escaping violence. However, some government programmes were used creatively to provide aid to the poorest women who could qualify for benefits, including housing in government schemes, food stamps and aid to dependent children.[32] The rationale for the study was to examine the various types of responses to the problem of domestic violence in order to consider how best to proceed as far as government provision was concerned. This research and demonstration approach to social problems is well established in the USA.

The 1977 survey of groups throughout the USA was conducted with 163 groups responding to a questionnaire focusing on the women, funding, staffing, services and organization. In addition, eight shelters, representing a wide variety of approaches, orientations and geographic locations, were chosen for detailed study and evaluation.[33] A brief summary illustrates the breadth of early ideas and practices in the USA. The 163 programmes came from all types of groups, mostly YMCA, National Organization of Women (NOW) chapters and church societies, with about 15 per cent from consciousness-raising groups, rape crisis groups or the National Coalition Against Domestic

Violence.[34] Each organization seemed to reflect its beginnings. Most were hierarchical in structure with decision making along lines of authority from boards of directors to programme directors, and sometimes included women who had been abused. At that time, about 15 per cent were democratic, non-hierarchical and included battered women on the staff.[35]

A few details provide a characterization of these programmes which were much more diverse than those in Britain. Of the 163 programmes, about 130 had shelters (about equivalent to the total number in England and Wales with its much smaller population). The average capacity was fifteen. In 1977 14,473 children were given shelter while 46,838 women were served in a variety of ways, some receiving shelter.[36] The average stay was two weeks with a maximum of one month.[37] Funding was primarily from individual donations of money, goods and services, followed by Federal funding which, as in Britain, was overwhelmingly job creation via the Concentrated Employment and Training Act (CETA), and welfare subsidies. Funding from private foundations, businesses and local and state government was far behind.[38] Staffing was overwhelmingly from volunteers augmented by CETA jobs. The ratio of volunteers to paid staff was three to one, and one-seventh of the staff were formerly battered women although they were three times more likely to be volunteers. Men comprised one-eleventh of paid staff and volunteers.[39]

Services were wide ranging including: shelter; social and emotional support and counselling; assistance and/or advocacy with medical, legal, employment and welfare needs; fundraising and clerical and administrative work; assistance with domestic work including food, cleaning and laundry; transportation; and child care including counselling, recreation, daycare and medical needs. Over a quarter of the programmes provided services for battering men consisting mainly of counselling and referrals.[40]

In general, the findings show many similarities between the two countries. Refuges and shelters were mostly supported through the volunteer labour of women and the rent from residents, often on social security benefits. Some received support from urban programmes directed at regional development in financially dis-advantaged areas. The few paid staff were supported by government job creation schemes and paid low wages. Government funding was meant to be temporary and neither country had a permanent source of funding for refuges from local or national government. Refuges were often poor, lacking in facilities and overcrowded although the spirit in them was one of dedication of workers, hope of the women and a general enthusiasm for change. The women who sought refuge in both countries found it beneficial at a time of crisis, and the British follow-up study was able to document the longer term, beneficial effects.

The findings also show differences between the two countries. From the outset, Britain had a substantially higher proportion of groups affiliated with the Federation which was clearly guided by feminist principles and striving to put them into practice. The small minority of groups outside the Federation were single, local groups, some aligned with Chiswick. This general unity provided a much wider political and power base facilitating further growth of the National Federation, strengthening the idea that refuges were the work of Women's Aid, and reinforcing their philosophy and approach to the problem. While this was by no means clear cut or uncontested, it was, by comparison with the USA at that time, much more unified. The extreme diversity in the early groups in the USA not only meant an initial image that was less clear, it also presented greater difficulty in building a unity within a national organization. Other differences include the presence of a substantial number of programmes for violent men in the USA and an almost complete absence of them in Britain. Most British groups were non-hierarchical and had no Board of Directors while they were commonplace in the USA. British refuges did not have wardens and the women set their own daily routines and undertook their own housework and cooking, with the only exception being 'play workers' for children's activities. Refuges in the United States varied, ranging from this pattern to one of fairly institutionalized regimes.

These early differences were important in the later development of refuges and the movements in each country and illustrate some of the diversity which characterizes the overall approach to abused women, the issue itself and proposed solutions. Since these early beginnings, some programmes have died, others have been radically transformed and the balance of the different types of shelters has changed, particularly in the USA. In them, however, it is possible to see much of what would become grist for the mill of future programmes and/or government policy, to observe subsequent changes in the movement and to get a glimpse of the variety of practices that sometimes approximate various strands of feminist as well as other orientations and practices.

Throughout the 1980s, even more refuges opened. Although some closed because of government cuts, the overall provision continued to increase, albeit more slowly than in the 1970s. By 1989, the number of programmes in the USA had reached 1,200 and existing shelters housed 300,000 women and children per year.[41] Also in 1989–90, Scottish Women's Aid had thirty-seven groups with thirty-two refuges and served 12,000 women and children, although 2,000 had to be turned away for lack of space. Wales had thirty-two refuges and served nearly 5,000 women and a similar number of children. England had just over a hundred groups with nearly as many refuges accommodating over twenty-three bed spaces per group.[42] The pattern is one of slow growth or stability; however, current threats to social services by the conservative governments in Britain and in the USA may affect this pattern in the future.

TYPES OF FEMINISM AND TYPES OF REFUGE

In considering the differences between the types of shelters/refuges, it is easy to view the building, quote the level of funding and cite the available services as a complete, or at least a necessary, description. This may be misleading, not because such details are inaccurate, but because the nature of refuges may be more clearly reflected in their philosophy and the relationships they seek to establish with and between women than in bricks and book-keeping. In examining the diversity in shelters, we seek to reflect on some of the underlying philosophies in order to highlight different approaches and regimes. The implicit or explicit philosophies of groups operating shelters are quite diverse, although many are based on feminist ideals. Examining the philosophical bases of shelters enables us to unravel the diverse orientations to women and workers as well as to wider issues of social action and change. We shall consider the foundation of various feminist orientations and then examine examples of different types of shelters which reflect feminist as well as other orientations.

The legacy

Several writers have characterized the different orientations within feminism using a variety of definitions and terms.[43] Anderson and Zinsser chart European feminism focusing on the changing discourses, sites of activity and specific goals and campaigns which range across the literary and philosophical, the political and the economic. The Renaissance of the fifteenth century developed new values emphasizing humanism, education and individual and civic virtue for men, and these were challenged to include women. Isolated women of letters, rather than a feminist social movement, entered the philosophical and literary debates about woman's basic nature as subordinate and driven by vice, asserting, instead, that women were fully human and had the capacity for virtue. Practical claims included education to ensure equality of the intellect and civilized treatment of women in courtship and marriage which could be brutal.[44] Feminist movements as such did not appear until much later.

Equal rights feminism sprang from the Enlightenment. Philosophers bequeathed Liberal ideas of the importance of human reason rather than power and authority based on tradition. They emphasized self-realization, freedom, autonomy and individual potential among men, particularly men of property. The revolutionary developments of the seventeenth and eighteenth centuries – the English Civil War, and the French and American Revolutions – brought new political rights for men and provided the context in which equal rights feminists emerged and made similar claims for women. They emphasized similarities rather than the differences between the sexes and the importance of environment rather than nature in shaping gender differences. They sought the end of male privilege which excluded women from their natural rights. Influenced by the French Revolution, Mary Wollstonecraft was a major proponent of equal rights feminism in England. In *A Vindication of the Rights of Women* (1792)[45] she sought changes in education for women and kinder treatment by husbands and lovers. She also ushered in a new phase in feminist discourse by looking to the state to secure women's rights and redress their grievances through legislative reform of marriage and education.[46] John Stuart Mill followed in a similar vein with *The Subjection of Women* (1869) and pleas for Parliament to reform the laws on divorce to allow women to divorce a husband for violence and cruelty.[47] In addition to wider claims for equal rights to citizenship, political participation and legal rights, equal rights feminists sought rights to child custody, personal property, the vote and education.[48]

In the 1830s, the same years that middle-class Englishwomen demanded the vote, working-class Englishwomen began to form unions and co-operative societies for the advancement of women's economic and political position.[49] Rather than concentrating on political and legal change as the equal rights movement, the Owenites concentrated on economic change campaigning around pay, working conditions and hours, and working-class women were recruited to socialist parties and trade unions.[50] They sought a fair distribution of products for their labour and criticized husbands and employers alike, linking the economy and marriage.[51] They believed that women would be liberated by the economic transformation of capitalism into socialism.[52] Focusing on women's labour, particularly in industry, they criticized the middle-class equal rights movement for ignoring the economic sphere in which working-class women had to earn a living in oppressive conditions. Under government pressure, accusations of atheism and sexual licence and the failure of the Revolution of 1848, the Owenites failed in 1850.[53]

The nineteenth century saw changing economic circumstances and the development of socialist movements seeking change for working people. Within them women sought a transformation of the economic order as a means of improving women's general position in society, and specific campaigns were aimed at equality for women in the workplace, access to better jobs, pay, conditions, choice of work, advanced and better education.[54] Feminist socialism, focusing on women's work, women's welfare and the vote, made new demands between 1875 and 1925, and built in Germany the largest working-class women's movement in Europe.[55] Feminist socialists had to steer their way through the indifference or antagonism towards feminist issues among socialist men and to translate the concerns of working-class women into socialist issues.

There was considerable antagonism between socialist-feminists and the middle-class equal rights movement concerning issues and tactics. In Germany, France, Russia, Italy and Austria the two movements loathed one another. Throughout Europe, feminist groups were divided between the equal rights movement of middle-class, liberal women focusing on the vote, especially for women of property, and the socialist women's movement of working-class women and their supporters focusing on the economy and the overturn of capitalism. Only in England and Scandinavia did feminists work in combination with liberal and socialist parties and equal rights organizations and unite middle- and working-class women.[56] Present socialist feminists thought emphasizes the importance of economic change and the role of the state and has borrowed more heavily from Marxism than from the original Saint Simonian and Owenite thinkers.[57]

Evangelical Christianity of the late eighteenth and early nineteenth centuries provided missionary zeal and a focus on social issues and moral reforms, such as slavery and temperance.[58] Within this tradition, women are viewed as naturally superior to men in characteristics such as kindness, gentleness and nurturing. A cult of pure womanhood supports ideas that women should be in positions of political power, education and leadership because they differ from, and are better than, men in these characteristics. The 'pro-woman' sections of radical feminism represent the modern variant.[59]

Olive Banks describes the ninetenth-century women's movement as a history of cross-cutting coalitions and cleavages within feminism and diverse alliances with groups outside. She examines factors that help explain the emergence of feminism as a social movement and define its diverse nature. She argues that the rise of the movement is associated with (1) ideas of liberal Protestantism with its emphasis on religious individualism, marriage and the family, and sexuality; (2) ideas of the Enlightenment philosophers and events of the French and American Revolutions which inspired notions cf natural rights and political democracy, and (3) structural changes that affected women's place in society, particularly the separation of home and work and demographic changes with greater or fewer women in the population.[60] Banks writes that the nature of feminism in the USA and Britain has been shaped by three intellectual traditions – evangelical Christianity, equal rights liberalism and socialist feminism.

The lull in feminism after the First World War and into the 1950s was partly precipitated by a belief among equal rights feminists and feminist socialists that they had won the battles for women's rights and marked by a turn away from feminism itself and on to causes related to feminism, particularly welfare work and women's issues associated with their traditional role within the family.[61] This adds a variant that is still relevant today.

The modern movement

It is this foundation of feminist discourses and feminist practice that provides the legacy of ideas and action prior to the re-emergence of feminism in the 1960s. The spectacular revival in the 1960s saw a re-entry of all three feminist orientations – radical, equal rights and socialist feminists – a renewal of political, economic and social dreams and demands, attempts to transform the basic institutions of society and specific campaigns for divorce reform, birth control, abortion, sexual freedom, and against physical and sexual violence.[62] Although the history often had to be rediscovered in the new feminist scholarship, many of the original ideas soon re-emerged and formed the context of campaigns for change. The battered-women's movement and the provision of shelters and refuges reveals this legacy.

Radical feminists have been most central in the orientation of the battered-women's movement in both countries. The pro-woman

orientation has lead to a concentration on the central importance of
gender, the intimate domination of women under patriarchy and a
consideration of its institutional and ideological forms. There has
been a concentration on the politics of the body and the politics of
the emotions and mind. Issues relating to the politics of the body
include rape, abortion, child sexual abuse, health care relating to birth
and reproduction, and violence against women. Campaigns in both
Britain and the USA have centred around each of these and concentrated on the violation of women's bodies as the cite of oppression
either by individual men or by institutions such as medicine (for
violations of the body) and criminal justice (for failure to protect
against violations). Concentrating on the politics of the mind emphasizes how the mind or emotions have been abused or distorted
through patriarchal beliefs and relations and must be regenerated in
another form. In both countries consciousness-raising groups
provided an early means of exploring these issues and emphasized the
need to become aware of the position of women in social and
personal relations and to reshape themselves and social institutions in
order to improve the position of women.[63]

In the USA, there has been a much greater emphasis both inside
and outside of the movement on the politics of the mind and
emotions. In Great Britain the emphasis has been on social and
material conditions. A cultural orientation of individualism and
therapy and powerful and influential therapeutic professions have
provided the climate in which the wider orientation to women's
consciousness and its social consequences could be shifted within
some groups towards greater emphasis on women's psychological
characteristics and the perceived need for therapy in recasting
individual women with the general aim of making them independent
and safe within the community. Although not articulated as such, the
general thinking is that if women become better equipped psychologically they will be able to ensure their own safety from male
violence. By becoming less 'helpless' they will be better able to handle
the men currently beating them. By securing mental and emotional
strength, as opposed to material and social means, women will be
able to escape and will, thereafter, be better equipped emotionally to
avoid choosing another such male partner. Thus, the solution to male
violence lies in female psychology and women's transformation
through therapy.

The movements in the two countries are further distinguished by
the additional importance of equal rights feminism in the USA and
the influence of Labour and left politics in Britain. There is a long

history of equal rights activism in both countries with British feminists seventy-five year campaign for the vote and changes in women's rights to property, child custody and divorce. In the USA a constitution with a Bill of Rights provides an overall context in which this approach is emphasized and shaped. Campaigns for equal rights before the law and law reform are particularly strong components of all of the new social movements in the USA, with civil rights providing a particularly important example. Similarly, the women's movement in the USA has been oriented to legal changes to facilitate equal access to education, work and wages. Following on, the battered-women's movement has placed great emphasis on campaigns to change the law and its enforcement so that acts of violence are treated similarly regardless of the relationship between the offender and the victim. This has been noted in the chapter on the movement and will be discussed in greater detail in the chapters on criminal justice, but the important point here is that the strong emphasis on equal rights before the law, with its basis in Liberal feminism, has played an important role in defining the particular character of the movement in the USA and the place of the shelter within it.

In Britain, the movement has been differently shaped by the combination of radical feminists within an environment of left and Labour politics, particularly at the local level, and, somewhat obliquely, by socialist-feminist concerns if not by socialist feminists themselves, who have largely remained apart from the movement. The emphasis is on the role of the state, particularly the welfare state, and its place in enabling battered women to escape from violence by achieving a certain economic independence through state provision of housing, social and health services and welfare benefits. Campaigns for equal pay and equal opportunity for wage work, while important in both countries, have generally been separate from the battered-women's movements although generally agreed to be important in the complement of factors affecting women's ability to escape from violent men. These facets of feminism form the wider context in which the movement and its shelters and refuges are shaped.

The characterizations of the different traditions in feminism exist only as general types, rarely found in a pure form either within individual refuges or in the movement itself, and are often modified by practice and blended through alliances. However, differences in foci do remain and help explain some of the differences in refuges, forms of organization and power, orientations to the problem and relations between the women who live and work in refuges. Any analysis of the different types of refuges and shelters must also note the role of orientations other than feminism, especially the therapeutic and bureaucratic/professional. The latter contain very different conceptions of social problems, of those who experience them and of social change. They are sometimes incorporated in the battered-women's movement through alliances, but also exist in their own right both inside and outside the movement. A mixture of orientations and organizations within and across refuges are thus threaded together in complex patterns of practical action and philosophical orientation, but styles and patterns can still be seen.

TYPES OF REFUGE

For our analysis, refuges and shelters are roughly categorized into four types, philanthropic, organizational and bureaucratic, therapeutic, and activist. While activists' shelters reveal numerous elements of the various strains within feminist discourse and action, the other three generally reflect different traditions. The examples have been chosen primarily from models that existed at the very beginning of the movement. As with Mathiesen's notion of the 'unfinished' the movement had many possible worlds from which it could initially choose. The direction in which it would develop was, at that stage, open and fluid. Everything was an experiment; anything seemed possible. Within a few years, the direction of the movement and the place of shelters within it would become more firm and fixed. But this early period before the movement had truly formed reveals the competing ideas and models for action extant at the moment of its beginning.

The philanthropic approach is more easily identified with the nineteenth-century view of benevolent, usually middle-class reformers, albeit without any particular professional qualifications, responding to the poor and those deemed inadequate by providing some form of material resources. There is usually a benevolent, hierarchical relationship between the philanthropist and the recipient of charity. Poverty and homelessness are of particular importance, thus following some of the moral and social reforms of the early evangelical Christian tradition within feminism but departing from much of modern, radical feminism. A contemporary variant involves the inclusion of professional counselling and therapy.

The therapeutic corresponds more closely to the modern mental health movement and the therapeutic professions in which individuals qualify to assist others through educational certification. Generally, they are trained to deal with personal and psychic inadequacies using therapy and counselling. They, and the delivery of their service, are most often organized in hierarchical channels of one-way communication and authority over their clients. Although such orientations exist within the movement, often through alliances, there is no close equivalent in the intellectual traditions of feminism.

The professional bureaucratic is more akin to the civil service, the administration of local government or a multi-faceted, private, voluntary or profit-making agency. It is staffed by professionals in a variety of areas and organized along bureaucratic lines. The primary orientation is towards the smooth and efficient running of the various agencies or professionals rather than the individual women *per se* and/or the wider social problem. The goal is to co-ordinate existing personnel, agencies, facilities and resources to deliver existing rather than new services, but to do so in a more efficient fashion.

The activist orientation is directed at grassroots action, self-help, involvement of abused women, and egalitarian relations within and outside the refuge. A wider and more political view is taken of the roots of the problem and the necessity for far-reaching changes to deal with the individuals concerned as well as the social supports underpinning wife beating in society. The target of wider change is sometimes cultural, focusing on ideologies and beliefs, sometimes material focusing on women's economic position, and sometimes institutional and/or political focusing on the response of organizations and the state. Often they include a mixture of all three. Depending upon the particular group, activists may draw on the Enlightenment or equal rights tradition, on socialist-feminism, and on the Evangelical ideas now translated into radical feminism. The creative combinations of ideas among activists often result in a pragmatic blending of traditions, but the foci and most strongly held principles still continue to place them roughly within these ideal types.

This variety of provision, politics and philosophy includes differing ideas about the women, the role of refuges and the solution to the problem of male violence. This, in turn, includes several continua: from self-help to enforced therapy; from notions of women's independence to practices reinforcing dependence upon new 'masters'; from viewing woman abuse as a problem linked to a wider political struggle for social change to that limited solely to service for victims; from emphasis on the community and/or the individual; from advocates working with abused women to therapists working on clients. Each idea or practice carries the baggage of a wider orientation, sometimes obvious to its users, sometimes not.

Much of the information about refuge provision in Britain and the USA is about local groups and has not been compiled to provide an overall view. The two government sponsored projects on refuge provision in the respective countries referred to earlier provide a basis for characterization of refuge types using basic information provided by the groups themselves, about their history, management, staff and volunteers, abused women and their children, the refuge or shelter, and relations with other organizations.[64] They show a range of beliefs, political approaches and organizational styles that provide variety and innovation as well as controversy. In outlining the variation among these groups, we shall focus on the structure, organization, philosophy, daily routine and relationships between women and workers. Let us begin by discussing architecture and regimes in order to illustrate how the material conditions of bricks and mortar, albeit of vital importance, do not determine the nature of relations conducted within them.

Architecture

Architecture is, of course, important in the development of routines of daily life. There is a long tradition of attempting to use architecture to affect human behaviour, be it through the design of churches, schools, convents or prisons, or through the development or control of the built environment. While much architecture and urban planning has been criticized for ignoring the needs of women or equating them with those of men, architecture has also been seen as a force for social change for women, as exemplified in the proposals for the kitchenless house.[65] But change cannot be achieved through design alone.

Differences in architecture, regimes and leadership, and some of their consequences, are evident in comparisons of refuges from London to Amsterdam, Alaska to Texas and points between. For example, the early refuges in Chiswick and Amsterdam had similar architecture and similar sounding feminist principles, but inside the refuges exhibited radically different styles of organization, leadership, daily life and routines or regimes.[66] Both had large Victorian houses described earlier, both were concerned about women victims and their children, and both used ideas of self-help and the like, but they varied considerably in translating general principles and ideas into practice. Visits to both revealed some of the main differences in practice not revealed either in architecture or basic philosophy. The open-door policy, a powerful tool in the political argument about the existence of the problem and the need for refuge, was adopted by

both but pushed to the limit at Chiswick resulting in extreme overcrowding, pressure upon residents and a sense of chaos. The
Amsterdam refuge was also full and the political point was made, but
it did not appear to be bursting at the seams and residents lived their
daily lives in a more ordered atmosphere creating a greater sense of
calm and well-being for all. Leadership also varied, with the hierarchical, top-down style of the charismatic personality at Chiswick
and a flatter, more horizontal, democratic and collective style in
Amsterdam.

Austin, Texas and Anchorage, Alaska, separated by thousands of
miles from the North to the South of the continental USA, also show
how very similar architecture can house very different approaches.
Both have had the almost unique opportunity to design and construct
a well financed, purpose-built shelter, attending to the details necessary to create pleasant, functional surroundings. In Alaska, the archi-
tect was commissioned to work in co-operation with Frances Purdy,
an activist with experience of working in buildings not suited for use
as shelters. The product of her vision is a shelter with several public
spaces of varying sizes for a range of activities from watching television to large social gatherings. A large communal kitchen contains
all the modern conveniences of a well appointed home as well as a
huge store for food including a pantry and walk-in freezer suitable
even for big game. Passive solar heating, full spectrum lighting, a
sauna and well-designed bedroom space for fifty-two persons all
make the shelter a pleasant place to live. Offices and small meeting
rooms are also a part of this well-planned multi-million dollar shelter
run by Abused Women's Aid In Crisis. Austin, Texas also had the
good fortune to build an expensive, well-appointed shelter but the
personal and political costs were high.[67] In order to obtain the co-
operation of local funders and influential members of the community,
the original group went through a purge of activists whose personal
politics or sexual preferences did not 'fit'. This narrowing of those
deemed 'appropriate' to work in the new refuge narrowed the
activists' base and took a high toll of personnel and inevitably
affected the orientation to the problem and the women.

As with architecture, shelters and refuges also vary in size, daily
routines, relations between workers and women, and views about the
women, the problem, the role of refuges and social change. A closer
examination of the four general types of refuges highlights some of
these differences. Examples of individual shelters/refuges are used to
illustrate the variation that was there from the beginning and to help
explain some of the general orientations that may be seen within the

detail of daily routines and stated philosophies. It is important to stress, however, that these are illustrative of more general themes that can be examined within the context of any refuge even as it changes over time.

Philanthropic

The philanthropic approach is illustrated by the House of Ruth in Washington DC. Located in the inner-city area of Washington with mostly black residents, it began as an offshoot of a soup kitchen which had a surprising number of women seeking food. In 1976, it was discovered that there were more than 5,000 homeless and destitute women in the city, and an emergency shelter was opened for them by an energetic women with four hundred dollars for the initial rent. During the campaign to gain public support for homeless women, many battered women and their children began to flock to the House of Ruth. In April 1977, House of Ruth Annex was opened specifically for battered women in a delapidated, old row house with three bedrooms, two paid staff, twelve volunteers who were mostly ex-battered women, and two para-professional women providing counselling, child care, job counselling and welfare advocacy. The board of directors included ex-battered women, business people, policy makers and politicians. The preference for private funding reflected the belief that government funding does not provide a secure future.[68] This may seem ironic, particularly in the capital city, but close proximity may spawn fewer hopes and more realistic expectations of government action.

Policy decisions were made by the board of directors, ongoing decisions by the executive director with input from staff and sheltered women, and daily administration by the programme co-ordinator and the resident with greatest seniority. Within the shelter, the regime included supervised daily resident meetings and scheduled house chores. Stress was placed on women's 'responsibility to the shelter, its program, their fellow residents, and their children'.

> House rules include times for wake-up, meals and curfew, daily chores, a daily meeting. No drugs, alcohol, or male friends are permitted. Upon arrival, women are directed to available community services for legal and medical needs, and the program is 'work oriented' with encouragement to search for work first and public assistance second.[69]

There was immediate explusion for curfew violations or failure to attend scheduled counselling sessions. 'A woman's progress within the program is evaluated weekly by her co-ordinator, who seeks to determine if she is using the resources available to her.'[70] With space for twenty women and children, the maximum stay was six weeks, but the average was only one week.

This organization of primarily lay individuals responded to abused women mostly in terms of their poverty and need for food and accommodation. In many ways it reflected its beginnings as a soup kitchen and a shelter for the homeless. The importance of focusing on the basic material provision of housing has been underscored by 1988 estimates of homelessness in the United States that ranged from half a million to three million and increasing. This certainly means plenty of work for organizations such as the House of Ruth and the National Coalition for the Homeless who blame the loss of decent paying jobs and massive cuts in Federal spending on low-income housing which fell during the Reagan era from $30 billion in 1981 to $7 billion in 1987.[71]

For the most part, such an approach is oriented to relief for individuals and the agenda does not include wider social change but, rather, the provision of a material resource to the most disadvantaged and deserving. Daily regimes are oriented to restructuring the individual in order to make her better able to compete for the material means of subsistence. The regimes of labour, discipline and personal reform to create the better worker are reminiscent of institutions established in the nineteenth century, such as poor houses, prisons and schools for the poor. Such an approach has its roots in nineteenth-century reformism. Although the connections with early feminism reflect the moralistic elements of Evangelical feminism, there is little correspondence with its modern inheritor, radical feminism, particularly with its emphasis on gender.

Organizational and bureaucratic

Further contrast was provided by CEASE, Community Effort for Abused Spouses, located in Alexandria, Virginia. Police data indicated a disproportionate number of domestic violence cases from the poorer section of the county, 'but lack of useful *nonarrest alternatives* was a major problem' (our emphasis).[72] The two-year demonstration project was a joint effort of NOW (National Organization of Women) and three professional agencies – mental health, justice and the social services. The hospital, social work and mental health centre were to co-ordinate existing services to provide a 24-hour emergency service. The most important goal was:

To develop an effective, replicable, multi-agency service model for diverting *couples* who are engaged in interpersonal abuse and violence from the criminal justice system to the human resources system [our emphasis].[73]

Management of this diversion scheme was by an advisory committee appointed by the board of the Center for Community Mental Health with membership from the county government agencies; women's organizations (Women's Legal Defense Fund, NOW and United Community Ministeries); and consumer/citizens. Paid staff included professionals and para-professionals from social services and mental health, with volunteers located in a staff hierarchy with clear lines of authority. The service included 24-hour coverage in the hospital emergency room and crisis intervention with counselling for individuals, couples and groups who came to the agencies during office hours. The poorest women able to demonstrate financial eligibility could receive some material assistance from the Department of Social Services (DSS) such as food stamps, medical assistance and job counselling. Shelter was another matter: 'Because the CEASE Program is based on collaboration of existing services, the *facility* [shelter] is nonexistent' [our emphasis].[74] Instead, referrals for emergency housing were made to a general emergency shelter or the County Women's Shelter (usually shelters for the destitute, alcoholic and mentally disturbed) where a woman could stay for a maximum of two weeks. The image is of a team of professionals working in social work offices or mental health centres giving counselling and advice during office hours or while on call at the hospital. It was the belief of this specialized service within the mental health system that the existing shelter for the homeless was sufficient for the few occasions when needed. They argued that:

categorical programs [i.e. shelters for battered women], although well funded in early years tend to suffer over time from decreasing public interest and government funding. Integrating services for battered women into the existing system is definitely one of the program goals. It is believed that sensitizing and training personnel in all human service programs, including the criminal justice system, will be to the long term advantage of the victims of domestic violence and their families.[75]

The general focus of such an approach is on the organization itself. Action is oriented to combining existing organizations to deliver, in a more co-ordinated fashion, much the same services as traditionally undertaken separately. Such an orientation would be of particular concern to the movement since they maintained that the need for, and successes of, their new responses arose partly because of the inadequate, and sometimes destructive, nature of the traditional policies and practices of social work, medical and law enforcement agencies. Attention to the individual was addressed to providing existing services only to those individuals able to seek assistance, with no attention on abused women in general or the social conditions that support the violence and help reproduce the next generation of violent men The focus on providing traditional services, albeit in a co-ordinated fashion, does not address the need for change of the traditional priorities, practices or orientations within agencies, does not provide advocacy or shelter in order to increase the independence and welfare of women, and therefore offers no agenda of social change.

Therapeutic

Rainbow Retreat in Phoenix, Arizona is basically therapeutic in oriention and regime, but also illustrates a mixture of the philanthropic and the bureaucratic with the contemporary variant of ministering to those viewed as psychologically sick.[76] It evolved out of an Alcoholics Anonymous programme for women and children living with alcoholic men. The residential home housed twenty-eight with additional space in an adjacent motel used as a dormitory, office space and 'treatment rooms, such as children's play therapy and counseling rooms'.[77] The house was managed by non-professionals and organized in a hierarchical, autocratic fashion. The Board of Directors, with over twenty members from the business and professional community, paid a corporate membership fee and served for two years. The Board was responsible for all final decisions and the resolution of resident's grievances or requests after they had first been through the 'housemother', resident treatment manager and director. Women and children were viewed as 'clients' with personal problems and inadequacies requiring therapy.

This treatment style programme offered women 'individual counseling, [discussion] sessions, group sessions, and transportation to community lectures'. It was funded by the Alcoholism Division of the Arizona Department of Health Services and planned to add 'outpatient counseling to the whole family unit'.[78] By 1980, funding from CETA, Phoenix divison of the Law Enforcement and Assistance Administration, Arizona Health Department, client fees and donations reached $350,000,[79] and a proposal to earn money from bingo was being considered. There were thirty staff (housemothers, cooks, counsellors and their aides) and about twice as many volunteers including student interns, students in practicum, former clients and members of the Rainbow Guild. The maximum stay was six weeks, with an average of two. Within the house:

> Clients can provide input at two weekly meetings or through a suggestion box.... [There is a formal grievance procedure and a structured, daily life.] After the crisis week, full participation in the structured program *is required* [our emphasis] by the client for the remainder of her residency [usually one week].... [Specific techniques included] confrontation, assertiveness training, grooming, self-exploration via Al-Anon meetings, and job exploration and development (although the latter was reconsidered because of difficulties in placing women in jobs).[80]

Batterers were allowed on the premises for counselling and visiting, and the diversion programme for them was an alternative to prosecution on misdemeanour charges for domestic violence.[81]

Such an approach is primarily focused at the individual level, using therapies meant to transform the individual woman through a focus on the violent man's alcohol abuse. Although unarticulated, such transformations must take the form either of making her better able to stop his violence, better able to cope with the violence or better able to leave the violence (although job-related services were abandoned as too difficult). Such therapeutic approaches are not oriented beyond the individuals who are their clients, to the wider group of abused women, nor do they have an agenda of social change directed at eliminating male violence or transforming the status of women.

In Britain, the early Chiswick Women's Aid refuge represents another variant on the therapeutic model. Although the original group began as a feminist collective, under the influence of Pizzey it soon eschewed such ideas and practices in favour of those of a distinct and in many respects idiosyncratic type of therapeutic community. Marjory Fields and Rioghan Kirchner, American lawyers, were early visitors to British refuges seeking to transfer to the USA the lessons already learned without reinventing the wheel. The lengthy quote from these observers provides considerable insight into the approach first taken at Chiswick:

> This is the grandmother of them all.... Chiswick is different from

all the other shelters in that it is run clearly by a large paid and voluntary staff ... is more of an institution ... [and] aims to keep the women for a long period of time.... It also differs from the others we have seen in that in Chiswick living is dormitory style in bunk beds and as many people as can possibly fit in a room are crammed in.

The shelter is managed and run by the staff.... The ground rules are established and maintained by the staff.... There is a house-mother who 'teaches women how to feed and bathe their children and how to put them to bed'. She 'teaches women how to play with their children'.... The staff believes that the children in the shelters are more violent than what they referred to as 'normal' children.[82]

The general approach was to create a therapeutic community to end the violence by 're-educating the women and the children out of the pattern of violence' in their lives, with the staff acting as therapists. The particular ideas about a therapeutic community espoused at Chiswick seemed to be taken from popular psychology. The therapeutic community was to be large and to recreate the chaos assumed to be part of the women's lives. Long-term care was thought to be necessary for women and children in order that they learn how to avoid inviting violence into their lives since women were 'violence prone' and 'addicted to violence' and would transmit violence to the next generation as boys automatically learned to be abusers and girls were imprinted through their mothers with the need for abuse.[83] It was suggested that the government should fund such a long-term institution. Fields and Kirchner commented that the staff created 'a dependency on the part of the residents' and did 'nothing to encourage the residents ... to make it on their own'.

they [the staff] are suffering from a severe case of rescue syndrome and that once they get a hold of the women and children they are unwilling to let them go. This did not seem to be the philosophy in the other places we visited.... The basic tendency is to treat them [the women] as though they were suffering from some form of pathology ... the paid workers clearly provide all kinds of services for the women and at the same time definitely control them and control the shelter. The result is that the paid staff destroys the women's role in managing their own refuge and destroys their self-determination.[84]

Chiswick's organization, particularly the uncontrolled open-door policy with its excessive overcrowding, created an even greater sense of chaos and constant crisis than in other refuges in Britain. The dominant influence of a single personality in every facet of refuge life mirrored Max Weber's description of the charismatic leader with the resulting unstable form of institutional order. Preference was given to ideas about cause that focused on the individual inadequacy of batterers and battered women alike, stressing notions of a chaotic lifestyle, intergenerational transfer of violence through family patterns, childhood learning through modelling adult behaviour and, somewhat later, biological inheritance among women of a tendency to seek abuse, called the 'violence prone woman'. Proposed solutions involved individual therapy, psychiatric intervention, and long-term institutional care.[85] This model of organization and regime did not embrace notions of social change.

Activist

Bradley-Angle House, in Portland, Oregon, provides an early example of an activists' shelter in the USA. It grew out of a shelter for women leaving prison and began a separate organization for battered women in 1975 with a CETA grant and $2,000 from the Women's Resource Center.[86] The early shelter was a multi-storey home in a residential area with a small office for staff and a bed for night staff. One-third of the staff were minority women who with other women worked in distinct areas, such as administration, outreach and follow-up, but in a generally non-hierarchical fashion. Volunteers, advocates, general shelter workers, employment counsellor, para legal counsellor and child care co-ordinators made up the complement. Volunteers included ex-battered women, women from grassroots organizations and professionals.

Decision making was based on feminist principles. Equality among staff and residents was stressed, and staff continually worked to develop more egalitarian administrative policies and to help residents develop a strong positive self-concept. Administration was by a working board of directors and an advisory board with members from all groups. Decisions were made by the Board and at house meetings with universal participation structured into the process. Residents helped make decisions about hiring staff, budgeting and organization, with consensus decision making based on experience and potential rather than professional training. The self-help group worried about institutionalization of shelters and created policies to defend grass-roots participation and minimize bureaucratic forms of 'professionalism'.[87]

In the daily regime, women were 'encouraged to become involved in the running of the household and make their own personal decisions'.[88] The collective made decisions at weekly meetings, group therapy was available, and cooking and cleaning were shared. The home advisor and housekeeper assisted daily routines and helped facilitate such activities as buying farmers' surplus food or obtaining discount prices since State law prohibited giving food stamps to anyone living and sharing meals in a residential programme except for alcohol and/or drug programmes. An advocate 'walked' women through the referral system to ensure they got the necessary services, learned their 'rights' and became more independent in dealing with agencies of the state.

At a more general agency level, a liaison person worked with the police, legal aid and other agencies to try to influence their policies and register complaints. B.A. House and the police each designated a liaison person to deal with the other organization seeking to facilitate good communication and mutual co-operation. Finally, B.A. House had a strong, working relationship with The Portland Men's Resource Center, which worked with batterers, provided public education and assisted with child care and typing at B.A. House. A monthly newspaper, *Changing Men*, and a film, *Men's Lives*, helped provide counselling for men. Batterers were self-referred since it was believed that this would avoid the justice system using the programme to divert men away from arrest.[89]

In Britain, the difference in approach between the early Chiswick and Women's Aid was profound. Fields and Kirchner observed:

> I think Chiswick is a pole apart from the other houses we saw.... The women we saw in England and Scotland who were residents of [other refuges] seemed quite capable of putting their lives together now that they were given a safe and peaceful place from which to reorganize themselves ... they all agreed that they were better off in the shelter than they were with their husbands ... [they] agreed that they could support each other and through discussing their problems together as a group help each other. They all agreed that they did not need psychiatrists.[90]

There are several sources of information about the self-help, egalitarian activists style of refuge in Britain. *A Refuge for Battered Women* (1978) is a case study of a Women's Aid refuge in Kent,[91] *Leaving Violent Men* (1981) describes a survey of 114 refuge groups throughout England and Wales,[92] and *Private Violence: Public Shame* provides an account based on in-depth interviews with eighty women living in a refuge in Cleveland, England.[93] Running through these and other accounts are familiar and consistent themes about the role of the refuge, relations between women and workers, forms of organization and working style, the goals of change and the political significance of the movement.

Refuges are viewed as important because they provide women with temporary housing, advice and personal support, and facilitate the use of agencies such as law enforcement and housing.[94] At Cleveland Women's Aid, the political significance of the movement involves many levels, most importantly:

> ... understanding the problem of men's violence against their partners as an aspect of the social subordination of women. This has a profound effect on the relationship between the group who run the Refuge (in a long term sense) and the women who use it. The sense of 'solidarity' on which this relationship is founded ensures that the autonomy of the women who live in the Refuge is respected and that their self-defined interests take priority even over the efficiency and smooth-running of CRAWC [the group] and the Refuge. The voluntary character of the organisation, as well as its single purpose and feminist basis facilitate this attempt to avoid the depersonalisation and displacement of aims often experienced in bureaucratic welfare organisations. While it is by no means inevitable that women coming to the Refuge share or are even fully aware of the underlying philosophy, they all benefit from it, since it both helps to avoid the stigmatisation and victim-blaming that often accompany the provision of help, and the tendency for the helping agency to define for itself and according to its own philosophy the problems and needs of its users.[95]

In running the refuge, women's autonomy is at the centre of daily routine and reflects a concern to 'avoid the contradiction of offering women an escape from one form of servitude, by inviting them into another in the shape of institutionalised, rule-ridden hostels'.[96] Life in the refuge is characterized by an absence of authority figures, no intrusions into privacy and few formal rules and regulations. There is little by way of a formal regime in Women's Aid refuges. None have resident wardens, women tend to organize their own daily activities and weekly meetings are often held, but attendance is voluntary. This is meant to create an atmosphere where women are treated as independent and capable adults who can talk freely with one another, support one another and gain from the exchange. The authors of the report on the Cleveland refuge note the paradoxes and dilemmas arising in trying to run 'an egalitarian, feminist, refuge in a hierarchical nonfeminist world'.[97]

The activists' refuge provides the opportunity for women to share their experiences of violence which unifies them, and women frequently praised this aspect of refuge life which allows them to realize that they are not alone and others are in similar circumstances. Women spoke of improvements in health, including sleep, appetite and relaxation, and of an increased sense of freedom. Research on activists' refuges in Britain shows that they are important in overcoming the isolation of womens' lives through shared experience and help facilitate the use of legal and social agencies which require public disclosure of a personal problem and often blame and shame the women for male violence.[98] Women are relieved that they are not unique, isolated or outside 'normal' society, and the chance to work through shared problems with other women reduces loneliness and restores self-esteem at a point when 'this is crucial for the struggle that lies ahead'.[99] For the women, the benefits of the refuge outweighed the difficulties associated with living with others in a world in which this is rarely practised. The difficulties most frequently mentioned are differing assumptions about child-rearing, household organization and privacy, as well as the physical amenities of refuges. Along with providing the basic needs of protection and accommodation:

> ... the combination of knowledge about resources available and the intimate but undemanding atmosphere of the Refuge seems to be effective in enabling women to confide their 'difficulties' and to face up to resolving them with renewed confidence and hope.[100]

Women indicate that it is better to have gone through a Women's Aid refuge and experience this process than simply to be rehoused in another home.[101] The importance of providing battered women with a place of safety and escape from violence and the pre-eminence of women and their children, rather than the institution of the family, are stressed. Accompanying ideas include self-help, assistance in regaining self-respect and making independent decisions about one's future, albeit in the context of institutional and ideological impediments to women's choices. The style of work and relationships between women who live and work in refuges follows ideas about working with, rather than for, battered women and horizontal, rather than vertical, forms of organization including collective decision making and the involvement of women who have experienced abuse.

While the improvement in women's self-esteem and well-being are of untold benefit, the Cleveland study notes, however, that translating this personal experience into 'full political and social awareness of the "public issues" involved is extremely rare'.[102] Thus, the question of wider social change is positively affected by the existence of feminist shelters and the personal experiences of change within them, but this is not sufficient. The agenda of social change must also be worked out in a wider context. [103]

The importance of refuge for abused women

The most powerful and supportive statements made about the importance of a place of escape from violence come from women who have found a haven within them. Their comments illustrate the enormous relief and numerous benefits provided. Safety, an end to isolation, companionship, solidarity, independence and mutual assistance are themes running through the comments of thousands of women from all over the world. Although almost any form of haven from violence is obviously welcome immediately upon escape, the routines of refuges, the nature of life and relations within them are also crucial, both to the women who experience those conditions and to those who benefit indirectly through the accompanying social and institutional changes that flow from them. Comments from women in activists' shelters in Britain, the USA and around the world reveal the significance of these factors to the women who have lived in them.

Refuges and change

Activists now run most of the refuges in both countries, and they are almost universal in Britain. The USA, however, still has a representation of the other three types, particularly the therapeutic. Within activist shelters, the ideal type of organization is democratic and egalitarian with a limited amount of hierarchy. For the women, the emphasis is on self-help, advocacy and individual empowerment. They are usually based in the community with grassroots membership. The types of feminist traditions represented are usually a pragmatic blend. Most prevalent is a blend of equal rights and radical feminist ideas, emhasizing equality and women's position in society. Themes from socialist feminism, emphasizing class and the economic and political order, are more likely in Britain although not completely missing from the USA. Emphasis is placed on provision of material resources, particularly those associated with state provision of accommodation and social benefits. In Britain, this forms an important part of economic support for a substantial number of women, and is a means whereby they can achieve a degree of independence from violent men. Support for individual women in crisis and advocacy for them within social, legal and medical institutions form the mainstay of activity in both countries. Wider social change, particularly of the status of women and of the institutions responding to violence, is very much on the agenda.

The organizational and bureaucratic approach often employs a co-operative, multi-agency model. The multi-agency approach is, no doubt, a useful model in responding to wife abuse. It will not, however, be effective in challenging male violence if it is concentrated solely in the hands of professional agencies using traditional methods and excluding abused women and activists whose innovative responses are directed at confronting men's violence by transforming institutional response rather than just diverting and/or containing it within existing agencies. Organizations have a tendency to resist change, to redirect the innovative proposals of activists' groups with whom they work and to re-establish the status quo after a period of experimentation. Thus, excluding or neutralizing activists and advocates for battered women would most likely contribute to the continuation, in a slightly new form, of the same responses found so wanting in the past. In the words of Mathiesen, the message would be a competing agreement, that is, the same old thing wrapped up in slightly new terms.[104]

Professionals also try to build and retain their own pre-eminence when faced with a challenge from outsiders. The attempt to keep the response to battering located within existing agencies has two effects: (1) supporting and expanding the position and authority of the professions involved and (2) defining those skills deemed to belong to the professions as the appropriate and preferred form of response to this problem. Thus, professionals often attempt to gain and/or retain exclusive control and access to any problem by creating a process of exclusive access to those who experience the problem through certification and licensing based on formal education required to enter the respective professions.

When a woman seeks assistance from a philanthropic or thera-peutic organization, she usually enters a relationship of dependency in which she becomes an object responding to the efforts of others rather than an independent subject acting in her own right and working with the support of others to manage her own life. The nexus becomes that of the manager or therapist working on 'their client' or that of the activist working 'with the woman'.[105] In refuges with these approaches women are subjected to regimes intended to tranform the individual, either in material or in emotional and psychological terms. Women are often required to attend counselling and/or therapy sessions which may be a condition of receiving shelter. In the USA, there is a widespread orientation towards the therapeutic even within some activist shelters. It must be stated that there is a serious problem of terminology in which some of these activities are clearly like traditional therapy sessions while others may be more like ordinary discussions which have simply been given the name of counselling or therapy. Only an examination of the content of such sessions on the local level can distinguish the crucial differences in terms of content and relationships within such sessions. It might be very useful, particularly for shelters who have an agenda of social change, to adopt terms which more accurately describe the activity, be it therapy, counselling or group discussions.

The orientation to the woman seeking assistance constitutes a crucial element in the overall process of seeking social change. There are three possible orientations to the person that distinguish philanthropic, therapeutic, bureaucratic and activist approaches. The woman becomes an object within the philanthropic and the bureaucratic approaches. That is, she is conceived of as the passive recipient of the intervention of others rather than an active creator within her own environment. Within the therapeutic approach, she is treated as an object/'subject'. That is, she is first treated as a passive or dependent person receiving direction from others, but their guidance dictates that she become a subject, acting to transform herself into an image provided by the therapist or professional. The woman's task is to become an object in order to receive advice which then dictates that she must turn herself into a particular type of 'subject'. Finally, within the activist shelter, the woman is treated as an independent subject acting on her own behalf. That is, she is allowed to create her own life as she sees fit and within the circumstances in which she finds herself. Assisted self-help is an important part of the woman's sense of self-reliance and ability to manage her own life. We would argue women must be treated as subjects rather than objects if meaningful change is to be sought, much less to occur.

A PERMANENT HOME

Beyond refuge is the rest of life. There must be some place to live. The refuge provides temporary accommodation and can be a personally supportive and transformative experience. It does not, however, provide a permanent home, and this can be one of the most crucial struggles for freedom from violence faced by women. As indicated earlier, housing is a basic material necessity of life. If a violence-free home cannot be found, a woman cannot be free from violence. Yet we live in a world in which women are still largely dependent upon men for this necessity, and many face the bleak prospect of a life of violence or homelessness. It is not difficult to see why the decision to stay or leave is a very difficult one in which the best route is not clear. Without a change in women's prospects of obtaining decent housing for themselves, those who leave home because of violence must usually become dependent upon another provider, a new partner, relatives or the state in order to have a home and be free from violence. This is tremendously difficult to organize, and it usually involves a drop in the standard of living, particularly for women reduced solely to the earning power of a woman's wage or state benefit. What has been done to try to redress this fundamental problem?

The importance of housing cannot be overestimated. Along with economic independence and viability, it ranks as one of the crucial factors affecting women's ability to find viable alternatives to a violent relationship. Women must have a place to live and they cannot escape violence as long as their home is occupied by a man willing to use violence or intimidation. As far as housing is concerned, a woman can only become free of violence under four conditions: (1) her male partner ceases his violence and lives peacefully, (2) the woman escapes to a refuge where she can live free of violence, albeit only temporarily, (3) the man is successfully evicted from the matrimonial home or (4) the woman is rehoused in another home. The refuge is essential but only provides temporary accommodation. To date, the overwhelming majority of men have not given up violence or managed to live without further harassment and intimidation of their partners. This leaves eviction of the man or rehousing the woman.

The British have been more active and innovative than the Americans concerning permanent housing for abused women, using legislation, public housing policy and second stage housing. From the outset, Women's Aid focused attention on the need for permanent housing as well as temporary refuge, and has actively campaigned for both. While refuge continues to be the priority and the political base of the movement, permanent housing is a crucial part of the movement's agenda of change and represents one of battered-women's most difficult practical problems. Legislation was passed early in the life of the movement. The Domestic Violence and

Matrimonial Court Act, 1976 set the scene for England and Wales, followed by The Housing (Homeless Persons) Act, 1977, which also applied to Scotland. Later, The Domestic Violence and Magistrates Act, 1978, the Matrimonial Homes Act, 1983 (England and Wales) and The Matrimonial Homes (Family Protection) (Scotland) Act, 1981 and the Housing (Scotland) Act, 1987 were added. They embody different remedies: eviction of the violent man, arrest for breach of injunction and rehousing the battered woman.[106]

The Domestic Violence Act (1976) allowed for temporary exclusion of the violent partner using a civil injunction with the possibility of attaching powers of arrest for subsequent violation. Many such pieces of legislation have also been passed State by State, within the USA (see Chapter 5). Problems arose immediately with differing interpretations of the nature of the law and problems of enforcement. Injunctions were difficult to obtain. Many judges demanded a severe level of violence before ordering exclusion from the home, and even more severe levels before attaching police powers of arrest for violation of the order. Problems of police enforcement were endemic. On the basis of their follow-up study of refuges and subsequent housing of battered women in England and Wales, Binney, Harkell and Nixon judged this approach to housing the least successful for women.[107] Women with exclusion orders were often forced to remain in refuges because men refused to move out of the matrimonial home and/or they were too afraid to return for lack of protection. Of the 411 women in their survey, only 8 per cent returned to the matrimonial home and only 4 per cent were still there a year later.[108] This finding was reiterated in the 1986 Report of the Metropolitian Police (London) Working Party into Domestic Violence.[109]

In Scotland, pressure from Scottish Women's Aid, along with Shelter, a housing action group, and the Scottish Council for Single Parents, culminated in the Scottish Law Commission's 1980 report on 'Occupancy Rights and Domestic Violence' and formed the basis of the Matrimonial Homes (Family Protection) (Scotland) Act, 1981 which came into force in September 1982. It deals both with the man's violence and the woman's housing, offering women greater protection from violence in their own homes and securing their right to remain there by (1) allowing wives – but not cohabitants – who do not hold the tenancy the legal right to remain in the home, (2) giving courts the power to transfer tenancy from one partner (almost always the man) to another and (3) providing protection through exclusion orders for an initial period of three months with possible extension and interdicts to which the judge might attach the power of arrest.[110]

The Housing, Homeless Persons' Act, 1977 and the Housing (Scotland) Act, 1987 approach the problem differently, providing rehousing for battered women in a separate accommodation apart from the violent man. In Britain, homelessness had historically been treated as an individual problem brought on by indolence, fecklessness and alcohol. 'Punishment' for such inadequacies was reflected in the Elizabethian Poor Laws introduced in sixteenth-century England and these were still very much in evidence in Dicken's portrayal of life in the nineteenth century. The National Assistance Act, 1948 heralded a new approach defining homelessness as a social problem and giving welfare departments the discretionary, but not statutory, duty to provide temporary accommodation for emergency cases of homelessness deemed 'urgent' and 'non-intentional'.[111] Throughout the 1950s and 1960s there was criticism of housing provision as inadequate, biased against single persons and single mothers, oriented to the nuclear family and at the same time willing to split poor families by providing temporary hostels for women and children only.[112] Government committees in the 1960s including Seebohm, Cullingworth and Finer all criticized housing policy as inadequate.[113] A powerful television documentary, 'Cathy Come Home', stunned the public and helped inform public opinion by portraying the housing plight of the poor in Britain.

The Housing (Homeless) Persons Act, 1977 was meant to address many of these problems and battered women were explicitly included by recognizing them as a special category in need of housing. The necessary criteria for obtaining a council house or being rehoused in a different one includes: (1) being homeless or threatened with homelessness, (2) being in priority need such as having dependent children, pregnancy, illness, old age, disability or violence, (3) not having made oneself intentionally homeless in order to obtain housing, and (4) having a local connection with the area of rehousing.[114] However, in order to quell the concerns of housing authorities about queue jumping and claims made from other areas, the bill was transformed from a 'rights based' measure to a 'discretionary' one. The clauses about intentionality and local connections created a 'prize loophole'[115] as women tried to escape from one area to another or to establish that they had not made themselves intentionally homeless but had left home because of violence. While women without children could in theory be considered when accommodation was available, the strain on resources made this rare.

With the Act, responsibility for rehousing was transferred from social work to housing departments and provision varied across areas given the attitudes and interpretations of officials and the type and amount of available housing. Other problems occurred when women were required to pay rent arrears built up by the man, sometimes while she was in a refuge, or meet stipulations such as seeking a divorce, obtaining custody of the children or trying to use the Domestic Violence Act to evict the husband or secure tenancy of the matrimonial home. The two pieces of legislation have often been used against one another in a Catch 22 fashion, with housing departments requiring the woman to seek an exclusion order before approaching them (and then assuming that rehousing is not needed because the man is no longer in residence); and courts suggesting that she seek rehousing under the Housing, Homeless Persons Act rather than exclusion of the violent man under the Matrimonial Homes, Family Protection Act (then assuming that exclusion is no longer necessary because she has another house). Scottish Women's Aid found that during the first year after the legislation, only 48 per cent of women made homeless because of violence were permanently rehoused under the Act.[116]

The Housing (Scotland) Act 1986[117] reintroduced the right of local housing departments to transfer tenancies, usually from husband to wife, provided suitable accommodation is provided for the other spouse. Transfer of tenancy of the home does not, however, suspend the violent person's occupancy rights which requires an exclusion order and only lasts for a limited period. An interdict must be obtained to prevent the man re-entering the home, removing items without the woman's permission or coming within a specified distance of the home.[118] The man may be arrested without a warrant for breach of an interdict. Despite serious failings and widespread criticism of housing legislation and its implementation, it has, nonetheless, provided some relief to battered women in Britain.

In the USA, there is no comparable provision for housing and the importance of permanent, affordable housing for women is now on the agenda. Rehousing is simply not possible without a stock of decent houses available for a fairly wide spectrum of the population. In recognition of this need, a bill pending before the House of Representatives in 1990 would require each State to provide at least 5 per cent of the annual public housing allocations for families made homeless through violence.[119] Despite the criticism and inadequacies of council housing for battered women in Britain, it is very advanced in comparison to the USA. Housing has been a part of state provision in Britain for so long that it is difficult to imagine the landscape without it. By contrast, public housing in the USA is generally of a very inferior standard and available only to the poorest citizens. This may, however, become the same in Britain with the policy of the present Conservative government to sell off council housing, particularly the best, leaving only the worst to be used for the poorest and those in greatest need. There is considerable alarm in many circles about government proposals further to reduce council housing and raise the rent of what remains, and about the policy concerning Board and Lodging Payments which eliminates a major source of funds for refuges. It is feared that fewer refuges will be available and those who do get in will be trapped in a bottleneck and unable to get out because of still fewer houses available for permanent accommodation.[120]

Other British innovations include the provision of second stage housing for women after leaving the refuge. Culdion, the Gaelic word for 'a place of safety', is an example. Scottish Women's Aid recognized that simply being rehoused on their own after leaving refuge was not always the best solution for many women who had come to enjoy and been strengthened by the companionship, mutual support and solidarity of the refuge, and wished to extend these social benefits to more permanent housing. The dream began soon after the first refuges were open. A steering committee was formed in 1977, the formal organization began in 1979 and, in co-operation with a housing association, the first house opened in Edinburgh in 1982. The 'House of Leith' has four stories with four bedrooms, three bedsitting rooms (combined bedroom and living area like a studio apartment) and communal kitchen, dining and living area.[121] The next house opened in May, 1988, a purpose-built three-storey house in Falkirk providing permanent accommodation for six women and their children in self-contained flats with large, shared living, play and storage space.[122] Six other projects are working to extend the development to other areas in Scotland.

Working with a Housing Association to develop second stage housing represents a new coalition for Women's Aid. New areas of knowledge and expertise have been developed in order constructively to participate in the process of designing, building and helping to manage new property. Along the way more fundamental principles have required defence. Communal space, so necessary for the mutual support, self-help and solidarity found in refuges, has had to be defended as a fundamental requirement of the community rather than an expensive and unnecessary addition to the nuclear units. The experiment is in its infancy but holds considerable promise for enhancing the lives of a few women and for extending the philosophy and influence of Women's Aid still further.

New ventures always present possibilities for social change and dangers of failure and/or a loss of wider vision and purpose. Second stage housing is meant to extend the grassroots movement, assist battered women and operate in concert with feminist ideals. In the context of landlords, housing corporations, housing legislation, legal property agreements, architects, builders and others who may not share the same goals or ideals, this is a major task and achievement. Activists continue to return to first principles as they work their way through this pragmatic process, and have emerged with another innovation that extends rather than dilutes those principles. However, new ventures are always a drain on time, energy and finances, and the effect on Women's Aid cannot yet be known.

Concentrating on housing for women, be it temporary refuge or permanent housing, contains within it one of the crucial aspects of the movement. Refuge provides a crucial material resource for women at a time of crisis. It provides women with a place to recover from injury, overcome isolation and begin the process of regaining confidence and greater control over their own lives. It provides the physical location for mutual contact between women living and working in their temporary home rather than contact with 'clients' in the business office of therapists and counsellors. It provides a source of inspiration and a vision about the problem which extends beyond an individual service to wider issues of changing women's social, economic and political status. It is a living laboratory of social change. Housing represents more than simply a roof over the heads of battered women. It points unequivocally to one of the fundamental indicators of women's status which leaves them dependent upon men for the material conditions necessary for life. This places them in a position that they may be left to choose between the unacceptable alternatives of homelessness or a life subjected to violence. Housing provides one of the vital keys in the wider context of change.

4 The state, public policy and social change

Since the beginning of the movement in the early 1970s, campaigns to change public policy, legislation and administrative practice have taken a variety of forms and met with varying degrees of success. In the next three chapters, we shall examine some of the more important changes and innovations in public policy and the justice system. Here we will witness encounters ranging from the more mundane accommodation of like-minded acquaintances to those more closely resembling the high drama, intrigue, plot and counter-plot of long-standing adversaries. In order better to understand the nature of these encounters and evaluate their outcomes, it is useful to place them in the wider context in which they occur. While it is possible to reconstruct these events in personal terms, focusing on who did this and who said that, this creates a false impression that encounters between activists and institutions of the state are simply about personalities working it out on the day. Instead, they are encounters between groups or institutions with histories, priorities and practices that form the backdrop to and set conditions upon the negotiations.

Without using this wider perspective as a guide, it is possible for the parties to the negotiation to have quite misleading ideas about the nature of their encounter and what can be achieved. For example, if activists enter a negotiation with an institution of the state concentrating almost solely upon the negotiation itself, they might easily believe that, at least in theory, virtually anything is possible. All that seems necessary is to make the theoretical possibility into a practical reality. A wider view of the history and nature of the institution may reveal that only certain types of outcome are likely. In addition, those inside and outside the movement who would evaluate the outcome of such encounters may naively be more harsh or unrealistic in their judgements of the outcome if, instead of being aware of the real constraints upon developing meaningful change structured into the encounter from the outset, they believe that virtually anything can be created by the individuals involved.[1] In this and subsequent chapters, we shall examine the process of achieving meaningful social change within the institutions of the state, and consider the very real hurdles imposed by institutional priorities and constraints. Perhaps, as a consequence, this may assist in evaluating more sensitively and accurately exactly what changes have been achieved and against what kind of odds. It may also assist in considering future developments.

Negotiations for changes in public policy, social services, legislation and law enforcement all take place within the framework of the modern state which governs the affairs of all western industrial societies. It is not our intention to examine the state in any detail, but any analysis of the attempts of the battered-women's movement to obtain social change should, at the very least, include a brief consideration of the nature of the state in order to consider its implications for such efforts. We shall consider some basic characteristics of the state in order to highlight factors affecting relations between social movements and the state, and to illustrate recent changes affecting the climate in which the movement has existed from its emergence to the present. From the outset, it must be stated that the nature of the state and its place in social life is neither agreed upon nor always completely articulated by those who have made it their major focus of study. As such, our task must be viewed as a tentative one.

SOME CHARACTERISTICS OF THE STATE

The state is a 'historical phenomenon', constructed through the 'association of men and women living together in an organized way'.[2] It has changed over time and with circumstances from the Ancient Greeks and the founding political philosophies of Plato's *Republic* and Aristotle's *Politics* to the 'modern state' which first emerged in eighteenth-century England. Each new state has differed in style, focus, dominant orientation and the relationship to civil society, including special interest groups and reform movements. The state has broadly been defined in terms of its authority, a rightful claim to obedience, the power to make decisions about 'general arrangements' for the whole group within its boundaries, the right to intervene in certain areas and the right to develop mechanisms to ensure compliance and punish deviance.[3]

Fundamentally, the state is a system of rules, based on 'its right to command obedience' and the power to enforce 'its rules, laws and regulations' even to the point of using 'force or compulsion'.[4] Thus there is a hierarchical relationship between the state and society. State power is exercised through different modes including administering to society and policing society.[5] Both modes will be examined in our analysis of public policy and the criminal justice system. Important issues include obedience and consent, coercion and co-operation, whether the state rules over the people or is the embodiment of their wishes, and whether it favours the interests of those who have property, wealth or status confirmed through class, gender or race.

The state in its modern form is meant to be a public and separate authority. Power is not secret but 'for all to see by public process'.[6] It is not capricious but backed by an established system of law. It is not personal but abstract and impersonal, defined in terms of the roles and functions of office rather than in terms of the person occupying that office. The rules should be known and knowable. They should be administered in a similar fashion for all. Thus, they should be subject to public scrutiny, criticism and change. As such, it should be possible, at least in theory, for the public to know what laws and policies exist to deal with the physical abuse of women in the home, to know how and to what extent they are enforced, and to engage in a process of attempting to change them. As later discussions will show, even obtaining information about the nature of laws and policies is sometimes difficult. Information about enforcement and efforts at change can be even more problematic.

In the modern state, it is not a powerful individual, like a feudal lord, who enforces the rules but an abstract authority that becomes concrete as it is vested in specific agencies and office holders, such as the position of chief of police or director of housing. Such a system is meant to provide greater uniformity in the enforcement of public policies and legislation despite the proclivities of individual office holders. The public nature of state power should have implications for victims and activists attempting to use institutions of the state to obtain changes or reforms. The impersonal, abstract nature of power should have ramifications for developing a type of law enforcement and administration of social services which is uniform, equitable and professional, albeit distant from the participants and their community.

The final characteristic of the state upon which we shall focus is the distinction between the public and the private. Especially in the liberal tradition, the public is that which is 'owned, organized or administered by the state', while the private is 'whatever is left up to the voluntary, non-compulsory arrangements made between private individuals', especially within the family and the economy.[7] Accordingly, the legitimate arena for state intervention is the public, while the private is left, on the one hand, to individual entrepreneurs and, on the other, to patriarchal control in the family. According to this account, the only arena in which women as a group may legitimately belong is the private world of the family, which, within this tradition, is cast in a patriarchal form. The only arena in which the state may legitimately intervene is that of the public world of political affairs. Hence phrases such as: 'A man's home is his castle', 'A woman's place is in the home', 'The family is a haven from a harsh world', and 'The state/police have no right to intervene in the affairs between a man and his wife', all ring a note of accord within this liberal conception of public and private. The public/private distinction is obviously gender based and patriarchal. According to Hall, it is

rooted in a particular sexual division of labour and one of the principal means by which the exclusion of women from public affairs has been constructed and secured. The maintenance by the state of the public/private separation is therefore sometimes taken to exemplify the patriarchal aspects of the state.[8]

Indeed, it has been generally noted that the modern state is based on the model of the patriarchal family, with the 'father as head of his people'.[9] All three arenas, the public world of the state and the private worlds of the economy and the family are ultimately male dominated hierarchies. The style of control may be either the impersonal, abstract and bureaucratic forms operating in the state and the economy or the personal form operating in the family. Although a few individual women may obtain positions of high office or status, this does not fundamentally alter the organizational form of the three hierarchies which remain male dominated.

Patriarchal control in the public and the private arenas coupled with the notion that it is inappropriate for the state to intervene in the private world of the family present serious problems both for the individual woman being abused within the family and for the battered-women's movement. The public/private distinction relates directly to those aims of the movement that call for intervention by the state on behalf of abused women and in opposition to male violence. Women seeking police protection for themselves and/or arrest of their abuser represent an attempt to obtain state intervention into what has been defined as the private world of the family. Seeking changes in legislation against domestic violence or sexual abuse, attempting to ensure their enforcement and trying to establish public policy for housing women and children escaping from violent men all represent attempts to obtain state intervention into the world of the family which, for the most part, has been deemed by the state as private and beyond its legitimate control. This call for state intervention in support of women dates back at least to the demands of Mary Woolstonecraft in the eighteenth century.

The distinction between the public and the private immediately raises questions. Does this mean that the movement is seeking a form of intervention in the private to which the state has traditionally had no commitment and, thus, for which the state has developed no mechanism for response? Does this mean that no change in state response to women in the private arena is possible as long as the state continues to be oriented almost exclusively to intervention in the public arena? On the other hand, does it represent an attempt to obtain forms of intervention which, no matter how well meaning, may result in a 'big brother state', prying and invading in so many aspects of our personal lives that privacy, liberty and freedom are lost or seriously reduced. In his examination of the expansion of state intervention into family life via the juvenile justice system in France, Donzelot[10] has referred to this process as the tutelary role of the state. Thinking about these dilemmas and the possible answers to them leads to the writings of those who have focused upon social reform and social change movements and to the different types of states which, over time, have been more or less oriented to such changes.

STAGES IN THE DEVELOPMENT OF THE STATE

The modern state has gone through several stages of development. The eighteenth and nineteenth centuries experienced several forms of liberalism (classical liberal, liberal-democratic and *laissez-faire*). The present century has witnessed the rise of collectivism, the welfare state of the 1940s and 1950s, the corporatist state of the 1960s and the 1970s, and currently the neo-liberal state. Liberalism began as an attempt to curtail the extensive and often arbitrary authority of the monarchy by narrowing the sphere of state authority and by defining a private sphere (personal, family and business life) outside of the bounds of legitimate state intevention. The term 'liberal' may be a bit confusing because popular, contemporary usage generally means 'open minded', tolerant, oriented to change or even egalitarian. While some of these terms are still used to describe the word 'liberal',[11] we should consider what was originally meant by liberalism and what it may mean today. The liberal state of eighteenth-century England was 'liberal' in contrast to the *ancien régime* with its almost absolute authority of patriarchs to intervene in all manner of personal, financial and political affairs.[12] It was the 'natural rights' and liberties of the individual, in opposition to the old patriarchal authority, that were to be defended by entering into a 'social contract' with the liberal state.

This early liberal state was no democracy. It was not intended to embody the political rights and civil liberties now thought to extend, at least in theory, to most of the population. Instead, the rights and liberties of the minority of male property holders were to be maximized by being allowed to conduct their personal and economic business free from interference from others or from the state itself.[13] While the rights of life, liberty and property were to be legally enshrined and protected for this powerful minority, the majority, including women, the poor and the working classes, did not have the right to vote, assemble as they chose, join a trade union or dispose of property. Struggles for these political and civil rights shaped the reform movements of the nineteenth century, which broadened the base and modified the liberal state but did not alter it fundamentally. 'In the end, "democracy" was grafted on to the liberal state, to create that hybrid variant the *liberal-democratic* state.'[14]

By the late nineteenth and early twentieth centuries there were increasing demands to improve the competitiveness of the British economy through the concerted action of a more interventionist state. The ability to plan organically on behalf of the whole society required an interventionist state. This move towards collectivism which demanded an enhanced role for the state was supported both by the dominant classes, who sought 'national efficiency' for improved production, and the working classes, the poor and unemployed, who sought reforms that would improve their lot and move towards greater equality.[15] The notion of the interventionist welfare state was first introduced by the Liberal government of Britain in 1906–11, but did not take shape until the Labour government of 1945 set forth their massive programme for post-war Britain. By the late 1950s some form of welfare state with an expanded vision of social and economic policy existed in all the large industrial countries in the western world, including the United States. It was during the later stages of this phase of the welfare state that the battered-women's movement was born and within this context that it rapidly developed into an international movement.

By the 1980s, however, there was a reversal in the trend with the 'New Right' moving away from an interventionist welfare state and towards privatization and a social world lead by the forces of the market. Under what has been called the neo-liberal state, considerable effort has been made to 'roll back the state' and to 'restore the ideal of the classical liberal state, but under the conditions of advanced twentieth-century capitalism'.[16] As we shall see, this shift in the dominant trend away from a welfare or interventionist state, with its emphasis on the community, quality of social life and some form of collectivism, to the neo-liberal state, with its emphasis on the market, the economy and individualism, helps us understand some of the changes experienced by the movement in negotiations with agencies of the state during these two periods.

STATE INTERVENTION: REPRESSIVE, CONTROLLING OR ENABLING?

Debate about the effects of state intervention can be intense and heated, with some maintaining that intervention is most likely to be intrusive, repressive and controlling and others that it can be enabling, empowering and protective. The issue of the public and private, the nature of the family and the integrity of the individual, including women, are all at issue. Those who view state intervention as 'repressive' and controlling focus on how it might limit opportunity and potential. Those who see it more positively focus on the potential to 'enable' individuals or groups to reach their potential or obtain protection from others either in the home, at work or elsewhere. Many stand somewhere in between. While this cannot possibly reflect the more complex reality, it is useful to think about the various orientations to the state in the process of considering some of the important issues that have been the subject of the relationship between the movement and the state as they negotiate around the problem of male violence in the home.

The repressive state

Classic Marxist analysis of the state suggests several themes including its functional, instrumental, ideological and cohesive nature, but most usually depicts it as repressive, stressing that 'the state and bureaucratic machinery are class instruments which emerged to co-ordinate a divided society in the interests of the ruling class'.[17] Given this perspective, no amount of state reforms can truly benefit subordinate groups (it should be stressed that the focus is on the working class and not on other groups such as women or racial minorities), as the state is viewed as ultimately organized to serve the interests of the dominant economic class. As such, a state that is the political instrument used to secure the domination of one group by another cannot, without utter transformation, be used to secure their emancipation. This would require 'a new form of political organization which ensures that the people control its own social life through direct and continuous involvement in all facets of government'.[18]

The relationship between the public and private is examined by Elshtain with a particular focus on the family and the state, and on modern feminist attempts to use the state to address issues of concern to women. She explores the writing of political philosophers for their treatment of the 'private' and of feminists for their treatment of the 'public'. Philosophers are found wanting for ignoring or denigrating women's lives in 'the private' sphere, while feminists are even more harshly condemned for ignoring 'the public' world of politics and criticized for not being political philosophers. More importantly, feminists are criticized in the strongest possible terms for seeking changes on behalf of women which would result in more state intervention in the family, the economy and the polity. Elshtain rejects state intervention in defence of victims or in order to obtain equality between women and men. This includes battered women, incest victims, efforts in support of equality at work (e.g. equal pay and equal opportunity legislation) and those in favour of establishing or equalizing women's status as citizens of the state (e.g. Equal Rights Amendment).[19] According to Elshtain, such intervention would interfere with the public/private division, the separation between the state and the family, and thereby destroy the benefits of the traditional family. Indeed, the picture she paints of state intervention is a nightmare so thoroughgoing and absolute that one expects Big Brother to march into the house, choose the evening meal, change the TV channel to the prescribed viewing and spank the children.

Although Elshtain maintains that she is not indifferent to the concerns of women and that any critique must be followed by a constructive alternative, she leaves only a few pages for scattered and unsystematic comments about what might be done. Basically, they amount to a reconfirmation of the traditional ideas of a strict public/private divide, eschewing state intervention and leaving the family to get on with it. In reality, this means leaving the most powerful to act as they choose with certain confidence that the state will not intervene. Basically, this is an unwavering support for a neo-liberal state and an equally fervent rejection of a welfare, interventionist or enabling state. While raising some genuine concerns about the extent and nature of state intervention in family affairs, the issue of male violence directed at women in the home, along with many other concerns of women, would seem to remain untouched in such a scheme.[20]

All abolitionists wish to see an end to prisons and some seek an end to the criminal justice system itself. They have also argued passionately, albeit for quite different reasons, against the claims of the women's movement for state intervention in response to male violence and in support of victims of domestic violence, rape and incest. Instead, abolitionists propose little or no intervention from the state, particularly the criminal justice system, in response to men who commit physical or sexual abuse. While Elshtain wishes to preserve the ideal of the traditional family by keeping the state out of its internal affairs, abolitionists do not want state intervention, particularly from the criminal justice system, because this will be repressive to the men concerned.

From the point of view of victims, this seems to represent a wish to protect men who abuse others from either punishment or control through institutions of the state. For their part, abolitionists accuse the women's movement of being reactionary and falling into the trap of supporting state intervention which they believe will be used to build up prisons and extend policing. For them, this unholy alliance means that the intentions of the women's movement to protect women will, no matter how well meaning, ultimately be used by the state in a heavy-handed way against men. These are genuine concerns, particularly as we witness proposals to expand prisons and policing throughout Europe and North America. There can be no doubt that this is a serious dilemma which must be addressed with great care and concern for both the men and women involved. However, in order to avoid this form of state repression, particularly by the criminal justice system, they propose that physical and sexual attacks upon women and girls should be dealt with by the community or by civil law but not by the criminal law.[21] For them, this would shift the focus away from a form of state intervention intended to punish and control the perpetrator of a crime of violence and towards the resolution of a disagreement between two equal citizens. In rejecting state intervention concerning such crime, many abolitionists implicitly adopt a neo-liberal conception of the state.

Neither abolitionists nor neo-liberals focus their attention or concern on the well-documented abuses within families, the victims of male violence or sexual abuse or, for that matter, the male abuser. To do so might make their defence of a non-interventionist state somewhat distasteful and difficult to sustain. Yet this is the challenge that feminists and the battered-women's movement have posed in their attempts to use the state to assist victims of family violence to reject male violence, and to challenge beliefs, social conventions and institutional practices which have traditionally supported or been indifferent to the abuse of women in the home. Perhaps it is this feminist challenge to the fundamental positions of neo-liberals and the abolitionists which helps explain the vehemence of attacks on those seeking state intervention as one aspect of obtaining meaningful change in the everyday lives of women.

It should be noted that activists have not sought state assistance for battered women blind to concerns about civil liberties, or indifferent to the possible abuses that may occur concerning the poor and people of colour.[22] Nor have they sought intervention in the form of government funding without a keen awareness of the dangers this poses to their own autonomy and the nature of their work. These issues have been debated within the movements on both sides of the Atlantic and, where possible, built into their strategies for change. However, the dilemmas faced by the movement are complex, some leading towards state intervention, others leading away. Male violence cannot be ignored, nor can agencies of the state trample over both victims and abusers in the name of protecting the one and/or controlling the other without really contributing positively to the problems of either. Responding to the violence presents serious dilemmas, but they cannot be resolved by being diminished or ignored since this is merely taking a decision in favour of the status quo which has so far failed both victims and abusers alike.

A more subtle variant among those critical of state intervention are those who do not see state intervention simply as repressive. Rather, they believe that while the purpose of intervention may be benevolent, it will, nonetheless, result in developments that tend to limit the expression of individual variation in lifestyles by encouraging and supporting a narrow definition of what comes to be viewed as 'normal' or acceptable. Foucault and Donzelot[23] have expressed this concern, particularly in relation to the family and sexuality. Unlike neo-liberals, they do not criticize or reject state intervention because it might change the position of men and women away from that of the traditional, patriarchal family, but for quite the opposite reason. They believe state intervention is a controlling and 'normalizing' force which will further reinforce traditional relationships and forms of behaviour. In this view, through the positive processes of education and support and the more negative processes of coercion and punishment, the apparatuses of the state intervene in private life in order to create and sustain a narrow and traditional definition of matters such as sexuality, family style and parenting. They do not fear that state intervention will change the traditional or dominant family patterns of the middle class in favour of some other styles of life; instead, they fear that such intervention will enshrine these dominant, traditional patterns and enforce them to the exclusion of other forms of individual choice and expression. For quite different reasons, all of these approaches are critical of state intervention. Each expresses different fears about the negative consequences that might occur when the state intervenes in the family for whatever reason. The solution for each of these protagonists is a non-interventionist state.

The enabling state

Many feminists writers have taken a position which is critical of the way in which the state has intervened in issues affecting women's familial and economic life but do not reject the notion of any form of state involvement in such affairs. In her work on women and the welfare state, Elizabeth Wilson is highly critical of how the state has related to the family in ways that support traditional, patriarchal forms, but she does not reject the notion of any form of relationship between the private and the public, between women and the state.[24] Mary McIntosh is similarly critical of how the state has contributed to women's oppression through support of the traditional family,[25] and, along with Michele Barrett, examines how the traditional style of family is supported to the point of excluding or diminishing other styles of life, but the state is not excluded from involvement in speculation about more positive arrangements.[26] Others have provided critiques of various forms of legislation and public policy affecting specific issues such as equal pay and opportunity, marriage and divorce reform, welfare benefits and poverty.[27] This is usually done, however, with an orientation to improving such areas of social, economic and family life within the context of a state more knowledgeable about and oriented to the welfare of women in the spheres of the family and the economy, and not with a view to a 'hands off' policy. This involves a newly structured relationship between the state and civil society, and not a complete separation between them.

Still others view the possible consequences of state intervention even more positively, although still not uncritically or without reservation, seeing the potential for 'enabling' a wider base of the population to achieve autonomy and reach their full potential.[28] Both liberalism and Marxism are criticized because of their narrow conception of what constitutes 'the political', maintaining that both have ignored equal rights and obligations in the household, while liberalism has also ignored those of economic life.[29] For Held, a broader view of what constitutes 'the political' is required if we are 'to grasp the diverse conditions necessary ... [to] institutionalize ... the principle of autonomy'.[30] For him, equality and liberty form the principle of autonomy, and this principle can only be realized by bringing into the political equation all facets of social life crossing the public and the private and including relations, institutions and structures that form the activities of production as well as reproduction.[31]

Asking how the state and 'society' or 'civil society' can combine to promote the principle of autonomy, Held states that we must first recognize the need for 'reforming and restricting state power and radically transforming civil society' and this must be done by enacting 'a "two-pronged" strategy of democratizing the state as well as civil society'.[32] His path to a new democratic order involves changing the state, by restructuring and democratizing its institutions, and civil society, through expansion of social autonomy. This would require:

> 1) curtailing the power of capital, patriarchal institutions and the state over civil society through struggles that enable citizens to equalize their power and, thereby, their capacities to act in civil society; and 2) making state institutions more accountable by recasting their functions as accessible coordinators and regulators of social life.[33]

Thus, state institutions are necessary for formulating legislation and new policies, for containing conflicts and for preventing 'new forms of inequality and tyranny'. A secure and independent civil society, including social movements seeking social change, are necessary to secure the goals of 'freedom and equality'. In addition, the state functions of protection, redistribution and conflict mediation are necessary in the transformation of civil society least they become fragmented or create new forms of inequality.[34] For Held, this 'two pronged' strategy of democratizing the state as well as civil society is necessary to obtain the principle of autonomy, and this is to be achieved through a process of creative reform involving 'innovation from below through radical social initiatives' and 'protection by state action'.[35]

Clearly, this definition of politics allows for a consideration of the issues of violence against women and private domination within the family by including the private arena of the family. By encompassing such facets of social life within the context of what is defined as

'political' but doing so in a way that puts them in the sphere of innovative, radical social initiatives from below that are protected rather
than directed by the state, the problem of violence against women
becomes an area of concern within the institutions of the state.
Accordingly, state intervention is viewed as taking a positive form
enabling the battered-women's movement to work for social change
that would, in turn, enable women to live violence-free lives and meet
their full potential.

The new social movements, focusing on race, gender, the environment and peace, are important since they are a new force 'outside the
system' for promoting an interest in welfare and in the 'authentic
needs' of the claim making groups.[36] The new social movements
provide new forms of representation and a new terrain for 'political'
struggles and, thus, are an important part in the transformation of the
relationship between the state and civil society. As such, the movement can be viewed as a promoter of the welfare of abused women as
well as a potential force in the shaping of new relationships between
the state and civil society. It is to the arena of these encounters and
political struggles to which our attention shall turn in examining the
response of state agencies to the change efforts of the movement.

PUBLIC HEARINGS AND THE LEGISLATIVE PROCESS

The original meeting grounds for the battered-women's movement
and the state were the national hearings about violence against
women held in both countries. They were the show-piece meetings
between the movement and the state at which explanations of the
problem, its ownership and proposed solutions were all at stake.
Before a huge public hearing in the USA or in several small sessions
in Britain, the recent past and proposals for the future were discussed
and debated. Examining this process of negotiation highlights in bold
relief the proposals of the movement and the responses of the state.
The hearings were forums for the movement to obtain further public
recognition of the problem and of their work. For government, they
were launching pads for legislation and meeting grounds for the full
spectrum of beliefs and myths, facts and fiction, new enlightenments
and old prejudices. In short, they were an important microcosm of
issues being aired and contested in society at large.

The process of negotiation between the movement and the state
was creative involving the emergence and continuation of a new
social movement and the prospects of innovative changes or retention
of the existing order. We shall consider several aspects of this process

including: the different ideas and discourses advanced about the nature and causes of the problem and those affected by it; which ideas were adopted by the government and elevated to the level of 'official' discourse and which were ignored or rejected and thus denied official recognition; the recommendations for policy and legislative changes proposed by government and their fit with the discourse; government action based on their own recommendations; and, finally, how the movement entered into the legislative process.

As we shall see, Britain and the United States took quite different routes through this process. As stated earlier, the hearings were showpieces for the new movements, arenas for increasing public recognition of the problem and launching pads for government legislation. In Britain, there was almost universal acceptance of activists' pragmatic solution for refuge and housing provision, and legislation was quickly passed, but feminist conceptions of the social and cultural causes of the violence were generally ignored or rejected in favour of ideas focusing on individual inadequacy and poor family background. The solution was adopted while the nature of the problem was denied or transformed. In the United States, the focus of the initial hearings was on civil rights and obtaining equal rights to legal protection from violence. This was a much more receptive arena for feminist ideas about the causes of the problem but the hearings were a much less successful launching pad for proposed Federal legislation. There were many developments in the dynamic process as the government and the movement progressed towards change.

NATIONAL HEARINGS IN BRITAIN

The first developments in public policy began in Britain with the Parliamentary Select Committee hearings on Violence in Marriage.[37] By 1974, the movement had gained considerable public recognition and there was sufficient public pressure for the government to consider action. At least thirty-eight refuges had already been opened, violence against women had become a public issue, Erin Pizzey and the Chiswick refuge were perceived by the media and the public as synonymous with the problem even though the movement had recently split into Chiswick and nearly all other refuge groups who formed the National Women's Aid Federation (NWAF). The atmosphere was charged. Pressure demanded that government respond to the problem.

It was a major achievement for the movement that the government had responded to activists' pressure by setting up a Parliamentary

Select Committee to take evidence and make recommendations for government action. The committee was created in February, 1975 and took evidence until July. Over five months, the thirteen MPs held twenty-three meetings, including fifteen where oral evidence was taken from selected, small groups of the public. In addition to hearing testimony in the House of Commons, they visited five locations in England, Wales and Scotland. Written and oral evidence were taken from Women's Aid groups, eight government Ministers and a wide spectrum of voluntary groups and social agencies. Much of this was reproduced in a government document over five hundred pages in length.[38]

Throughout the meetings, Women's Aid groups pressed the case for battered women and refuges and stated their criticisms of social and legal services. Social and legal services presented their positions. Some viewed the problem as serious and widespread; others denied its extent or severity; still others preferred personal beliefs about why violence occurred or what kind of individuals are involved. The final report of oral and written evidence is filled with a cacophony of voices reiterating evidence, ideas and myths.

The construction of information and the contest of ideas

The content of evidence is largely shaped by the style of Parliamentary hearings. Unlike the Civil Rights Hearings held four years later in the USA, the witnesses called to give oral evidence before the Select Committee of Parliament were neither requested nor allowed to give a presentation, no matter how brief, which would serve as a foundation for systematic discussion. Instead, the Committee, sitting at a table in front of the handful of witnesses called on the day, used an inquisitorial style, somewhat like a judge or prosecuting attorney, with MPs asking whatever questions happen to come to mind, often jumping across topics and witnesses, sometimes with little or no systematic thread. Through this process, MPs remain in firm control of the information given and the ideas and proposals presented to them. While any interested party may submit written testimony in advance, and this may or may not inform questioning or be published in the final account of proceedings, the controlled way of taking oral evidence is crucial in shaping the discourse about the nature of the problem and the recommendations for government action that finally emerge.

Those ideas, information or opinions which MPs wish to emphasize may be pursued at length, with many witnesses and over several sessions. Those they do not wish to entertain are less likely to find their way into oral or written evidence, or may appear in a fashion so fragmented that the meaning or impact is lost. If MPs choose to ask unrelated or even irrelevant questions, it is difficult for those who respond to present a coherent picture or proposal. If written evidence is excluded from the published report or ignored in oral questioning, it simply disappears. Since all committees manage agendas and control testimony in some fashion, it is important to acknowledge this part of the process of constructing a social problem and to consider how it may affect the 'official' discourse and recommendations eventually developed from the deliberations.[39]

There were some crucial differences in focus between the three sources of discourse meant to recount the process, the *oral evidence* taken in the public hearings (published verbatim), the final, summarized report and the *recommendations* for action. Taken together, they present a curious puzzle requiring explanation. In the verbatim oral evidence, a wide diversity of explanations and solutions is presented; in the brief summary, called the Report, individual rather than social explanations are embraced; and in the Recommendations for action, material rather than individual solutions are proposed. Before discussing this outcome and possible explanations for it, let us consider in some detail the contest of ideas and the process of arriving at the final recommendations for change.

Chiswick and psychiatry

The discourse of oral and written evidence was greatly influenced by Chiswick which was the focus of public attention at the time. The overall process was initially shaped by setting an agenda for the twenty-three meetings which began with Erin Pizzey and her psychiatrist, J.J. Gayford. The Committee of MPs seemed particularly interested in ideas about the intergenerational transmission of violence, immature couples and alcohol abuse, and these concerns continued to be raised throughout the hearings. This particular concern had an ethos reminiscent of ideas often associated with the culture of poverty, multiple deprivation, intergenerational deprivation and the popular notions of problem families. Indeed, at that time, a Conservative government minister, Sir Keith Joseph, had initiated a massive research programme funded by the government and sponsored by the Social Science Research Council (SSRC) to study intergenerational deprivation. Although this caused a stir among those who thought it reactionary, it clearly reflected thinking among some politicians and civil servants at the time.

A few observers have commented on the seeming connection between Sir Keith Joseph, Erin Pizzey, J.J. Gayford and, indirectly, the Select Committee.[40] Sir Keith, although not on the Select Committee, was indirectly involved in several ways. He was the Conservative Secretary of State for Social Services, owner of Bovis, the construction company which provided the Chiswick refuge, and initiator of the government research programme on intergenerational deprivation – embodying the notion that inadequate parents rear the next generation of problem people and families – and an influential thinker in the House of Commons. Without adopting a conspiracy theory, it can easily be seen how like-minded people may associate and support a general climate of ideas inside and outside of government. The focus on an intergenerational link between violence and other kinds of family problems and/or deprivation mirrored earlier ideas about 'social genetics', multiple deprivation and the poor which had, at various times throughout the century, gained considerable popularity and, at others, met with searing criticism. An uncritical adoption of ideas about intergenerational deprivation was reflected in the comments made to the Select Committee by Gayford and Pizzey, many of which were enthusiastically pursued in questioning by members of the Committee.

Three of the first four sessions of the hearings were given exclusively to representatives from Chiswick Women's Aid and to Gayford, who had the unique opportunity of being recalled on two additional occasions and, on one occasion, to be the sole witness giving evidence to the MPs. Within minutes of opening the first session, the Committee was told that:

(Mrs Pizzey) – We see mostly, ... the women who have been involved with men who have been violent before they were married ... what we see, which is terrible violence – the violence that actually transforms a generation of children into another generation of wife batterers.[41]

Attention was focused on individual characteristics. The women were viewed as pathetic, immature, inadequate, provocative and violent to their children; the men as alcoholic and/or psychopathic; the children as disturbed, violent and the next generation of abusers. The problem was defined as a psychiatric one. The solution was institutionalization for all.[42]

The women:

(Dr Gayford) – Many of these women have a degree of inadequacy, whether this is something that has been a result of their poor genetic endowment, a result of their poor environmental upbringing or a result of the battering is very difficult to see. It is noticeable even in the more intelligent.[43]

(Dr Gayford) – A few women present as extremely damaged personalities who will need long term support with their children. Often they need protection against their own stimulus-seeking activities. Though they flinch from violence like other people they have the ability to seek violent men or by their behaviour to provoke attack from the opposite sex.[44]

(Mrs Pizzey) – We have as much work with the mothers who are violent towards their children and who have multiple problems as we do in the initial stages of just offering refuge.[45]

The solution:

(Mrs Polaine, housemother of Chiswick) – I would like to have doctors, psychiatrists, and remedial teachers there so that we could really see the degree of damage to our mothers. Because it does not always become apparent; it takes weeks and weeks. They do not tell you the truth.[46]

(Mrs Pizzey) – ... as far as the mothers are concerned there is a high percentage of women who go from one marriage into another. She herself needs a time in community care because her next relationship must be a good relationship for the sake of her children.[47]

The men: alcoholic or psychopathic.
The solution: institutionalization under psychiatric care.

(Sir George Young) – We were all struck by the disparity in incidence of wife battering between immigrants and UK citizens.... I do not wish to lead you on to dangerous ground, but is there not something about the Irish, some characteristic that makes them exceptionally prone to this.... [48]

(Dr Gayford) – The simple answer to your question is one word – drink.[49]

(Mrs Pizzey) – By taking the man into a hostel it would be a great relief and it would help him.... It would almost have to be a prison-like condition, because the men are extremely violent.... For instance, Henderson Hospital has a unit for psychopaths....

They will not take an aggressive psychopath. But their work could be used to help and perhaps to set up such a unit.[50]

(Dr Gayford) – There is a proposal that there will be regional secure units so that there are mini Broadmoors [hospitals for the criminally insane] all over the country; this has been promised; but we have unfortunately seen nothing of it.[51]

The children: violent and disturbed.
The solution: institutional care.

(Gayford) – The pattern of the children is extremely disturbed indeed. Many of the males are very violent.... When you reach this situation there is only one thing that can happen: they have got to be in an environment where they will be subject to the right sort of influence ... they need a very good surrogate father....[52]

A link between childhood experiences of violence and later violent behaviour was assumed and affirmed by Chiswick and repeatedly taken up by the Committee in their questions.[53] MPs enthusiasm for these notions was not daunted by knowledge of the unconfidential and haphazard way in which the questionnaires were handed to women upon arrival at Chiswick, and although it was revealed to MPs that one-third of the questionnaires were simply discarded without reason, the 'findings' seemed, nonetheless, to be accepted without challenge.[54]

The ideas presented by the Chiswick representatives, and enthusiastically received by the Committee, were those stressing the individual inadequacy or pathology of batterers and battered alike and the unquestioned belief in the intergenerational transmission of violence. Hence, the great concern about the children least they also grow up to form violent relationships. The Chiswick solution for these damaged individuals was to medicalize the problem and provide institutional care for men, women and children alike. They did not wish to see refuges for battered women all over the country and suggested about five 'sanctuaries' with 'facilities to deal with the problem' rather than '400 of an indifferent level'.[55] The idea is reminiscent of the large, Victorian hospitals and asylums then being shut down in Britain and the USA. More psychiatric and therapeutic intervention was proposed. Indeed, Pizzey, Gayford and McKeith, also a psychiatrist, were soon to propose that the government fund an institution where the whole family/battered women and children could go for long periods to be cured of this problem.[56] Such ready acceptance of these reductionist, and sometimes racist, ideas and

Victorian solutions is resonant with widely accepted conceptions of
social problems and are thus more easily grasped and adopted than
wider cultural and structural explanations and solutions that focus on
women's position in society and in the family.

Women's aid

This was not the only form of discourse presented to the committee.
The definition of the problem, its causes, nature and extent, and
suggested solutions as well as the role of government, were seen quite
differently by Women's Aid groups from the newly formed Federation. Instead of concentrating on the characteristics of the individuals and their childhood, Women's Aid focused on the material needs
of women and their children, and what the government could do
through social and legal provision. They proposed changes in policy
and practice to assist with the material needs, particularly through
refuge, housing and financial assistance for single parents and dependent children. They also recommended changes in the law concerning
injunctions and suggested the introduction of exclusion orders. The
need for research carried out in conjunction with Women's Aid was
briefly mentioned. Comments about individuals took a different
form, stressing their difficult circumstances and the need for mutual
support, better services and protection.[57]

The woman:

> Women's Aid – (written memorandum) – A woman entering a
> refuge is brave and desperate.... The decision that she must leave
> home has not been taken lightly, but over a length of time she has
> come to realise that the level of physical violence used against her
> is intolerable. In many cases she leaves because she thinks the
> children are in danger – she leaves her interests until last.[58]

The failure of traditional sources of help:

> She has usually been to her General Practitioner [medical doctor],
> or several agencies both statutory and voluntary, but the help
> offered has not been adequate.[59]

The solution:

> Refuges provide safe, supportive surroundings where women can
> overcome their fear and isolation.... It has been found that women
> who have been battered gain a great deal from sharing their experi-
> ences with others who have suffered the same treatment.[60]

The children:

> There are inadequate nursery facilities all over Britain, but
> children have a special need for extra care at times of stress and
> change. Money should be provided for the staffing and facilities
> available to children in refuges. Obviously we would wish for quick
> easy communications with Social Services in cases of suspected or
> actual non-accidental injury to children.[61]

Little was said about the men, *per se.* The concern was with
protecting and supporting women, and legal remedies to stop
violence were seen as part of that process. Proposals were made for
injunctions to prohibit further violence and powers of arrest for
violations of injunctions. Criminal prosecution of men was mentioned
but not pursued either by witnesses or the committee.

Feminist ideas about social rather than individual causes of
violence were not so easily embraced by the committee as Glasgow
Women's Aid learned in an exchange about 'male supremacy', the
positions of men and women, and the socialization of chidren.[62] They
put their heads over the parapet and were taken to task in an
antagonistic fashion markedly different from questioning around
ideas about individual inadequacies, pathologies and alcohol abuse.
Sex roles and the socialization of all children, not just those from
violent homes, were mentioned by Women's Aid but resisted by the
Committee.[63] One MP even made reference to 'our Dr. Gayford in
London' when pursuing his point about the causal effects of alcohol,[64]
and a similar stance was taken in comparing Gayford's research to
that of our own.[65] Glasgow was one of the few Women's Aid groups
explicitly to put this position to MPs. Most other groups concentrated
on policies and pragmatics even though they held strong feminist
views. Perhaps this was a tactic based on a belief that MPs would
reject proposals for change if they were seen to be embedded in
feminist ideas. Indeed, Glasgow's experience would seem to justify
such a notion.

Six Women's Aid groups from England, Scotland and Wales gave
evidence at hearings thoughout the country.[66] Refuge and permanent
housing for women and children were central to their practical proposals for material changes. They stressed the urgent need to provide
temporary accommodation in the form of refuge for battered women
and their children and to change tenancy arrangements so that
women, rather than batterers, would have the right to occupy the
marital home. They viewed the problem as one of male violence and
sought changes in the law and law enforcement to protect the woman

by controlling violent men. They challenged most of the existing agencies, particularly the police and courts but also social work, housing and medicine, claiming that they ignored the problem, failed to respond effectively and blamed the victim, often in order to rationalize indifference or inaction.

Individual women were of paramount importance, but both the woman and the problem were viewed within a social rather than a psychological context. Rather than seeing the immediate solution in 'curing' individual inadequacies, Women's Aid saw it in providing the material resource of accommodation and legal protection. For them, the women were not viewed as inadequate and incapable but as struggling to make a better life, often against tremendous odds. Women were not viewed as helpless, a phrase that was soon to be embraced in the USA, but as actively struggling within a context that was often pretty hopeless. The task, therefore, was not to transform the women but to change the conditions in which they were trying to construct violence-free lives: conditions that directly and indirectly supported rather than unequivocally rejected violence; conditions that often made women choose between continued violence or homelessness; conditions that ignored their active attempts to stop the violence or escape and live autonomous lives; in short, conditions that blocked rather than facilitated women's own efforts to stop or escape from male violence. Self-help and assisted self-help, similar to the North American concept of advocacy, were important concepts characterizing the women as able, but in need of assistance as they worked for change against considerable odds. This contrasts with the Chiswick characterization of women as inadequate and in need of personal transformation managed by medics and psychiatrists.

Other groups

Government bodies, statutory agencies and a wide variety of voluntary organizations also gave evidence. They ranged across voluntary agencies like Marriage Guidance, Church of Scotland Moral Welfare Committee, The Salvation Army Women's Social Services and The National Council for Civil Liberties. Statutory agencies included social work, the justice system and housing. Representatives of institutions of the state included an impressive array of high ranking officials from The Scottish Office, The Home Office, the President of the Family Division of the Supreme Court of Judicature,[67] and heads of government departments such as the Secretary of State for Social Services.[68] For some, the problem was seen as outside the remit of their agency. For others, the definition of the problem and proposed solutions were framed in terms reflecting the philosophy and remit of their organization. Some were supportive and innovative in outlook, others resistant to the issue and the need for change. For most, the nature of the new social problem and its solution were repeatedly cast and recast, not in a new mould but in the shape of responses that already existed within each agency.

The positions taken depended on areas of responsibility and the demands for resource. The police were strongest in denying the extent or severity of the problem or the need for any change in their service. Social work and housing departments acknowledged the problem but were quick to note that they could not meet the demands for council property for refuges or permanent rehousing. The Committee later noted, 'We have been disappointed and alarmed by the ignorance and apparent apathy of some Government Departments and individual Ministers towards the extent of marital violence'.[69] In all, 141 individuals gave oral evidence and forty-nine memoranda were published.[70] While all were welcome to provide evidence, and the full spectrum of opinion was represented, some ideas were more resonant with the Committee than others. This shaped the 'official' discourse about the problem.

Official discourse and government recommendations for action

The mass of over five hundred pages of oral and written evidence (vol. 2)[71] was summarized in twenty-one pages referred to as the Report followed by twenty-eight Recommendations. Together, the Report and Recommendations (vol. 1)[72] form the compressed and concentrated version of five months of deliberation, and they, rather than the fuller account of oral and written evidence, represent the 'official' shaping of the problem and the government's proposed direction for change. They are important because they distil the discourse and delineate government proposals for action and change.

In retrospect, the shape of the final Report can be seen to emerge fairly early in the hearings as some lines of questioning are dropped, new ones added and others pursued across several sessions. While the summarized Report is meant to reflect and stand in place of the overall proceedings, it actually reveals those innovative ideas and practices MPs were, in the final analysis, willing to adopt and highlights the tendency to use tried and familiar approaches, familiar agencies and experts, and familiar solutions even when addressing new problems. As in this case, real innovations can sometimes break into this process and, willingly or unwillingly, be accepted as part of the response. It seems unlikely, however, that a real alternative or radical innovation could prevail as the sole response. The question is not whether activists' ideas and programmes succeed or fail in this process but how much becomes accepted or established and how much is lost or compromised, and whether this represents a loss of original principles or practices.

As already mentioned, there is a curious lack of fit between the oral discourse about the nature and causes of the problem and the subsequent government Recommendations for its solution which take a shape that would not have been predicted based on the Committee's apparent enthusiasm for individualistic and psychiatric explanations. Instead, feminist practices, along with some, although certainly not all, of their ideas, were embraced in the Recommendations. The provision of refuge using voluntary labour and the principles of self-help received great praise and support, albeit within a context of a desire to limit government expenditure. Women's Aid pressure for change in social and legal services was acknowledged and there was an orientation to changing legislation although there were no recommendations for changes in the response of the police.

Proposals for action and change

Sections on 'Alleviation' and the 'Law' constitute the major thrust of the Report. Activists received great support for their practical programmes for assisting victims of violence, even though their explanations about cause and their proposals for change in police practice were not embraced so enthusiastically.[73] Refuges and housing were the alleviating factors receiving most attention in the Report and Recommendations. The committee expressed admiration for the practical work in refuges, emphasizing volunteerism, the principle of self-help, practical assistance and the provision of needed services with little financial assistance from local or national government. Some MPs congratulated Women's Aid on their supreme effort in opening refuges and developing working relations with existing agencies,[74] concluding:

> We accept the evidence given to us by so many witnesses that the first and most urgent need is for more places of refuge. ... We recommend that one family place per 10,000 of the population should be the initial target.[75]

'One place for every 10,000' signalled government support for the expansion of refuges and this was used by Women's Aid groups in campaigning for more refuges throughout Britain. The Committee also embraced the local autonomy of Women's Aid in running refuges and encouraged expansion.[76] The activists principle of self-help was endorsed, 'a new stereotyped hostel service is not what is envisaged.... The self-help idea should be retained as far as possible, so that the wives themselves are fully involved'.[77] Establishment of a national network of Women's Aid refuges was encouraged,[78] as were their efforts to form housing associations in order to provide second stage housing for women after leaving the refuge, stating that,

> although many women will wish to live alone with their families, many may well wish to continue with some form of communal living, perhaps in units of two or three families per house.[79]

While the principle of communal living seems a pragmatic and useful arrangement for those who wish it, its acceptance is perhaps a bit surprising in light of MPs resistance to proposals for changes in sex roles and family arrangements. There was also praise for the Women's Aid workers and reiteration of some of their basic ideas about refuge provision.

> They will remain places of refuge where a woman can go for temporary safety, where she can have some time to assess her position, think over her problems, discuss them with others and then – not unduly hurried but not staying too long – leave to resume life in her old, or if necessary a new, home.[80]

The sting in the tail of praise for enthusiastic voluntarism was the implication that little might be expected from government funding so urgently sought by Women's Aid. On the other hand, the Report contained an endorsement of Women's Aid's basic philosophy of refuge provision, supported their repeated rejection of the myth that women accept violence and rebuffed those who believed change was impossible.

> We believe that [urgent] action will make a substantial contribution to reducing the level of violence in the United Kingdom, and may well contribute to a reduction in the murder rate. We reject the views of those who think that battered wives 'must enjoy being battered' or 'can look after themselves'. We also disagree with those, including at least one Home Office Minister, who think that nothing much can be done. With this attitude we contrast that of the Judges of the Family Division.... Her Majesty's Judges, at least,

recognise the scale of the problem and are eager to take up the challenge it presents.[81]

MPs briefly raised the spectre of statutory agencies taking over the response now that activists had completed the pioneering work of 'discovery' and raising public awareness. Jo Sutton, the first National Co-ordinator of the Federation, responded that it would be very difficult in terms of the resources available to statutory bodies, and, more importantly, Women's Aid felt that the problem should remain in the voluntary field.[82] Five recommendations were made about refuges: (1) they should be readily and rapidly available; (2) a grant for NWAF should be 'sympathetically and urgently considered'; (3) Chiswick should continue to receive funding temporarily; (4) the Department of the Environment 'must ensure that more refuges are provided by local authorities and/or voluntary organisations'; and (5) the 'One family place per 10,000 of the population should be the initial target'.[83]

Permanent housing was also emphasized as an important aspect of alleviation. Three recommendations were made: to introduce legislation, if necessary, clarifying the responsibility of local authorities to provide battered women who leave home with temporary accommodation;[84] to implement previous proposals on local authority and private tenancies;[85] and to give magistrates power to exclude violent men from the matrimonial home.[86] The importance of temporary refuge and of a secure right to occupy the matrimonial home unmolested was pressed by activists and then recognized by government as crucial in alleviating the problem.

In the following sessions of Parliament, legislation concerning housing and safety in the home were passed for England and Wales, and, later, for Scotland. This involved some negotiations between the state and the movement, but they were not nearly as problematic or time consuming as those that would later be required in the USA. For England and Wales, The Domestic Violence and Matrimonial Proceedings Act (1976) gave women the right to occupy the matrimonial home and provided for exclusion orders.[87] The Housing (Homeless) Persons Act (1977) made battered women a priority category for rehousing if they had to leave home because of violence.[88] The Magistrates Court Act 1978 facilitated the use of injunctions to prevent further violence in the home.[89] Scotland followed somewhat later with The Matrimonial Homes (Family Protection) (Scotland) Act 1981 confirming the right to occupy the matrimonial home upon a spouse, usually the woman, who does not hold the tenancy and thus preventing her ejection by a violent husband, and providing for the civil remedy of an interim exclusion order to prohibit the violent man from occupying the matrimonial home.[90] The primary purpose of the Act is to prevent homelessness through violence.[91] Later still, The Matrimonial Homes Act, 1983, for England and Wales, further clarified and streamlined powers to prohibit or restrict the right of a violent spouse to occupy the matrimonial home.[92] Together, these laws are meant to reinforce civil orders of protection (injunctions and interdicts), introduce exclusion orders with the possibility of attaching the power of arrest for breach of the civil order, to define battered women as a priority category for housing, and to facilitate the enforcement of the law on injunctions.

The initial legislation was fairly quick on the heels of the Parliamentary Hearings. One reason legislation can be passed rather quickly in Britain, and particularly in relation to what we shall see happened in the USA, is because there is effectively only one house to consider the legislation, although the Lords can and sometimes does alter legislation from the House of Commons, and all committees are controlled by the party in power. Once the government in power is committed to an issue, the procedure for passing legislation is much more straightforward than in the USA with its two houses and diverse committees often controlled by the opposition party. In addition, some legislation in the USA, such as legal injunctions, must be passed on a State by State basis requiring fifty different laws, rather than on a national level, as in Britain, thus requiring only one law.

It is important to note that despite criticism of law enforcement stressed by activists, and some fairly pressing questioning of the police by MPs when taking oral evidence, this concern virtually disappeared in the text of the Report and from the Recommendations. Instead, all that was recommended was that the police keep statistics and Chief Constables review their policies for approaching the problem.[93] Passing mention was made about training for new recruits and regular written advice leaflets from the Chief Constables, but even these rather lukewarm proposals for educating law enforcement officers were not translated into formal recommendations. MPs noted sympathetically the reluctance of police to intervene because of their 'embarrassment' if a woman withdrew charges (police and court records show that this is not common, representing only 5 to 6 per cent of the cases),[94] and invoked traditional ideals about domestic privacy and the 'well established attitude of the home being beyond police surveillance'.[95] The Report contained sympathetic support for non-interventionist procedures from police and made no proposals for change in practice while, at the same time, reaffirming that the assaulted were due the full protection of the law. This contradiction between non-intervention and legal protection seems to be acknowledged verbally but ignored in practice.[96] The legal response to the violent assaults and policing shall be discussed in the next two chapters.

This represents the main orientation of the Report and Recommendations and generally shows the extent of the influence of the pragmatic action, if not the causal explanations, of Women's Aid. Lest this provide a misleading picture of wholescale adoption by the Committee of activist orientations, let us illustrate some of the issues dealt with more briefly, but which, nonetheless, show diverse and sometimes contradictory orientations. By comparison to the sections on alleviation and legal issues, the Report contains only brief statements about definition, causation, prevention, the Finer Report on single parent families, research, publicity and finance. Brief coverage, however, does not mean that crucial ideas and proposals are necessarily missed. For example, the brief coverage of the definition, scale and nature of the problem emphasized the activists' position that violence in marriage is about violence against women in their position as wives, and that this is more serious and widespread than previously known or imagined. Under 'causation', however, it is first stated that little is known, then the opinion is expressed that there is 'no evidence that the husband alone is responsible for his violence. The behaviour of the wife is relevant' as is environment, housing, employment, physical and mental health, sexual relations and other factors.[97] Also mentioned as 'causal' are characteristics stressed by Chiswick, such as early marriages and pregnancies, short courtships, alcohol, a childhood in a violent home, psychiatric problems and the inability to communicate.[98] No mention is made of the subordinate status of women or male dominance despite their introduction into oral evidence by Women's Aid.

The discussion of 'prevention' contains a brief three-point plan about education for marriage and parenthood, alcohol and the special needs of children from violent homes 'to break this cycle of violence'.[99] Implementation of the neglected Finer Report on single parents and social services was proposed in order to streamline advice services, change attitudes of the Supplementary Benefits Commission (welfare provision), establish Family Courts and change housing provision.[100] This not only reiterated a previously recognized need but also served as a warning about the possible neglect of recommendations from earlier select committees. It was noted that only one government sponsored research project existed in the UK and that there should be more.[101] Seeking to save government funding for research, admittedly already very low, they ruled out 'the usual panacea of large scale research programmes' and proposed that one or two crisis centres become action research projects to evaluate effectiveness and value.[102] The importance of publicity in raising public awareness was briefly noted, and a five sentence paragraph on finance emphasized that the recommendations would not involve much public expenditure, but urged a quick decision by the government on the principle of whether any finance was to be provided.[103] Conferences were to be held throughout the country during the nine months following publication of the Report to consider the Recommendations, and, shortly thereafter, the government was to report to Parliament on local and national action taken and further plans for action and change.[104]

Some of these proposals for alleviation have come to nothing while others have only begun to develop in the late 1980s and early 1990s. Brief attention was given to 24 hour family crisis centres, needs of husbands, financial support for battered women and social and medical services.[105] The first did not materialize, but this should not be surprising since innovative action usually requires a group or constitutiency to organize the response, some form of funding, and, in the case of existing organizations, the motivation to change established practice. The 24-hour crisis centre had neither a constitutency nor funds. No formal recommendations were made about violent men, and the constitutency for men's programmes only began to develop in Britain in the late 1980s. Little has been done to change procedures to ensure uniform, considerate and helpful responses for giving benefit to battered women who need financial resources. Despite deeming it insufficient 'just to treat physical injuries and dispense tranquillisers', the medical fraternity have been very slow to develop training, referral systems, and to adopt procedures of 'vigilance at an early stage of the violence'.[106] In 1990, the Department of Health began to consider a UK-wide initiative of research and demonstration projects to examine early forms of interention by health providers and voluntary groups.

Children were seen as a crucial part of efforts to alleviate the problem and singled out for 'special attention' because of the negative effects of witnessing violence, removal from their homes and being 'unsettled' while in a refuge. The Committee recommended that special attention be given to 'breaking the cycle of violence by attention to the welfare and special needs of vulnerable children'.[107] Children were seen as so important that a subsequent select committee was to consider their needs. Indeed, it might be said that the needs of the children were seen as even more important than those of battered women. The concluding comments of the Report read: 'For what is involved is not the plight of a particular category of unhappy women, but the future of families, involving men, women and – most important of all – their children'.[108]

In summary, it can be seen that despite the MPs' persistence in the oral evidence about individual 'causes' of the problem and psychiatric explanations, little attention was given to them either in the summarized Report or in the Recommendations. Thus, the official discourse and government proposals for action minimized an area receiving considerable attention in the oral evidence. Instead, the Report concentrated on material provisions, refuges, housing and the law. Perhaps this should not be surprising. Parliamentary Select Committees are meant to gather information and move from an issue of public concern to public policy and legislation.[109] Certain organizations, such as law, social services, education and the economy, are more accessible for policy development and experimentation than the more amorphous area of personal traits. So, while MPs may have exercised their concern and curiosity about the causes of violence which they appeared to see as located in individual attributes, their proposals for change were primarily directed at organizational responses. They offered material provisions, not changes in ideology or beliefs. In doing so, MPs employed two of the institutions already available to the government for change (law and housing) as well as the new alternative provided by the women's movement (refuge).

NATIONAL HEARINGS IN THE UNITED STATES

In the United States, government responded to the rising groundswell of pressure from the movement and growing public concern by organizing consultations with activists. The first White House meeting, held in July 1977, was designed by activists and government representatives to bring together battered women, service providers and Federal personnel to put the case for battered women and provide support for grassroots activists. It was brief, including the testimony of one battered woman and twelve papers, each lasting three minutes. However, the content had been co-ordinated by activists to focus on the abuse of women, the provision of autonomous, community run shelters and a multi-cultural approach accessible to all women.[110] Activists maintained that attention should not be diverted nor the nature of the problem distorted or confused by focusing on alcohol, drug abuse or child abuse. This concern, as we shall see, was not misplaced. This was one of the first coalitions of women inside and outside the Federal government working for change. No decision was taken by government, but Federal legislation to authorize funding for shelters had been introduced during the preceding month and had begun what was to become a long and difficult process of seeking legislation.[111]

Within six months, the US Commission on Civil Rights held full hearings to consider whether battered women were receiving equal protection under the law. This was the show-piece meeting between the movement and the state. The US Commission on Civil Rights was established by Congress in 1957 as a temporary, independent, bipartisan agency to gather information, investigate complaints, serve as a clearing house for information, and submit reports and make recommendations to the President and Congress concerning denials of equal protection of the laws.[112] While the centre of attention was on legal protection rather than refuge provision, the meetings also served as a launching pad to press for Federal legislation to fund shelters. In Britain, there is no such body within the agencies of the state wherein issues of the rights of various groups within civil society might be considered. It is significant that in the USA this was the first main forum of government in which this issue was addressed. While at a later date hearings would be held in the Senate, a body more comparable to that of the British House of Commons, the Civil Rights hearings are the focus of attention here because they provide an important contrast.

Similar to the British hearings four years earlier, the US Commission on Civil Rights invited written and oral statements from activists, academics and representatives from legal, medical and social agencies. This resulted in a seven hundred page document containing the presentations as well as a lengthy list of shelters, state statutes and proposed Federal legislation.[113] The Commission's basis for studying the problems of battered women came from 'its statutory mandate to study and collect information regarding the denial of the equal protection of the laws on the basis of sex and, in particular, in the administration of justice'.[114] The agenda included 'law enforcement and justice, support for shelters and statutory social services, causes and treatment of wife abuse, and the Federal role'.[115] It was hoped that the consultation would inform the public and facilitate communication among activists, researchers and policy makers.[116] Unlike the

Select Committee, which had not recommended change in police practice, the Commission's jurisdictional basis for studying the problem meant a strong focus on the law and law enforcement.

The construction of ideas

On the last two days of January 1978, thirty formal presentations and responses were heard before an audience of over six hundred observers and activists who had come from all over the USA to listen and lobby. Using Betsy Warrior's directory to find one another, activists shared information about emerging shelters, hotlines and models of state and local laws for use in testimony. The Consultation opened with an overview of the scope of the problem presented by Del Martin, a well-known feminist organizer and activist, and some very lively exchanges took place.

The agenda and method of presenting and debating ideas and evidence helped shape the discourse. Since the object was to identify issues and possible solutions, testimony was presented in a way that allowed ideas to be developed and debated by presenters and formal respondents. Invited speakers were given about twenty minutes each to present prepared papers, two or three others served as members of a panel and presented their prepared responses which were followed, in turn, by questions from Commissioners.[117] Such a style allows for fuller development of the topic by presenters and a freer exchange of ideas than is possible with the inquisitional style used by the Select Committee in Britain. Listening at length also provides Commissioners with a greater opportunity to learn. The material presented is determined by the presenters, not controlled by an inquisitional style of questioning from politicians. This style encourages a more interactive form of discourse between government and the public.

The style of presenting information and ideas, along with the equal rights remit of the Commission, resulted in important differences between the two countries in how the problem was initially discussed at government level. The differences were not so much in the particular issues raised, but in the language used, the ideas about causes and, to a lesser extent, the solutions proposed. The focus on equal rights allowed activists to deal with the obvious point that women are not treated equally. In stark contrast with Britain, Commissioners supported this position and actively encouraged its inclusion in the hearings. The opening comments of the chairman made this very clear and the selection of Del Martin, a well-known activist for battered women and women's issues, set the tone.

Del Martin's opening presentation covered the historical acceptance of wife beating, present indifference or ineffectiveness of the responses of social and legal agencies, and the importance of the grass roots, feminist groups and their provision of shelter. The causes of wife beating were clearly examined in terms of women's inferior position in society, the economy and marriage.[118]

The problem:

> I deliberately called my book *Battered Wives* to focus on marriage as the institutional source and setting in which the violence is initiated and carried out ... domestic violence cannot be fully understood without examining the institution of marriage itself as the context in which the violence takes place.[119]

She noted that the widespread incidence of wife beating meant it could not reasonably be seen simply as a problem of individuals or of 'personal interaction'. A wider analysis was required in order to understand the roots of the problem and to address them effectively. This included power, personal interaction, the history of marriage, present attitudes towards women, sex role stereotyping, acceptance of the violence and the response of helping agencies.[120] The non-arrest policy of police was criticized for denying women the right to equal protection under the law because it is a breach of duty and 'does not result in men resolving to give up beating their wives but is more likely to reinforce his behavior as he quickly learns what will be "tolerated by the system"'.[121]

The response:

> The shelter network, established by grassroots women's groups with its 'underground railway' by which battered women can be transported from one State to another, affords the only real protection to the victim.[122]

> Solutions to the problem, therefore, call for nontraditional measures and radical change in approach, the impetus for which has come from women.... What the women need is advocacy: ... someone to listen nonjudgmentally; secondly, assurance and support; third, someone to help them through the bureaucratic maze of legal and social services.[123]

On therapy:

> Some see therapy rather than law as a solution. But what kind of therapy? ... Psychotherapy, feminists believe, is based on patri-

archal assumptions which are the cause of the wife/victim's plight and therefore is inappropriate to solving her problem.[124]

Social change:

> Clearly the problem of domestic violence cannot be solved without addressing the foregoing economic issues or without revolutionary changes in attitudes towards the roles of women and men in our society. Without such changes we cannot ensure women 'equal protection under the law', and without such protection they will remain vulnerable to their husbands' abuse.[125]

Nothing could differ more from the opening session of the Parliamentary Select Committee. Martin's testimony about the problem and its roots in marriage, male domination and women's subordinate status, and the sympathetic hearing this received from Commissioners, stands in stark contrast to the Select Committee's initial embrace of the psychiatric explanation of individual inadequacy.

The contest of ideas

Despite having a committee basically sympathetic to the activists explanation of causes and solutions, there was still considerable controversy. Most of the presentations concentrated on legal responses and on the importance of shelters run by grassroots activists with a feminist analysis of the problem. However, activists expressed fear and concern about funding and research, and there were exchanges about the police and crisis intervention, and about whether beaten husbands outnumbered beaten wives.

Law enforcement and programmes for crisis intervention, mediation and diversion were debated.[126] Police, prosecutors and judges were criticized for ineffective responses.

Presenter – Marjory Fields (attorney):

> The legal system fails to protect battered wives. It assumes that battered wives are guilty parties who have provoked, deserved, and wanted the attacks that they have suffered. Having no recourse on the law, battered wives are forced to flee and hide from their assailants. As a result, they are deprived of their liberty and their property without due process of law. The offenders are usually free to remain at home among friends and relatives....
>
> Unfortunately, [police] training was and is designed to encourage mediation to reduce police injury, and secondarily to help the

parties. Much of this [training] material is sexist.... [In the New York City training manual on Police Response to Family Disputes] emphasis on the guilty, rejecting wife as the cause of family conflict is further developed in four family dispute skills for officers to watch in training. In all four skits the women are presented as dominating and forceful, except one who is a heroin addict.[127]

Respondent – Juanita Kidd Stout (Judge):

It seems to me that it really serves no useful purpose to blame police as much as you're blaming them. I am not excluding them from blame altogether, but it certainly serves no useful purpose to blame police for the policy of nonarrest when there are limitations imposed on their power and authority to arrest. I think it might serve us better if we review the various statutes throughout all 50 of the jurisdictions ... and approach a remedy from a legislative viewpoint.[128]

Along with pressing the case for funding of shelters, fears were also expressed about the possible negative effects of Federal funding and proposed Federal legislation. This also touched on the issue of activists versus professionals.[129] Fear was expressed that much-needed Federal funding of shelters would change the focus of the work or squeeze out activists and their principles in favour of research and professionals with a different agenda. Those with experience of the anti-rape movement spoke from bitter experience.

Lisa Leghorn (Transition House, Boston):

There are close parallels between the two movements in the analysis of the problem, and in the alternative institutions which have been developed by grassroots for addressing it. As private and government monies were allocated for anti-rape services which the grassroots groups had labored years in freeing up, most of these monies were not to these groups, but to various profes-sional agencies with little or no experience with the problem, who have been notorious for changing the focus of their work and the social problems they deal with as the flow of monies changes.[130]

Dr Flitcraft (medical doctor):

I think that the history of mental health in this country is not one which primarily provides a healthy image for program develop-ment, and I think funding through the mental health agencies is a very ambivalent process.[131]

The most desirable type of research was debated, with activists stressing that it should be community based, responsive to battered women and oriented to discovering causes directed at finding solutions instead of establishing what was already known to be a large problem. Some raised the question of whether money should be spent for research or for shelter.[132]

The issue of battered husbands also became the subject of debate. Murray Straus presented in written evidence to the Committee his case for 'husband beating', but completely avoided this hottest of topics in his oral presentation before the audience of hundreds. The method used to measure this violence will be examined in the chapter on research, but what is important here is the political process whereby the topic would have gone into the public record through written evidence unknown to the audience and thus unchallenged and without debate or critique had it not been raised by the few who had actually seen the written paper, members of the Committee and the two formal responders. It was, however, queried, particularly about whether equal numbers of battered husbands and wives actually existed and whether violence by women was actually in self-defence. If so, could such men be called battered? It was noted that the press was giving considerable coverage to this issue, which not only denigrated the violence experienced by women but was also being used to withdraw support for women's shelters.[133]

The possibility of changing violent men was discussed. Although there was considerable pessimism about change, some cautious hopes were expressed, referring to what was then a new programme for violent men, EMERGE, with its feminist analysis of the problem and clear vision of 'addressing and changing the power relations between men and women'.[134]

Dr Hilberman (Assistant Professor of Psychiatry):
> I want to add that when we talk about treatment for the batterer, treatment implies that there is sickness, that somebody wants to change that behavior, or that that person is uncomfortable because of his behavior. I don't think we have any evidence that half of the population is sick or mentally ill or that men want to change their violent behavior. So at this point we have very little to offer them. My focus in working with battered women is to help them get themselves together so that they can get out of the violent relationship and stay out.[135]

Ms Leghorn (activist):
> The commitment towards not tolerating violence has to happen within everyone's community, as well as within families, where

people who know what is going on hold the batterer accountable for his behavior and expose it and state publicly and strongly that they will not accept or condone the behavior. Until that kind of response takes place on all these levels, I don't think men are going to change.[136]

Commissioner Saltzman:

Apparently, what we are talking about is some fundamental changes in our social structure, which up to now perpetuates violence.[137]

Permanent housing, welfare benefits and employment opportunities were discussed by the relevant government departments. Health, Education and Welfare (now Health and Human Services and roughly equivalent to the British Department of Health and Social Services, which became two agencies in 1988) had no mandate to address the problem. The only resource was aid to dependent children, a welfare provision available only to destitute women with young children, along with other provisions for protecting children.[138] The Department of Housing and Urban Development (HUD) had no specific programme for shelters although one group in Minnesota had been able to overcome the political and bureaucratic obstacles to obtaining Community Development money for a shelter. HUD was in the process of revising its regulations concerning eligibility for funds, largely because of participation of the women from Minnesota.[139] Again, the Department of Labor reported having no special programmes for battered women.

The only avenue of direct assistance to programmes was the job creation scheme, CETA, The Comprehensive Employment and Training Act, which enabled the employment of refuge workers for one year.[140] The Legal Services Corporation provided legal aid to battered women and was currently bringing a class action against the police which shall be discussed in the next chapter.[141] Basically, there was very little in the way of government programmes to assist battered women or the shelter movement, and discussion of interagency contact represented little more than a willingness to try to make contact.[142] By comparison, the British already had in place more developed institutions for providing housing, social services and health care either to the entire population, as with the health care, or to a much broader section than just the poorest, as with housing and social services. This allowed greater possibilities for providing material and social resources to a wider section of women. It also allowed for involving state agencies more directly and fully.

Commissioners heard evidence and considered written submissions illustrating beyond a doubt that in the USA battered women were treated unequally before the law.[143] The hearing legitimized the needs of battered women as a matter of national concern and an arena for public policy, and provided the opportunity for activists to take the first steps towards forming the National Coalition Against Domestic Violence.[144] The hearing ended with an expression of admiration from the Chair:

> ... may I say to you that your presentations, ... have been one of the most exciting experiences I have had during a long period of service in the Federal Government.... I have never experienced this kind of a response. You made a deep impression on me, as I know you have on my colleagues. Your commitment is obvious, your concern is obvious.[145]

Federal legislation and the movement

In Britain, national legislation flowed more quickly and directly from the Parliamentary hearings and provided material resources and some legal protection for battered women as well as some financial provision for shelters. This was not the case in the United States. Consequently, one of the largest and most sustained efforts of the newly formed National Coalition Against Domestic Violence (NCADV) was the attempt to obtain Federal legislation to provide funding for shelters. While laws against the violence itself were being fought for and passed in each State, there was also a massive national effort to pass Federal legislation to fund shelters on a national level. The effort to secure Federal funding was spearheaded by activists and innovative legislators and began against a backdrop of widespread public interest and concern and within the context of a state more oriented to such issues. It would end in an era marked by a very different climate.

In response to pressure from the movement, and immediately preceding the Civil Rights Consultations, two separate bills were introduced in the House and the Senate meant to provide Federal funding for shelters. They differed in orientation. The *Domestic Violence Prevention and Treatment Act* [bill] was introduced in the House of Representatives by Republican Newton Steers and Democrat Lindy Boggs, and in the Senate by Democrats Edward Kennedy and Wendell Anderson.[146] It proposed the familiar model of a research and demonstration programme within the Department of Health, Education and Welfare (HEW), now Health and Human Services (HHS).[147] The *Family* Violence Prevention and Treatment Act [bill] was introduced in the House by Democrat Barbara Mikulski, proposing community based action involving the creation of a National Center for Community Action Against Family Violence within ACTION, the Federal Agency incorporating the Peace Corps and its home-based equivalent, VISTA.[148]

The bills embodied different orientations to government funding of service provision. Research and demonstration (R and D) was the usual approach to running a programme through HEW (the Domestic Violence bill). Mikulski's Family Violence bill provided a community based alternative to the R and D approach to public policy, noting that HEW, and especially its branch of the National Institute of Mental Health (NIMH), had previously used rape funds for research rather than services. Mikulski saw this as a community issue, believed ACTION would be more amenable to grassroots influence and doubted that HEW was capable of running a good community based programme.[149]

The bills also embodied different government approaches to social problems: one focusing on responses managed by professionals and the other focusing on community action. The first providing jobs and funds for members of the social, psychological and medical professions to develop and manage services for battered women and to academics to study the problem. The other envisioned a response developed by members of the community, including battered women, advocates and activists developing programmes to suit local conditions and needs. The community approach did not exclude the use of those with professional training, but the overall programme was not conceived as one shaped by the orientations of psychologists, social workers or lawyers nor staffed primarily by them. Funding would be more oriented to services than to expensive clinical salaries or research. Neither of these bills passed, but they remain important because they illustrate two different orientations to the relationship between social movements and the state. They also show very different approaches to social problems themselves, one embracing the notion of wider social change while the other moves towards ideas of individual inadequacy and solutions based on therapeutic interventions.

The process of getting a bill through the House, the Senate and Presidential approval is complex, involving many points of compromise, amendment, transformation and possible defeat. Each stage can be the subject of intense lobbying by different interest groups. In this case, an amended and synthesized version of the Mikulski and Boggs–Steers Bill soon emerged. The government response began rather smoothly and with unprecedented speed for a grassroots initiative. Activists organized and lobbied but, in May 1978, the bill failed in the House by a margin of only four votes.[150]

Activists were disappointed and exhausted. One can imagine their surprise when, just before summer recess, the Senate, without major debate, passed their own bill by voice vote.[151] With only one day of business left in the session it went over to the House where the House Rules Committee took unprecedented action and reconsidered the legislation, moving it out of committee for a vote in the House. With adjournment looming only hours ahead, months of intense negotiation and lobbying just behind and a bill that had moved through the process faster than any other of its kind, it is not difficult to imagine the excitement and anxiety among legislators and activists alike. At the eleventh hour, a persistent Republican critic read thirty-five amendments into the Congressional Record, effectively killing the bill.[152] During this same session, The Child Abuse Prevention and Treatment Act (1978) passed with ease,[153] reflecting not only a different orientation to these two forms of violence but also laying a foundation for some future twists in the fortunes of funding for abused women.

The 1979–80 session of Congress saw even greater activity and more intense and sophisticated negotiations as activists applied the lessons learned and attempted to increase their influence on another new bill. The Legislative Committee of the Coalition offered extensive critiques of the The Domestic Violence Prevention and Services Act [bill].[154] They lobbied for earmarked funds for advocacy and services in community based groups; minimal Federal, State and local bureaucracy; a Domestic Violence Council within HEW provided policy and decision-making responsibility remained within community based, women-centred groups; a rejection of NIMH as the Federal bureaucracy managing funds and programmes; research funding only for the purpose of assisting local groups with specific needs; and maximizing grassroots control of the review process of programmes as much as possible.[155] At the very least, the Coalition wanted provisions to include all women, not just the legally married, confidential record keeping, free shelter space and no licensing requirement for shelters.[156] The latter was seen as a means of squeezing out activists in favour of professionals.

These proposals for legislation represented an attempt by the social movement to retain control over the social problem they had identified and the response they had developed. This might be seen as a struggle between civil society and the legislative arm of the state reflecting Held's 'two pronged' strategy of creative reform, with 'innovation from below through radical social initiatives' emerging and continuing through 'protection by state action'.[157] Activists' efforts also represented an attempt to broaden the democratic base of the state through their participation in the legislative process and to ensure that legislation was responsive to the needs of the community and implemented under its management. These efforts represent an attempt to recast the relationship between the state and the movement.

What happened? Again, surprises and intense lobbying and negotiation were in store. The House bill was heard earlier than expected, once again necessitating intense activity if activists were to play a part in the democratic process. They set up a plan of action to poll members of Congress, organize a nation-wide letter and telephone campaign and obtain support from over sixty other organizations, mostly women's groups. President Carter personally endorsed the bill which passed the House by a margin of two to one. But this time the debate in the Senate was to be long and difficult.[158] The better part of a year passed and the wider political climate changed before the final fate of the bill was known.

New social and political developments were to affect the outcome. There was the growing backlash of conservatism, including a criticism of state provisions of social services in favour of the market economy and monetaristic social policy under *laissez-faire* capitalism; a move to a neo-liberal form of state; a revival of fundamentalist religious thinking and vigorous attempts to introduce this into political decision making; and a growing backlash against the notion of equal opportunities and the women's movement. Finally, the election of Ronald Reagan to the Presidency lead to a lame duck legislature at the time the bill was to be heard. The administration that initiated the legislation and provided its ideological support had been voted out of office. Legislators work in a state of political limbo during the short period after a November election defeat and before the January inauguration when the new President and Congress enter office bringing philosophical and pragmatic changes. In this case, the sweep of change was considerable. Federal funding of services was not to be the new approach to any social issue; women leaving home for any reason, even temporarily and even because of violent treatment from their partners, was not the new approach. With the threat of a

Republican fillibuster if the bill came to the floor, it was withdrawn.[159] After such a sustained drive, activists' disappointment may have been lessened by the knowledge that the bill had gone further than most of its type in a shorter period of time, and, in the end, was lost because of wider political changes beyond their influence. For the time being, funding for shelters had to continue to be a local and State issue.

The Mikulski bill continued to be introduced each year, but each year saw defeat. Finally, in the 1983/84 session of Congress, a different tactic was taken. Still based on the original philosophy, the bill was condensed and converted into an Amendment and attached to the Child Abuse Prevention and Treatment Act as it came up for re-authorization.[160] As mentioned earlier, both the shelter bill and the Child Abuse Act had been introduced in 1978; the first failed while the other passed with ease and was now up for renewal. With the shelter Amendment riding on its back, the Child Abuse Act received its expected overwhelming endorsement from the House (voting 367 to 31) and needed passage through the Senate and the President's signature before becoming law.

The passage in the House was credited to the activists campaign co-ordinated by the Coalition who organized popular support, lobbied politicians and developed an informal coalition of Washington-based women's organizations,[161] illustrating what Sapiro has described as the truly professional skills of American feminist electoral participation in the 1980s and its ability to transcend partisan loyalty as they entered 'big-time politics'.[162] The family violence Amendment was to provide individual States with $65m over three years for prevention and services for victims and $2m each year for police training.[163]

Once again, all was not well. During the debate on the floor of the House, the Amendment was so radically transformed by further Republican amendments that the new social movement was now in danger of having expended years of energy and increasing political sophistication to obtain funding from which it might be wholly or partially excluded, or be left providing a service with which activists might fundamentally disagree. Six changes were of prime importance:

1 increased emphasis on prevention (with shelters not viewed as preventive);
2 expansion of types of organizations eligible for funding (religious, charity, voluntary, drug and alcohol programmes and self-help counselling);
3 requirements that shelters do not require a maximum stay, censor

mail or telephone calls, or interfere with reconciliation efforts unless requested to do so;

4 using a definition of the family that disqualifies cohabitants not legally married;

5 requiring each state to provide an eviction procedure for abusers sharing a residence;

6 a definition of 'related assistance' which may include food, clothing, child care, transportation, emergency medical care, counselling, alcohol and drug abuse treatment, and self-help services to abusers, victims and dependents.[164]

The expanded definitions of eligibility, provision and service providers would seem to lead inevitably to a reduction in the amount available for the grassroots movement as established shelters would compete for funding with new and different organizations to provide shelter and other services. This could lead to a transformation of philosophy, policy and/or practice as activist organizations attempt to meet the criterion of funding bodies. The third provision may seem both strange and irrelevant since coalition shelters do not use such practices, but the language implies that such coercion is used, thus further reducing their ability to compete for funds. Such a discourse fits the common, negative stereotype of feminists 'kidnapping' women away from their husbands. It ignores the reality of thousands of abused women desperately seeking, on their own accord, a place of safety for themselves and their children. In October 1984 the Family Violence Prevention and Services Act was, at last, signed into law as an amendment to the Child Abuse Prevention and Treatment Act, with appropriations of $8.3m for 1985 and 1986 and $8.5m each year for 1987–8.[165]

Finally passed, what might the legislation mean for abused women and for the movement? How closely does it approximate the five points for which the Coalition lobbied in 1979? It is sobering that legislation for abused women took so long, was so difficult and, in the end, was not achieved explicitly for women but attached to the more popular and acceptable cause of child abuse. This combination further adds to the possibility of conflating the two problems, further subordinating the issue of violence against women and enhancing intergenerational theories about cause. Attention is thus drawn still further away from the violence itself, from issues of male domination, power and control and from men's ultimate responsibility for their behaviour. Other legislation has been passed, particularly the Victims of Crime Act (VOCA), also in 1984, authorizing the use by shelters of fines for Federal violations of State victim compensation programmes.[166] In 1990, four bills and one resolution to help battered women were pending before Congress, covering issues of immigration requirements for foreign residents who are battered, restricting custody of children to the non-violent parent, provision of some public housing for those made homeless through violence, training for State judges, and creating new Federal misdemeanour crimes for domestic violence when the abuser crosses State lines to commit the act. Included in the latter are proposals to double-fund shelters and to fund the development of special spouse abuse units by police and courts.[167]

THE DYNAMIC OF PARTICIPATION AND CHANGE

At stake in the negotiations between the movement and the state are definitions of the nature and causes of the problem, who will respond to the problem, and what form that response will take. While the possibilities seem almost endless, at least in theory, the form of organization and established practices and interest usually limit the innovative in favour of the familiar. A part of this process involves the discourse used in shaping notions about the problem; another involves the responses in the form of recommendations, legislation, public policy and government funding. Ironically, government proposals for change often differ from the discourse initially used in outlining the problem. The discourse of the Parliamentary Select Committee in Britain varied from that of the Civil Rights Commission in the United States. The discourse of the former cast the problem in individual terms and emphasized psychiatric ideas, but when it came to public policy they recommended material responses in the form of refuges, housing and legal protection. The USA adopted a discourse of equal rights for individuals and was much more inclined to accommodate notions about the unequal status of women in society and changes in the justice system, but later government proposals often differed from this discourse. In the final analysis, both countries opted for some form of change in the areas of temporary shelter and legal protection, and both adopted some of the activists' agenda for government action.

The British were quicker to legislate at the national level, partly because the legislative process provides the party in power with the advantage of leadership on all committees, but also because a more well developed welfare state means that government agencies are generally more active in providing a wider variety of social services to a broader spectrum of the community. Areas such as housing and health care can more easily become a part of the state response to a new issue simply because they already provide a service to the wider community. In the USA, the system may also have been an important conributing factor in the slower response to Federal legislation. The division of power and leadership between the two political parties throughout the system of committees, the two Houses of Congress and the Presidency, while serving other purposes very well, nonetheless makes the passage of legislation more difficult unless an issue has bipartisan appeal. In addition, welfare provision is often only for the poorest and the destitute, thus leaving the state without agencies with which to address problems affecting women across the class system.

Although feminist discourse and analysis have often been ignored or denied by government, this was strongest in Britain. The ironic twist is that while British politicians denied feminist discourse they moved quickly to legislate for many of their proposed changes. In the USA, the discourse was much more readily adopted but Federal legislation to provide funding for shelters proved difficult to achieve and, in the end, may have taken a shape more likely to squeeze out activists and their agenda for change. On the other hand, the equally enormous efforts in the USA to change State, rather than Federal, laws in order to provide better legal protection for women have met with much greater success, as shall be seen in the next two chapters.

It is not easy for a new social movement to enter into the political arena or to obtain change at all, much less to do so quickly. The process involves much more than a good idea, powers of persuasion or even a well-documented case of injustice. The nature and speed of change in legislation and public policy must proceed through resistance to new cultural beliefs and attitudes as well as through the mechanisms for developing policy and legislation which tend to be balanced towards the status quo and established interests. The invisible conduit through which discourse passes into recommendation is composed of political allegiances, existing institutions, previous policies and priorities, and established interest groups delivering existing services. These routes are less likely to be trod by 'outsiders' carrying the banners of new groups with less familiar or immediately acceptable messages. The new social movement and the new activists would not have an easy route to participation in the government process and to bringing their voice to the seat of government. That path is already occupied by others, more familiar travellers, who have trodden the path before and will usually be given priority at crucial turning points. Both the established travellers and their destination are familiar to government, even if not completely routinized. Professionals, bureaucrats and academics who have traditionally been a part of the government process of 'connecting' the government institutions with civil society often propose established and familiar solutions even as they address new problems and demands. We shall see this pattern of familiar participants and established solutions reappear in the subsequent responses of policy makers, legislators and criminal justice.

Beginning with resistance to the acknowledgement that a problem exists or warrants public concern, several other routes may be taken upon which government resist rather than embrace change. Sometimes public hearings may be used to diffuse protest and delay rather than facilitate demands for change. Government may also make recommendations without providing resources, fail to accommodate new organizations or unfamiliar constituencies, and/or attempt to roll a new problem into the routine responses of existing agencies which may have helped create the problem in the first place.

How can we understand the contradiction between discourse in the show-piece public hearings and the proposals for government action? The British embraced a psychological discourse, then recommended material provision. The USA more readily adopted a feminist discourse but were painfully slow to legislate for the material resources of shelter and financial support. This would appear to be understood at least as much, if not more, in terms of the process of implementation through the channels of existing policies, institutions and practices as in the nature of the discourse used on the journey from evidence and ideas to recommendations and practice. Although British politicians shaped the discourse about causes around psychological explanations, this discourse, unlike in the USA, is not such a part of the popular view of life and social problems, nor are there large numbers of practitioners or organizations for delivering such responses. It is perhaps curious that the politicians gave such a slant to this view since it played little part in their final recommendations, most of which might be more easily predicted from the nature of existing policies, institutions and practices. Yet the British also embraced the innovative, pragmatic response of the battered-women's movement even as their explanations were ignored.

In the USA, feminist discourse was more readily adopted, although not without resistance, but the welfare state is not so highly developed to provide material and financial resources to citizens other than the poorest. Thus, existing government policies provide less scope for such response. New and innovative policies were required but were thus more difficult to develop upon existing responses to social problems affecting a broad spectrum of the population. Even so, this was very nearly achieved in the first attempt at Federal legislation when public interest was high, the women's movement was in ascendency and the state was more community and welfare oriented than it was soon to become. The struggle to obtain the legislation continued in a climate which began to alter radically and in ways that obviated against, rather than for, women's issues. It is a monument to energy, hard work, increasing political sophistication, alliance building and tactics that legislation of any type has been passed within the conservative agenda and *laissez-faire* social policies of the 1980s.

The negotiations between the state and the new social movement have certainly resulted in change. It has done a great deal, albeit not nearly enough, to meet the short-term goals of providing relief to women who are abused. The verdict on the long-term goal of eliminating male violence is still not out.

5 Challenging the justice system

One of the earliest targets of protest for the battered-women's movements in Britain and the United States was the unresponsiveness of the criminal justice system (CJS), especially the police. In the early 1970s, activists discovered what battered women had long known, that the CJS failed to protect the victim or to act against the offender. Police did not usually arrest men for assaulting their wives or cohabitees, rarely offered assistance to women and sometimes denigrated them for seeking protection within the law. Judges, prosecutors and other criminal justice personnel also failed to deal with the violence in a meaningful manner. Attempts by women in England, Wales and the United States to file complaints against their husbands in lower courts were usually deflected by prosecutors who did not see such complaints as worthy of criminal justice sanction (this option was not available to women in Scotland). The end result was that women were denied assistance and their legal claims were rejected.

Activist's in the battered-women's movement recognized the importance of the CJS in dealing with the problem and attempted to bring pressure aimed at changing established patterns. The story of this struggle, its successes and limitations, will be recounted in this and the next chapter. An understanding of the struggle for change and the persistence of established practices requires a consideration of the historical and contemporary contexts in which these social processes occur. Here, we shall consider the feminist discourses associated with the use of law as an instrument of change, chart the historical background to the challenges and changes and analyse the nature of changes in statutes and policy. In the next chapter we investigate the way these changes have affected criminal justice practices.

LAW AND JUSTICE AS INSTRUMENTS OF CHANGE

Historically, oppressed groups have often used the principles of natural justice as goals of their struggles and foundations for legitimizing social protest. In this century they have attempted to employ the law as a means of achieving equality and in order to redress inequities in social and economic conditions. Alternatively, governments have traditionally employed the law and the legal institutions of the state in implementing various measures of change as well as retaining the established order. State apparatuses as embodied in the police, courts and prisons play a crucial role in implementing the political, social and economic agendas of both democratic and authoritarian regimes. Both social movements and governments attempt to use the law in order to implement change and/or retain the status quo.

Demands for equality, justice and rights have played an especially important role in recent social struggles in North America. The civil rights movements of the 1960s used the law as a significant instrument in confronting government and society, and when the Federal government eventually enacted civil rights legislation it in turn was enforced through law and criminal justice. It is not surprising that contemporary feminists have followed the examples of the civil rights movement of the twentieth century, feminist reformers of the nineteenth century and early thinkers such as Mary Woolstonecraft who first proposed that women use the state and the law as a means of securing change for women. They have sought to confront the law and criminal justice as a means of improving the lives of women and children. These efforts have been mounted around a wide range of issues, including battering, rape, marital rape, child sexual abuse and pornography.

Some feminist activists and scholars have argued that it is impossible to use the law and legal apparatus to confront patriarchal domination and oppression when the language and procedures of these social processes and institutions are saturated with patriarchal beliefs and structures. They have sought to construct a feminist jurisprudence as one means of challenging established law. Tove Stang Dahl has proposed a parallel system that would operate alongside or in conjunction with formal law. She urges a reduction of emphasis on the formal discourse of law in favour of a focus on 'law in practice'.[1] A more feminist jurisprudence would, she argues, stress the importance of legal guidance from below relying more on custom and public opinion, and be more responsive to women's needs.

Other feminist academics have argued that women's justice should be based on an alternative moral discourse, thus leading to very different ways of dealing with social evils such as crime. Gilligan has argued that women's sense of justice is expressed in a 'different voice'.[2] She proposes that legal practice presents itself as gender-neutral, whereas it is, in fact, thoroughly male centred. Male 'justice' stresses abstract moral reasoning, first principles, autonomy and impartiality. She asserts that a female sense of justice is expressed in a 'different voice' stressing attachment, affiliation, interdependence and contextual understanding of human behaviour. Following the logic, that '... in the different voice of women lies the truth of an ethic of care ...' she proposed responses based on 'the premise of non-violence – that no one should be hurt'.[3] Stressing the feminist themes of 'caring, sharing, nurturing and loving', other commentators have urged that responses to crime should be based on '... a process of ongoing communication and involvement that considers the needs, interests and motivations of all involved'.[4] We should never, these theorists propose, 'return evil with evil'. Justice should follow principles which lead us to '... seek to forgive, reconcile and heal ...' striving 'to find within ourselves outrageous love, the kind of love that extends even to those it is easiest to fear and hate ...'.[5] Given this vision, a femininst jurisprudence means a more personalized approach rooted in an 'ethic of reform.'[6]

In a more fundamental assault on justice and in the face of what they see as the futility of attempting to change it in order to serve the needs of women, a few feminist commentators have proposed the near abandonment of the struggle around justice. Carol Smart has presented the strongest case for abandoning or radically reducing efforts to transform justice.[7] Concentrating on the discourses of justice – the language, methods and procedures of law – she argues, that feminists should not be too quick to turn to law. Offering apparent solutions it is, she argues, so saturated with masculinity that it can never be a solution to violence against women. Using the law simply traps feminists in its discourse, elevates legal functionaries and, in the end, concedes more power to the legal system. Feminist jurisprudence does not reduce or challenge the power of law, it merely gives greater legitimacy to law as a route to 'truth and justice'. For Smart, using law can also cause a backlash of hostility and is 'therefore, hazardous'.[8] In the final analysis, although she qualifies her remarks, Smart argues that law bears 'no relationship to the concerns of women's lives', and feminists should concentrate on constructing alternative 'resistant discourses' through women's groups.[9]

These commentaries present a framework for considering the struggles and innovations of the battered-women's movement. Following these proposals we must ask whether activists' efforts have made a difference in the lives of women and consider the form these innovations have taken. In this chapter and the next, we will show how the movement has not rejected a struggle around law in its efforts to assist women. From the very beginning law and criminal justice have been seen as significant targets of struggle and it is not at all clear that this has been done using a 'different voice'. We must ask, however, whether the results of these struggles have altered discourses and practices associated with justice, or have they merely been encompassed by and reinforced the usual operation of criminal justice? As Stang Dahl has suggested, we must go beyond the level of discourse and explore law in action, the way criminal justice innovations have affected the actions of police and prosecutors and consider the way these have made a difference to the lives of women. In analysing law we certainly need to consider discourses and the symbolic messages they embody, but if we are concerned about the way the movement's efforts have affected women we should pay particular attention to mechanisms associated with confronting, implementing and practising new laws and policies. In the final analysis we must consider whether it is possible for criminal justice to embody enabling discourses and practices for women who have been the victims of violence. To begin this analysis we consider the way in which the movement first confronted criminal justice.

PUBLIC HEARINGS AND CRIMINAL JUSTICE

The first major national forums for articulating the accumulated grievances against the criminal justice system were the hearings of the Parliamentary Select Committee in Britain and the Civil Rights Commission Hearings convened in the United States. Battered women, activists and committed professionals recounted numerous examples of inadequate criminal justice response and proposed various solutions. The evidence and proposals for reform were remarkably similar. In Britain activists and feminist lawyers argued for 'more vigorous intervention' by the police who should protect women by upholding the law, especially through the enforcement of injunctions. One legal advocate urged:

> What I do not want to see for battered wives is what we saw with battered children: the only way the law in this country will protect

is when it is faced with a corpse.... Certainly, women have died through this sort of attitude, and if this Committee can in some way recommend that the police ... prosecute, I would ask them to do so.... One of the first things we would like to see is that injunctions should be backed by a warrant for arrest.[10]

The report of the Civil Rights hearings contained a very strong statement about the unequal treatment of battered women.

Women who complain of abuse often are treated cavalierly by the police, the courts, and other elements of the criminal justice system. Little effort has been made in most jurisdictions to provide the necessary specialized facilities to serve victims of domestic violence.[11]

Marjory Fields, at that time an attorney from Brooklyn Legal Services (a US government funded free legal service for the poor), with extensive experience of cases of battering, proposed that violence against women should be treated as a crime, men must be arrested and prosecuted, and there should be an immediate end to systematic discrimination against victims.[12] Through such actions the criminal justice system would be sending a strong and unequivocal message of disapproval of violence against women. Fields's statement was the most explicit in identifying the need for two forms of response: one associated with the protection of the victim and the second concerned with confronting violence through the use of arrest. In both hearings, most representatives and advocates primarily argued for the use of civil law measures to protect the victim and to control violent men.

Representatives of the criminal justice system responded mostly by denying complaints and deflecting responsibility. Witnesses for the police indicated that a criminal justice response was appropriate only in exceptional circumstances. The Police Superintendents Association of England and Wales stated that, 'In the great majority of cases we believe that we deal with such cases without any degree of reluctance'.[13] The representative of the Chief Police Officers Association concurred and claimed that existing legal provisions '... are adequate to deal with this problem'.[14] Police and judicial representatives argued that violence in the home was an insignificant problem compared with more serious matters, such as traffic offences and theft, claiming that police responsibility was minimal. Social services and family counselling agencies should take the major responsibility for such problems, although police officers take '... positive action at the time, to give advice, to keep the peace, and most of all to prevent injury' and '... as often as not play a conciliatory role ...'.[15]

Police and judicial representatives concluded there was no need for significant change. The Lord Advocate, the highest law officer in Scotland, claimed there was no need to change substantive law: police powers of arrest were adequate and increased penalties were unnecessary. More severe penalties might exacerbate the problem:

Sentences of imprisonment could well have an adverse effect upon a family by removing of the 'breadwinner', and imposing heavy fines will likewise reduce the 'purchasing power' of the family and place the burden of subsidizing such families on the taxpayer.[16]

Police in Britain were extremely reluctant to expand the powers of injunctions by attaching the power of arrest and rejected an extension of their involvement in this 'civil' matter. The London Metropolitan Police claimed it would be '... a dangerous step to involve the police within the civil process ...' placing '... an intolerable strain on manpower resources and be to the *detriment of safeguarding other members of the public'* (our emphasis).[17] Injunctions were viewed as too time consuming, and to pass such legislation would be giving preferential treatment to women, an anathema in the present 'egali-tarian' society, '... the equal status of women in society today precludes any preferential treatment for them; otherwise the law could fall into disrepute'.[18]

Representatives of British criminal justice were strongly opposed to expanding their role, pointing out, for example, that they were at that very moment seeking to shed some existing responsibilities. The best place for this problem was with social services or refuges, but not the police. Although refuges were endorsed by some CJ witnesses, abused women and advocates commented on the irony of police co-operation with refuges yet their reluctance to assist individual women. Other witnesses from law enforcement expressed reservations about refuges, believing that they precipitated the break-up of families. In their view, an important role for shelters was the provision 'of assist-ance to bring about a reconciliation and re-unite the family'.[19] Family unity was paramount for the Chief Police Officers Association; their representative argued, 'Every effort *should be made to re-unite the family'.*[20] Only the Lord Advocate of Scotland explicitly supported divorce as a solution, indicating it should be more readily obtainable.

The resistance of criminal justice representatives in Britain was strong and unified. Either there was no problem or it was trivial. Police work devoted to such cases was '... very time consuming and a distraction to the overall police effort'.[21] They further argued, that the CJS had to protect men from the false claims of women. According to the Home Office witness some 'wives were uncooperative', 'positively hostile'. The representative of the Edinburgh police pointed to the 'possibility of malice, a wife and daughter may conspire to make false allegations against a husband'.[22] For representatives of the justice system, the claims of women's groups about failures in the law and law enforcement were either erroneous; fabrications or, at best, distortions, and proposals to strengthen injunctions were unnecessary or misguided. They rejected the need for changes in laws and practices and argued that continuation of existing practice was more than adequate.

In the USA, the Civil Rights hearings in Washington DC, and subsequent on-site hearings in two States, produced similar debate between advocates and law enforcement representatives. Witnesses testified that police and prosecutors failed to respond in an effective manner and that arrest was a rare occurrence. Most representatives of criminal justice did not deny the existence of a problem, but opposed the use of criminal justice sanctions. It seemed that for many of the witnesses from criminal justice agencies the major problem was physical danger to officers. One police official indicated, '... more officers are killed in family situations than probably anything else ...'[23] (a widespread misconception which is refuted by a closer examination of actual police contacts in these cases and of nation-wide statistics on violence against the police).[24] Even if this were true, it would be an extraordinary rationale for not intervening.

Preferred solutions included police dispute resolution and civil legal remedies and criminal court diversion to mediation and counselling.[25] A police official from Harrisburg, Pennsylvania stated,

> once the [officers] arrive, they are instructed to calm the situation, to keep control, to protect participants, and to keep it out of the legal field and to recommend outside [social] agencies to handle the problem.[26]

Cases should be dealt with by requesting or requiring one of the spouses to leave the residence. Police department guidelines in one city advised, 'the best solution ... is generally for one of the spouses to leave the home until the next day'.[27] If the justice system became involved, prosecutors should use 'orders of protection' or diversion to social service agencies for conciliation.

The Chair of the Civil Rights Commission was especially keen on such civil 'solutions', He argued that the police were 'managers in disputes' and declared himself 'very, very much interested in the mediation functions' of police and courts.[28] Witnesses from the Law

Enforcement Assistance Administration (LEAA), a branch of the US Department of Justice specifically responsible for innovations, testified that the problem was a focus of concern but indicated there was no commitment to enlarging the responsibility of justice.[29] For the CJS, the way forward was integrated services based on a model of victim/witness programmes involving neighbourhood centres staffed by community volunteers engaged in mediating disputes.

THE LEGACY OF CRIMINAL JUSTICE

In both the United States and Britain, the majority of criminal justice representatives rejected the need for radical change in existing responses. Representatives of criminal justice in the USA appeared, however, to be more willing to accept the existence of a problem and the possible need for renewed efforts. Civil injunctions, social service intervention and private solutions were the accepted solutions in both countries, and, in the USA crisis intervention, mediation and diversion were the preferred responses. Change, if needed, would only involve developments incorporating existence responses. These positions were challenged at public hearings. Battered women, legal advocates and members of the movement rejected such views and defined them as complacent.

In order to understand the legacy of neglect documented by activists and reflected in the orientations of representives of criminal justice, it is necessary to locate contemporary criminal justice response in the context of their historical development, starting with a brief examination of the nature of community based justice in the eighteenth century and moving to a consideration of the emergence of abstract state justice in the nineteenth century. It is then necessary to trace developments, in the late nineteenth and early twentieth centuries in the United States, of unique forms of responding to family problems associated with therapeutic professionals and family courts.

Women once played an important role in European community justice. In eighteenth-century Europe, they organized and participated in popular protests and demonstrations against economic and social injustices.[30] For example, they sought to bring down the price of bread, to force grain on to the market and to alter the most exploitative activities of traders and retailers. In early nineteenth-century Scotland women were at the forefront of community efforts to protect the traditional rights of crofters (small tenant farmers) against the attempts of landowners to eject them from the land.[31]

Women were also prominent in community efforts to curb the excesses of patriarchal domination and violence. Men who flaunted their contempt for the accepted conventions of marriage by engaging in flagrant forms of adultery, or by overstepping the wide boundaries of legitimate patriarchal chastisement by beating their wives to excess, were sometimes subjected to community chastisement. In communities in Britain and Europe women and men employed public rituals and sometimes more direct actions in attempts to shame men into behaving more decently towards their wives.[32] Processions, recitation of verses and the banging of pots and pans were one way that communities attempted to use public shaming and disapproval to try to transform private, unspeakable issues into public ones worthy of condemnation and control. In this way the community supported the victim and rebuked the offender. Whether this stopped the violence is impossible to say, but it certainly provided a voice for the concerns of women and public support and recognition of the plight of individual women. Whatever the benefits of this justice, it was deeply patriarchal. Curtailing only the most obvious and flagrant forms of abuse left the usual patterns of patriarchal control unfettered and merely set the boundaries of what was considered 'normal'.[33]

Mechanisms of formal justice played only a minor role in the regulation of family affairs during the eighteenth century. The peace bond was the major relief for women subjected to violence and severe abuse at the hands of their husbands.[34] Peace bonds, first introduced in the fourteenth century, applied judicial restraints on an abusive husband, sometimes requiring the payment of a surety which might be forfeited if he continued to abuse his wife. Only a very few women of noble rank were able to use this form of civil relief.

With the emergence of abstract bureaucratic justice in the nineteenth century, women were increasingly excluded from the processes of justice. In the late eighteenth and throughout the nineteenth century in Britain and the United States, laws were codified, new courts created and the powers of existing ones strengthened, and police and penal systems were set in place. Traditional community based methods of responding to public and private injustices were condemned and repressed. With these developments, the mechanisms of contemporary criminal justice were firmly established.[35] Women played only a minor role in this process: primarily working outside of the criminal justice system as critics or moral adjuncts.[36] Operating outside the formal mechanisms of 'justice' meant that the concerns and protests of such women were often ignored or rejected. Thus, women and their perceptions and concerns played only a minor role in shaping the new legal codes, police procedures and penal reactions. It is no exaggeration to say that the laws were made by men for men primarily for the protection of property and the prevention of public disorder.

The prerogatives of men and the subjugation of women were firmly enshrined in this new system of justice. In Britain and the United States, married women were unable to enter into contracts, had few legal rights to property after marriage or claims to their children, and were barred from certain professions and trades.[37] Statutes pertaining to married women made them dependents, subject to patriarchal control within the home and community. Men's rights over households were further reinforced through the emerging social ideas of true womanhood and the cult of domesticity.[38] The rights and privileges of husbands were supreme. In turn, husbands were legally entrusted with the responsibility to protect and support their wives and children. Whether the law granted men supreme control of paternalistic protection, the outcome was the same: male domination was enshrined in the legal structures of the two countries. Legal developments in the nineteenth century continued to reflect and reinforce a patriarchal order. The moral and material authority of husbands was upheld by legal statutes.

Within this context it is not surprising that the problem of violence against women in the home was considered of no particular importance in the usual course of the application of 'justice'. Indeed, it was nearly impossible under such a system to contemplate the possibility of rape in marriage.[39] Occasionally, judges would hand out harsh sentences to men who severely assaulted their wives, but this was unlikely in societies where male dominance was applauded and male violence ignored or condoned. In the late eighteenth century, Blackstone, the most influential English legal authority of the time, reaffirmed the rights of moderate chastisement in his commentary on English common law. Although statutes passed in early nineteenth-century Britain included violence against wives as an assault, judges apparently clung to the dictates of Common Law and did little to challenge the patriarchal privilege of legitimate chastisement of wives.[40]

A prominent London magistrate, Edward Cox, articulated the dominant judicial orientation to crimes against women in his book, *The Principles of Sentencing*, which was the definitive guide to sentencing in the late nineteenth century.[41] Cox offered numerous recommendations, usually punitive, for sentencing: boys should be whipped, burglars sent to repressive prisons and violent offenders treated to long prison sentences. His punitive fervour was not evident, however, when he wrote about violent crimes against women. According to Cox, rape was a 'rare and exceptional' event and he thought that men who beat their wives should not usually be subjected to judicial sanctions. Cox thought that the men who appeared before him for beating their wives were often 'tortured and taunted to the verge of madness' by women, and he indicted that it was only understandable that they should use violence. Women, he implied, often exaggerated the violence in order to condemn innocent husbands. As such, women rarely needed protection and when judicial reaction was necessary, he recommended the peace bond and deferred sentencing. Like his twentieth-century counterparts, Cox felt that criminal justice intervention would disrupt the domestic order: 'After a husband has been placed upon the treadmill on the complaint of his wife, is it possible that he can love her, or is she likely to honor and obey him?'[42]

Although these views appear to have been strong within the judiciary, they did not go unchallenged. By the last half of the nineteenth century, the problem of violence against women in the home was being placed on the public agenda in the United States and Britain. It was placed there, not by concerned judges, the police or politicians, but by women who raised their voices outside of the institutions of the state. Early feminists, such as Frances Power Cobbe in England and Lucy Stone in the United States condemned such violence and championed reform in legal responses. Cobbe was probably the most influential and effective nineteenth-century campaigner for battered women. Her campaigning and pressure on parliamentarians in the 1870s was very influential in bringing about improvements in civil law as relief for women.[43] Her concerns were taken up by male parliamentarians who were able to engineer the passage of new legislation, generally known as the Matrimonial Causes Acts.[44] Beginning with the enactment of the first Act in 1878, women who were victims of violence were able to obtain legal separations from violent husbands, and were entitled to custody of their children and retention of earnings and property secured during separation. A woman could only obtain a separation order if her husband had been convicted of aggravated assault on her and if the court considered she was in grave danger. Like the peace bond, these injunctions provided civil remedies for violence in the home.

The campaigns for battered women in the late nineteenth century emerged in the context of the concerns of social purity leagues and temperance groups (such as the US Women's Christian Temperance

Union) and a growing middle-class fear of the public violence of the 'dangerous classes'. In Britain and the United States there emerged a growing antagonism towards working people and a near 'panic' about crime and the criminal classes.[45] Public concern for assaulted and murdered wives was never as strong or as vehement. However, a few campaigns were waged in both countries to introduce flogging as a punishment for wife beaters. In 1874 a parliamentary committee gathered evidence from legal authorities and criminal justice personnel on violence against children and wives and considered whipping as punishment.[46] Witnesses expressed some concern for brutally assaulted wives but voiced little concern for women experiencing 'ordinary' assaults. There was almost universal rejection of flogging as an appropriate sanction for ordinary assaults. Bills proposing the introduction of flogging for wife beaters were introduced on four separate occasions into Parliament; none were successful.[47]

In the United States, flogging for wife beaters was first discussed in the 1880s at which time a number of state legislatures debated the issue.[48] President Theodore Roosevelt referred to the problem in his fourth annual address to Congress in 1904 and recommended corporal punishment. After much debate over a number of years, apparently providing an excellent opportunity for lawmakers to express their prejudices against women by ridiculing the problem and belittling its consequences, only a handful of States passed laws directing whipping for men who beat their wives.[49] These laws had little impact; only a few men were ever whipped for the offence of wife assault.

Moral panics, subsequent debates and legislation were not so much about protecting women as they were about concern for public order. Assaults on wives were incidental to the more general debate and concern. With this background of growing concern for the immorality and violence of the working classes, individual women and women's groups were able to raise the issue of wife beating, to argue that it affected many working-class women and successfully to pressure male parliamentarians and state legislators to enact legislation aimed at providing greater protection for married women. Activist women published accounts of the violence, rejected arguments that blamed women and proposed legal remedies. Most of the campaigners focused their concern on the 'lower orders'. Cobbe, one of the most enlightened and radical of these reformers, nonetheless wrote of the concentration of wife-beating in the 'kicking districts ... among the lowest labouring classes'.[50] Unlike Stone, she did not endorse whipping or flogging as a punishment for wife-beating, arguing that it would not improve the situation for women and might even make matters worse. The lessons of the late nineteenth century in both countries point to how the demands of activists may be shaped, co-opted and/or absorbed within an existing legal system.

PSYCHOLOGY, SOCIAL WELFARE AND FAMILY COURTS

If legislators and judges often ignored or slighted the problems of women, new professional groups emerging in the late nineteenth century would make these problems one of their primary concerns. Psychiatry, psychoanalysis and criminology were emerging disciplines during the late nineteenth and early twentieth centuries. These new professions offered explanations of victims, crime and criminals, which conceived of females as ruled by their biology and sexuality.[51] Criminal women were conceived of as over-sexed, under-sexed, overly masculine, morally and mentally inferior and a serious danger to public morality.[52] Female victims were thought to be irrational and prone to illusions, fabrications and exaggeration.[53]

Freud's conception of incest as an expression of unconscious female desire is probably the best known example of the transformation of female experiences into fantasies.[54] Female victims of crimes such as sexual assault, rape and violence in the home, who had in the past been characterized as prone to exaggeration, were now 'confirmed' in these perceptions. Psychiatric discourse identified them as suffering from delusions, hysteria and sexual fantasies. Women were conceived of as the cause of the violence against them. 'Nagging' wives precipitated beatings and 'seductive' daughters provoked their fathers into incestuous acts. According to these new 'scientific' accounts, women usually made fanciful accusations about violence. By the 1930s psychoanalysis had enshrined the myth of masochism into its conceptions of normal female psychology. Based on these speculations presented as scientific truths, it was argued that women derived sexual gratification from the violence they experienced.[55] These professional discourses filtered into judicial thinking of the time both in Britain and in the United States, reinforcing and legitimating conventional perceptions of female victims.

As a result of their inclusion in new institutions in the United States, such as juvenile and family courts, therapeutic professionals and their views began to have an important impact on the conceptions and treatment of female victims. This happened at the turn of the century, when US cities embarked upon new social experiments combining social welfare and justice.[56] The first family court was created in Buffalo, New York in 1911, and in 1914 the first adult psychiatric clinic directly linked to a court was established in Chicago.[57] By 1920, over ten major cities had juvenile, family or domestic relations courts. Fuelled by the advent of the new behavioural sciences and its allied professions, clinical psychology and social work, reformers set about creating mechanisms for aiding children and families. Similar concerns and interests were expressed in Great Britain but they did not result in the creation of new judical institutions. These US courts and their allied professionals were extraordinarily ambitious. A few embraced radical ideals and sought to apply new techniques to social problems. One of their major ambitions was to make immigrant and working-class families 'respectable', 'moral' and 'industrious'; free from violence like 'normal' American families. To create this healthier society, they urged both state and private social service intervention in families through institutions such as family courts.

Family courts held out the promise of solving marital problems through timely intervention, patient concern, and social investigation, followed by the application of psychological and social remedies. Judicial experts agreed that domestic disputes, troubles regarding children and other contentious matters should not be solved through the antagonistic procedures of criminal courts. Domestic relations courts would be able to solve family problems in a setting which emphasized discussion and reconciliation engineered by social service intervention. Legal procedures and solutions were intended to play only a minor role. As one judge wrote about his court, it would be 'a great social agency'. In most locations, physical assaults on wives became the most frequent basis for complaint and referral.[58] This was the beginning of the systematic official diversion and exclusion of violence against wives from the criminal justice system in the US.

Nineteenth-century justice had often ignored violence against women in the home, excused and sometimes tacitly supported men who beat their wives based on the idea that they were merely following an established patriarchal right. In the twentieth century, new rationales would emerge and intermingle with the old. As one Philadelphia judge remarked, assaults on wives are 'not really a crime; it is a matter of laziness or shiftlessness or indifference or incapacity or negligence or mental or physical deficiencies on the part of the husband'.[59] Women were also the focus of explanation. Wives were thought to be extravagant, and immigrant women were seen as poor housekeepers and mothers which provoked men to violence.

Social workers and judges usually recommended reconciliation, advised women to improve their housekeeping, cooking and child care and to cope with their husbands' violence.[60] Similar notions were evident in Britain, but they were less likely to be reinforced by therapeutic professionals working within the CJS.

Domestic relations and family courts are still thriving in the United States, attempting to settle family problems through social or psychological means. In the 1960s the ideals of the mental health movement penetrated these courts, further expanding the therapeutic conceptions of the problem of violence against women. Long-term psychotherapy was considered the ideal, followed by short-term couple counselling emphasizing problems of family interaction. Despite this promise, the usual response of such courts was an avoidance of intervention.[61] One of the most common responses was a summary dismissal, a 'go home' order. Sometimes such decisions were preceded by judicial admonitions addressed to the husband and wife, involving directions for the husband to refrain from violence and for the woman to be a better wife and mother. Common judicial responses included lectures, mediation, peace bonds, short-term counselling and continuances to provide a period of 'cooling off' for the couple.[62] By the time of the rediscovery of the problems of battered women in the early 1970s, family courts and psychiatric and social work approaches had reduced these criminal assaults to problems of individual or social pathology. The CJS was not considered the appropriate institution for dealing with violence against women within the home; it was now defined as a family and personal problem best dealt with through social and psychological solutions.

CRISIS INTERVENTION

In the late 1960s these ideals were extended into police work in the United States through the introduction of programmes of crisis intervention and mediation. The criminal justice establishment conceived of crisis intervention as a humane programme that would aid the police and courts and assist victims. Psychologists and criminologists working in conjunction with the police urged the introduction of new behaviourally based intervention techniques into police responses to problems in the family. Police officers were over-burdened and court calenders and city jails were bulging at the seams. Using crisis intervention to deal with 'family disputes' was one method for dealing with these problems. Family crisis intervention was another strand in the growing web of psychiatric interventions into the community (see

Chapter 7).[63] As one of its early proponents argued, 'Family crisis intervention provides an opportunity to offer brief emergency psychiatric services, identify unmet needs and act as a referral source to other community agencies ...'.[64] By 1978, millions of dollars had been invested in crisis intervention programmes throughout the United States.[65]

According to the therapeutic professionals who urged crisis intervention, domestic disturbances rarely involved violence. Arrest was inappropriate for solving the complex social and psychological problems evident in these non-violent 'family squabbles'. 'Family fights', they argued, were dangerous events, apparently not for women, but for police officers. Police officers, they pointed out, often inflamed these conflicts and increased the risks of injury to themselves by 'forming protective–seductive alliances' with women and thus 'contributing to the emasculation of male disputants'.[66] Instead of arrest, which they incorrectly argued was frequently used, police officers should become counsellors and mediators, trained in the skills of crisis intervention. Once intervention had occurred couples could be referred to the appropriate social or psychiatric agency.

In order to demonstrate the efficacy of these approaches, Law Enforcement and Assistance Administration (LEAA) created 'model projects' in six cities.[67] The projects involved a number of specific goals, including attempts to reduce the number of recalls to the police regarding domestic disputes, to increase the quantity and quality of referrals, to reduce family violence and homicides, and to reduce injuries to the police and members of the public.[68] Goals such as these were to be achieved by training police officers in communicative and interactive skills that could be used when intervening in 'domestic disputes'. Training programmes would increase police officers' repertoire of responses and sensitivity to and knowledge of the component parts of family conflict, increase multi-cultural awareness, change attitudes in order to 'facilitate human helping', and enhance police officers' understanding of their own feelings in dealing with other people.[69]

The language of these proposals and training materials obscures the usual problem to which police are responding when they go to the scene of a 'domestic dispute' by abstracting and/or distorting their usual features. Academics, therapeutic professionals and police managers write about 'family fights' and 'domestic squabbles' in which 'normal patterns of communication have broken down'. For them, solutions should not include arrest and official sanctions. Instead, police officers aided by psychologists will help 'families' search for behavioural alternatives and promote 'the family's functioning as a stress mediating system'.[70] In order to achieve these goals police officers must learn to use the apparently well-established techniques of clinical crisis intervention. Training involves learning how to assess the 'needs' of disputants, creating a greater awareness of non-verbal communication, and developing appropriate styles of intervention and crisis management. The words 'woman', 'man', 'victim', 'aggressor', 'offender', 'violence', rarely if ever appear in this literature.[71] It is a discourse without concrete substance, riddled with abstract, unconnected, allusions such as, 'disputants', 'combatants', 'citizens' and 'mediators'. Crisis intervention was and is touted as a boon to all. It will eliminate choked court calendars, prevent police line-of-duty injuries and deaths, help families in crisis, reduce violence in the community, aid police work by reducing the need to return to family 'squabbles' and enhance police officers feelings of self-worth.

Research designed to evaluate these efforts was primarily conducted by early proponents of crisis intervention.[72] The New York evaluation conducted in the late 1960s which was used to justify the introduction of most innovations was surprisingly modest. Eighteen officers initially trained in crisis intervention techniques carried out the programme in selected areas. Bard's initial reports on the results of this evaluation research are glowing. According to his account the programme was effective in improving police officers' skills in inter-personal communications and reducing call backs and violence.[73] With these early results, Bard and others became even more committed to crisis intervention and strongly supported its introduction through the publication of papers in police journals and the presentation of talks to criminal justice audiences.[74] In 1974, LEAA designated crisis intervention an exemplary programme suitable for introduction on a large scale throughout the United States. Bard and Connolly concluded,

> This program, indicating the commitment of the National Institute of Law Enforcement and Criminal Justice to the notion of training in family crisis intervention, must have had an enormously persuasive effect on police departments throughout the country....[75]

By 1977, over 70 per cent of police departments with over 100 staff were training police officers in crisis intervention.[76]

Research results have played only a minimal role in the intro-duction of crisis intervention in the US; a correspondence with traditional beliefs and practices was far more important. Subsequent assessments of the initial studies and additional research reveal that in most respects these programmes were dismal failures in dealing with violence and disputes in families. Re-evaluations of the New York study showed it actually failed on several counts. Crisis intervention did not deter violence. Instead, disturbance calls rose three fold, there were more repeat calls to the police and a subsequent increase in family homicides in the research area.[77] In fact, Bard's own final evaluation of effectiveness showed that intervention made no difference.

> The evaluation failed to detect significant changes after training in the number of family-related homicides, the number of arrests for family-related assaults, or in the number of family-connected injuries to police officers in the cities studied.[78]

The most frequently cited positive finding from this research is a change in participating officer's attitudes and orientations. They appear to be slightly less dogmatic and better informed.[79]

This does not mean that such programmes made no difference in police perceptions and responses. There was some indication in the research results that 'family-related' crimes were becoming a decreasing proportion of all arrests as revealed in criminal statistics.[80] We might surmise that this was the result of attempts to convince those police officers who had previously treated violence in the family as a crime worthy of the legal sanction of arrest, that it was not serious and should simply be mediated. Probably the most important impact of these programmes was not radically to change police perceptions and practices but to reinforce established ones. LEAA training materials taught police officers that most family disputes were *not* violent and therefore not crimes.[81] Training Manuals sometimes depicted the women and men involved in such disputes in a manner which reinforces sexist and racist attitudes. Women are presented as depressed, menopausal, dominating and 'likely to resort to physical violence' and it is claimed that 'physical force is the common response among certain ethnic groups'.[82]

Recent research on the use of crisis intervention and mediation by the police shows that it has had an important impact on their responses to family violence. For example, on the basis of research carried out in the mid-west in the 1980s, Oppenlander concluded, 'Mediation appears to be a way to avoid arrest in the majority of domestic assault cases in which it is used', and is related to 'an avoidance of the law enforcement function of the police'.[83] Yet having failed to arrest violent offenders, officers do not attempt to mediate between a husband and wife. According to Oppenlander, police 'have an aversion to mediation in man–woman quarrels as well as inter-action with a lone woman'.[84] In the light of police training in crisis intervention, we might expect them to refer couples to other agencies if they do not mediate and arrest. Ninety per cent of officers claimed they knew about other agencies and 80 per cent said they routinely or sometimes made referrals, yet Oppenlander's observations of police action revealed that only 4 per cent made referrals and officers rarely mentioned shelters to women.

A research evaluation of mediation projects funded by Neighbor-hood Justice Centers revealed a very poor rate of success in cases of violence in the family.[85] Promises made through mediation are rarely kept, 'agreements between disputants in intimate relationships were found four times more likely to break down than agreements between parties with more tenuous relationships'.[86] There was also a larger per-centage of dissatisfied respondents among those involved in family disputes than other types of disputes.[87] The 'one-off' session of mediation conducted in a fashion that assumes two equals meeting to resolve their differences with a neutral third party – a very unlikely scenario given the imbalance of power achieved and maintained through the use of physical force – was found to be largely inappro-priate. According to the authors of the evaluation of Neighborhood Justice Centers, the types of cases appropriate to crisis intervention and mediation are those in which 'the dispute is not tremendously complex or deeply rooted.... The solvable dispute is typically one which requires only the relatively brief intervention of a skilled third party'.[88]

The successful introduction of crisis intervention into so many US police forces must be understood against a backdrop of traditional police response stressing non-intervention, a need to reduce pressure on courts and police, a history of the entrance of psychological orientations and professionals into the criminal justice system and a political need to appear to deal with problems of violence and conflict within the family. In crisis intervention we have what is an apparent success story for criminal justice administrators and policy makers. They successfully introduced a new, 'radical' programme into the police, notoriously conservative and resistant to change. The reason for success is that crisis intervention did not urge new action but basically reinforced and legitimized existing police practices of non-arrest, diversion and minimal response to the problem. Historical evidence suggests that the police have usually treated the problem as a private matter requiring personal and civil solutions. Here was a new 'professional' response which legitimated these practices, providing a novel language and ideological justification. Crisis intervention and meditation served the purpose of negotiating the offender away from the CJS and appeasing the growing moral concerns for protection of the victim by providing a supposedly effective means of stopping or reducing future violence. The fact that it did not work was conveniently ignored by all except, of course, the repeat victims and their abusers, and, somewhat later, by activists in the battered-women's movement.[89]

Taken together, the indifference or antagonism to the plight of battered women, and in the USA the operation of the Family Court, systematic diversion and mediation, amounted to a near abdication of legal responsibility.[90] It is, therefore, not surprising that with the rising awareness of the women's movement and the emergence of the issue of battering in the early 1970s, the practices of the justice systems in both countries should become the source of protest and pressure for change. In Britain, the public hearings helped focus this concern and encouraged new laws but without recommendations for changes in police practices. In the USA, attempts to change the justice system were complicated by the widespread existence of crisis intervention and mediation which gave the appearance of responsiveness Activists and advocates initially had to argue against these new, apparently helpful innovations as well as against the more traditional perceptions and reactions. One of the very important tools for challenging law enforcement in the US was the use of the law itself in the form of class actions against the police.

CRIMINAL JUSTICE INNOVATIONS

The United States

One of the early catalysts for change in the CJS response to battering in the United States was the class action lawsuits brought on behalf of battered women against police departments in New York City and Oakland, California for failure to protect women from physical abuse. With the growing awareness of abuse and the outcry coming from the movement, feminist lawyers joined the effort to ensure provisions for legal safety, which had so frequently been neglected. Legal action was necessary because law enforcement agencies were extremely reluctant to change policy and practice. A written request to meet with the New York City Police Commissioner to discuss the problem was not even acknowledged.[91] Within this context of resistance, lawsuits were extremely important; they raised public awareness of the problem, publicized institutional forms of injustice, led to changes in State laws and set a precedent for police response all over the country.

In October 1976, the case of Scott vs. Hart was filed against the Oakland Police; two months later the case of Bruno vs. Codd was filed against the New York City police. In New York, the Litigation Coalition for Battered Women charged police and courts with gross failure to comply with the New York State laws.[92] The case was brought on behalf of twelve women all of whom had received no action from police when called to respond to a physical attack upon them by their male partners. One of the plaintiffs, Carmen Bruno, told of how the police once witnessed her husband attempt to strangle her and yet refused to arrest him.[93] Such inaction must, of course, be understood against the context of a historical legacy of inaction and the practice of crisis intervention that was operating within the New York City Police Department.

On 26 June 1978, nearly two years after the case was filed, the New York City Police Department settled out of court.[94] Without admission of guilt, they agreed to change their practice by: arresting men who commit felonious assaults, misdemeanours and for violations of family court protection orders; sending officers to every call from a battered woman; assisting women in receiving medical help and pursuing men who have left the scene of the assault.[95] The Oakland Police Department also capitulated with a similar settlement. With successes on both the East and West Coasts, the precedent was set and could be used in any city or state as a model of action and, more importantly, as a lever against police resistance to local pressure for change.[96] Leverage provided by these lawsuits was very important to other groups who sought to persuade their local police to enforce the law and assist women. As lawyers responsible for the Bruno case stated,

> The impact of the police agreement is being felt all across the country. Police departments in Chicago and New Haven when threatened with lawsuits modelled after Bruno, agreed to adopt policies similar to those achieved in New York.[97]

The era of crisis intervention, family court diversion and police inaction appeared to be ending.

Following the successful New York and Oakland class actions against the police, there was a flurry of activity. New legislation was

introduced, increasing pressure was brought on local police departments and innovative experiments appeared to spread throughout the
CJS. The initial period of reform from 1976 to the early 1980s,
witnessed the creation of research and demonstration projects in law
enforcement and police training in several states, often under the
auspices of the LEAA. Innovative criminal justice programmes and
new law enforcement legislation was often the result of local and
national pressure by activists.

As the movement began to pressure for changes it was confronted
in each state with a seemingly bewildering variety of laws, procedures
and practices. Yet there was considerable commonality across jurisdictions: orders of protection (injunctions) were often useless and
only available to women who filed for divorce; crisis intervention,
mediation and diversion were widespread; few men were being
arrested for wife abuse and even fewer cases ended in court. Keeping
the peace and keeping the family together, even a violent one, took
precedence over arresting violent offenders and protecting victims.
Legal changes required the introduction of criminal justice legislation
in each of the fifty state legislatures; these efforts were often aided by
the publication of model legislation in movement publications. The
acts proposed new laws and new directions for all segments of the
CJS. One of the most important areas of concentration was on the
introduction of new or improved protection orders. Two of the first
model forms of legislation focusing on protection orders were
successfully introduced in Pennsylvania and Massachusetts.[98]

The provisions of the 1976 Pennsylvania Protection from Abuse
Act defined abuse as bodily injury, serious bodily injury, fear of
serious bodily injury and sexual abuse of minor children. The definition of the family included spouses and people living as spouses as
well as others related by marriage or consanguinity, thus providing
protection for cohabitants. Protection is provided after filing a
petition with the court alleging abuse, and attempts to overcome the
usual causes of delay and ineffective enforcement include: allowing
justices to act when the court is closed, immediately notifying police
of the issuance of an injunction, and permitting emergency injunctions prior to a full hearing which must be held within ten days of the
issuance of the order. At the hearing, abuse must be proved based on
a 'preponderance of evidence' rather than beyond a reasonable
doubt. The forms of relief can include issuing protection orders or
consent agreements directed at cessation of the violence, granting
possession of the residence to the victim and/or excluding the abuser
and decisions regarding custody and visitation rights pertaining to

children. If the husband breaches these provisions he may be judged to be in contempt of court, arrested and subjected to a $1,000 fine and six months in jail.[99]

In 1983 only seventeen states provided protection orders, but by 1990 forty-eight had enacted or revamped injunctions that enabled courts to refrain men from abusing, harassing and assaulting the women with whom they live.[100] In many states these statutes only apply to married couples while others also include cohabitees. Forty-eight of the fifty states also provide powers to exclude the man from the household for a specified period of time. As a means of reducing harassment and intimidation, other provisions allow for exclusion of the man from the woman's business or place of employment or the children's school. Orders may require men to make temporary support payments to the family, to pay restitution for lost earnings, moving expenses associated with abuse and to compensate women for medical and legal expenses arising from violent attacks.[101] Twenty-eight states and Washington DC also authorize mandatory counselling at the discretion of the judge, although there appears to be a wide variation in the sort of counselling offered.[102]

Approximately forty states now consider a breach of injunction either a misdemeanour, criminal offence or criminal contempt and therefore include the power of arrest in their enforcement. In West Virginia such contempt might result in a sentence of thirty days in jail and/or a $1,000 fine.[103] As a result of such changes, injunctions are now theoretically easier and faster to obtain; most states allow emergencey protection and exclusion orders issued *ex parte* (without a formal hearing with the man present) when there exists immediate or present danger. Twenty-three states provide emergency protection orders outside of normal hours of the court. The state of Colorado '... permits police officers to telephone a judge for an emergency order from the victim's home whenever the courthouse is closed; the officers then serve the order on the batterer on the spot'.[104]

Measures such as these are primarily civil responses, intended to provide relief and protection without invoking criminal justice sanctions. Some states have also acted to improve responses by emphasizing the criminal nature of violence against women in the home and reiterating that existing assault statutes do indeed include this violence. A small proportion of states have enacted specific 'spouse abuse' statutes. The Arkansas criminal code now specifies three degrees of wife battering and four degrees of assault of a wife. California law specifies incarceration for two to four years in county jail for 'corporal injury resulting in a traumatic condition'.[105] The majority of jurisdictions continue to identify such assaults as mere misdemeanours, and in states such as Tennessee, a man can only be charged with a misdemeanour regardless of the seriousness of the attack.[106]

One of the most significant developments is a change in the requirements of arrest. In twenty-three states, police officers are now able to arrest on 'probable cause' in cases of simple or minor assault within the home.[107] In many states similar provisions apply to the violation of a protection order. Probable cause refers to a situation where a police officer observes conditions – injuries, a frightened dishevelled woman, damaged property – that leads to the conclusion that a crime has been committed. Prior to the enactment of new laws police officers were unable to arrest without a warrant in instances of simple assault unless they actually witnessed the attack. Probable cause arrests were only possible in serious or felony assaults. Further criminal justice action was possible, though apparently not very probable, if women themselves sought redress directly from the courts. If judges accepted their accounts they might issue a warrant for the arrest of her attacker. In the past, such procedures rarely resulted in the issuance of a warrant or an arrest, nor did they bring relief to the victim.

In addition to expanding the authority of the police to make probable cause arrests, a few of the new state and city statutes go even further by imposing a *mandatory* duty to arrest the violent offender. Connecticut, Maine, New Jersey, North Carolina, Oregon, Utah and Wisconsin now 'mandate' arrest for domestic assault usually by extending the concept of probable cause.[108] According to Lerman, the introduction of mandatory arrest creates the potential to increase arrests, reducing 'police discretion to treat family violence as trivial, and makes it an offence for police to fail to make an arrest where probable cause is present'.[109]

States have also enacted legislation mandating police and courts to provide greater assistance to victims. Massachusetts law requires officers to stay until imminent danger has passed, to help the victim obtain medical treatment and to advise her of her rights. Officers are also required to carry and dispense cards providing women with information about their rights and possible avenues for gaining assistance and telephone numbers of hot-lines, shelters and social services. Some states mandate legal counsel for women seeking protection orders and provide legal advocates to assist women in their attempts to seek such orders.[110]

Efforts have also been directed at changing attitudes and actions through mandated training of criminal justice personnel. Alaska, for example, has created a systematic programme aimed at familiarizing officers with techniques of intervention, laws and procedures pertaining to violence in the home, available resources and the nature of information that must be given to victims regarding their rights.[111] Materials on wife abuse regularly find their way into police training, albeit often on an *ad hoc* basis. In some localities women's groups have had considerable success in being 'allowed' the opportunity to give lectures and distribute materials in police training programmes. By the end of the 1970s there were even signs that members of the police establishment were beginning to treat the problem as a serious matter requiring police action. In 1976 a training manual issued by the International Association of Chiefs of Police, a predominantly American organization, proposed that the police should begin to make a distinction between domestic disputes not involving violence and assaults. The manual indicates:

> wife beating is foremost an assault – a crime that must be investigated. A policy of arrest when the elements of offence are present, promotes the well-being of the victim.... The officer who starts legal action may give the wife the courage she needs to realistically face and correct the situation.[112]

Great Britain

By comparison, the initial changes in British law and its enforcement have, until recently, been very meagre. The major developments in Britain have been in civil law, with no new specific criminal justice legislation and very few innovations in enforcement. Legislative action was initiated at a national level, primarily as a consequence of the deliberations of the Select Committee and pressure from Women's Aid. This resulted in acts to strengthen the civil protection for women attacked by a male partner. For England and Wales these are the Domestic Violence and Matrimonial Proceedings Act, 1976 (MPA), the Domestic Proceedings and Magistrates' Court Act, 1978 and the Matrimonial Homes Act, 1983.[113] For Scotland, the Matrimonial Homes (Family Protection) (Scotland) Act, passed in 1981, is the Scottish equivalent of the MPA.[114]

Wider changes have occurred in the administration of justice in England and Wales which may have an impact on cases of violence in the home. In 1984 new legislation made spouses compellable witness.[115] Two years later, an independent Crown Prosecution

Service was established in England and Wales.[116] Both of these developments while not explicitly intended to deal with the problem of violence against women might have made it easier to achieve prosecutions of violent partners. There has also been continuous local pressure and lobbying directed at particular police forces resulting in a few local developments, especially *ad hoc* training of police officers. Periodic Directives regarding police procedures have been issued by the Home Office in England and the Lord Advocate in Scotland primarily urging greater assistance for victims but with little interest in the offender. A few police forces, particularly the London Metropolitan, West Yorkshire and Welsh forces, have taken a more pro-active stance on arrest of violent spouses. Significantly, the Directives which urge firmer and more meaningful action are merely advisory and Chief Constables are not obliged to follow them. Furthermore, directives are not public documents and the public and the movement can only learn about their specific intent if Chief Constables are willing to make the information public.

Prior to the enactment of the British legislation in the 1970s, women were able to obtain a non-molestation order only if they were already engaged in civil action such as seeking a separation or divorce. Once action was filed it was theoretically possible to obtain relief through an injunction against a violent husband. Procedures for serving notification and methods of enforcement were the responsibility of court bailiffs and not the police. The Select Committee of 1974 and a Law Commission report on family law considered these provisions and procedures inadequate. The Select Committee concluded, 'If the enforcement of civil law could be made more satisfactory, a man who had beaten his wife once might well be prevented from repeating his crime'.[117]

The most basic improvement arising from these laws was the provision enabling women to seek an interdict in Scotland (injunction in England and Wales) without having first started proceedings for a divorce or separation. The Acts also extended the powers of judges and magistrates in England and Sheriffs in Scotland in several ways: to issue emergency protection, to apply a restraining order to prevent a husband from molesting his wife and her children, to exclude him from the home or an area which included the home and to force the husband to allow his wife back into the home if she had been forcibly ejected.[118] What was truly innovative was the possibility of attaching a power of arrest without warrant for breach of these injunctions. These provisions, it should be pointed out, were enacted despite the vigorous objections of criminal justice representatives throughout Britain.

Introduced into Parliament in 1976 by Jo Richardson, MP, shortly after the Select Committee Report on Violence in Marriage, the Domestic Violence and Matrimonial Proceedings Act, 1976 is intended to provide speedy relief for the victms of domestic violence regardless of their marital status. It is considered an emergency measure which can be backed up by exclusion orders and provisions for arrest if the order is broken. The Magistrates Court Act for England and Wales was intended to allow for inexpensive, immediate and swift local action by magistrates who administer the vast majority of justice in England and Wales. Because magistrates are more accessible than county judges they are meant to be able to act in an expeditious manner to issue personal protection through non-molestation orders. Magistrates can also issue exclusion orders (though not emergency orders) and attach powers of arrest if the husband has actually injured his wife and/or children. According to its proponents, this Act would provide inexpensive, immediate assistance to women being attacked and threatened by their husbands. The limitations of this Act are the requirement that applicants must be legally married, its strong requirements regarding arrest and an inability to protect from harassment. When the husband breaches the restrictions and a power of arrest is not attached, the woman is required, as in the past, to pursue enforcement of injunctions directly through the court. The latest piece of legislation, the Matrimonial Homes Act, 1983 is not, strictly, an injunction nor can it be used to meet immediate needs. Rather it is intended to be used to exclude a violent partner and provide long-term solutions for disputes between husbands and wives. Criteria for deciding on exclusion include, '1. the conduct of the spouses in relation to each other and otherwise. 2. the respective needs and financial resources of each spouse. 3. the needs of the children. 4. all the circumstances of the case'.[119]

Public pressure and legislative lobbying in both countries has certainly resulted in changes in traditional policies and the implementation of new statutes. The movement has been able to confront and alter some of the assumptions and structures created in the nineteenth century and begun to make abstract justice more responsive to community demands. The concerns of women have been reinstated into the structures of justice, at least on the level of discourse and policy. Changing policy is a crucial step in securing improved responses to the problem, yet the justice system, as we have shown, is resistant to widening its role in dealing with violence in the home. Changing practices involves altering not just laws and policies but also the structures, perceptions and cultural practices that are deeply embedded in the system of justice. We must ask if these developments have affected traditional perceptions of female victims and the culture of indifference and the practice of diversion. Questions such as these are particularly important since it is the responsibility of judges, prosecutors and police officers, and not of activists, to enforce new laws and policies.

6 New laws and new reactions

In some respects, the new laws and innovative programmes brought about by the challenges of the movement can be seen as predictable extensions of the changing political and social concerns of the late 1960s and early 1970s. The 1970s was a decade of expanding criminal justice; more police, more prisons and more community forms of policing and sanctioning. In an era with a strong progessive ethos, expansion and alteration of criminal justice was construed as an attempt to create and distribute improved services and improved justice to offenders and victims alike. During this period, schemes were created in both countries, for expanding the social service role of the police: through community policing and juvenile liaison in Britain, and crisis intervention in the United States. Especially in the United States, considerable effort was directed at diverting community problems away from the justice system by creating neighbourhood dispute resolution and mediation centres.[1] Sanctions were often redesigned to 'treat', 'rehabiliate' or 're-educate' offenders inside and outside prisons, occasionally through radical experiments.[2] While in retrospect these developments can now be seen as part of a progressive agenda in the area of justice, at the time they were criticized by both the right and the left. Many on the left noted how the new alternative sanctions were not truly alternatives, but merely additions to the complement of criminal justice responses, further widening the net of state control into the community. The right complained that the new approaches were not real sanctions and would do nothing to eliminate crime and disorder. At the same time as these developments were being introduced for offenders, victims were also identified as in need of improved services and assistance, and, in the USA, a burgeoning programme of victim assistance developed primarily through the financial support of Law Enforcement Assistance Administration, LEAA.[3]

Ironically, during the same period there were social and political forces stressing criminal justice solutions which were not part of this progessive agenda. A climate of widespread fear of crime developed in reaction to popular and student protest, disorder and unrest in the cities of the United States and Great Britain. Much of this fear centred on the young: students protesting the continuation and escalation of the Vietnam war, young people expressing alternative lifestyles and cultures and youthful members of minorities protesting about inequalities. These were the folk devils of the late 1960s and 1970s. Media reporting focused and intensified public fears and prejudices, inflaming moral panics in both countries.[4] Crime, student protest, urban disorders and alternative cultures were often equated with a breakdown in public and private morality. There were demands for repression aimed at reducing these problems through various institutional responses, including, of course, the CJS. These developments also fed the expansion of the CJS.

Today, the progressive elements of criminal justice are sparsely represented in political agendas. We now live in societies saturated with the rhetoric of law and order, a rhetoric long used in political agendas in the United States and now prominent in Britain. The rehabilitative ideal is given little credence today and the police are now clearly mandated to get back to the fundamentals of enforcing law and order. In both countries the justice system continues to expand, though now in a more repressive direction with longer prison sentences, ambitious schemes for building prisons, and more rigid penal regimes.[5]

The movements' struggles to introduce new laws and procedures began during the transition from the relatively progressive era of the 1970s and has continued through the law and order societies of the 1980s and 1990s. The early efforts of the movement to change practice in the justice system occurred in the context of the waning of the old progressive order and the beginning of the new. This is particularly marked in the USA where many of the early developments were achieved under the auspices of LEAA programmes, an agency established to improve justice in the community. In this chapter we chart the translation of new laws and policies into practice, giving special attention to innovative community based multi-agency programmes.

LAW ENFORCEMENT ASSISTANCE AND ADMINISTRATION INITIATIVES

LEAA was created in 1968 as a result of widespread concern about the operation of the justice system. From its creation to its closure in 1981, and subsequent replacement by the National Institute of Justice (NIJ), it was the funding branch of the United States Department of Justice meant to centralize and professionalize the widely dispersed and unevenly developed local criminal justice systems. LEAA was an integral aspect of the 'war against crime' in the US. It provided community groups concerned about victims, such as battered-women's activists, with a specific organization for introducing experiments into local criminal justice systems. Concern about protecting victims intersected with LEAA's own agenda emphasizing more efficient and effective law enforcement. While activists in the rape crisis and battered-women's movements were mainly interested in improving responses for women, LEAA was oriented to improving the efficiency of the CJS. Supporting victims was seen as a method for securing more effective witness participation in order to increase rates of prosecution and conviction.

The LEAA also sought to reduce costs by shedding some of the burdens facing criminal justice. Police departments could not handle the volume of crime they were encountering, prosecutors could not process all of their cases and it was impossible to clear court calendars. One answer to this backlog was to keep some offenders out of the criminal justice process by diverting them out of the system at an early stage. Crisis intervention and diversion were techniques for achieving this goal. Diversion was not seen as a failure of police work but as a means of improving it by eliminating those cases seen as less serious. This would reduce costs and improve efficiency by concentrating police and court efforts on the most serious crimes and offenders. By 1979, LEAA had established approximately 220 victim/witness assistance programmes.[6] Most were located in prosecution offices and were primarily oriented to generating more effective witnesses and, secondarily, to supporting victims. LEAA programmes provided one important means for feminist lawyers and activists within the movement to gain entry into an often reluctant justice system as a means of implementing new laws, policies and practices.

In 1977, the LEAA established a Family Violence Program as an outgrowth of the Victim/Witness Assistance Programme.[7] While representing only a very small part of LEAA's overall funding, it was, nonetheless, the first Federal response to battering with a programme ostensibly created specifically for battered women and other victims of family violence and sexual abuse in the home.[8] Through matching grants local governments were encouraged to improve their response to victims and witnesses and give special attention to victims of rape, sexual abuse of children (including incest) and physical assault. These were labelled 'sensitive crimes', seldom reported and difficult to prosecute because of the feelings they provoked in the victims.[9]

Congress mandated LEAA to focus on 'the role of the criminal justice system in preventing and controlling violent and abusive behavior in the home', using a 'comprehensive' approach including social service agencies and community based groups. They emphasized that this focus did not imply an enlargement of the role of the CJS, but rather an attempt to define its relevant responsibilities in order 'to improve the response to crimes in the home'.[10] Thus, LEAA defined the experimental Family Violence Program in a broad context, as addressing both social and legal problems requiring a comprehensive community effort involving a partnership between the CJS and other community services.

By the end of 1980, the LEAA Family Violence Program had supported a total of twenty-eight local action demonstration projects, three national-level projects and two grants to major medical centres working on sexual abuse of children.[11] The local projects were oriented to a comprehensive approach including public, private and grassroots organizations oriented to 'planning, co-ordination and data collection, as well as new justice-related and or social service and mental health agency components'.[12] In addition, three national projects were supported: (1) The Police Executive Research Forum meant to examine the police role in the area of domestic violence; (2) The American Home Economics Association for development of family violence public education materials focused on prevention; and (3) The Center for Women Policy Studies to provide technical assistance to the Family Violence Program involving on-site assistance to the regional experiments providing services to battered women; to distribute information in the form of a national newsletter, RESPONSE, and to establish and maintain a national resource centre, co-funded by the newly created and short-lived Office on Domestic Violence.[13]

COMMUNITY APPROACHES TO CRIMINAL JUSTICE IN THE USA

LEAA experiments with prosecution of cases of family violence, coupled with more efficient and meaningful police and judicial actions, were developed in several locations in the United States, notably Westchester County, New York, Philadelphia, Pennsylvania, Miami, Florida, Cleveland, Ohio, Los Angeles and Santa Barbara, California, and Seattle, Washington.[14] The principles of these programmes were firmly planted in the agendas of LEAA's victim/witness programmes, aiming to reduce case attrition and assist victims by improving prosecution, increasing police response and providing better, more co-operative witnesses. Despite the emphasis on prosecution, many of these programmes were linked to pre-court diversion programmes which mandate offender counselling prior to final court disposition. Possibly reflecting LEAA ideals, such programmes sought to limit the 'burdens' on the court system while enhancing criminal justice response. LEAA-supported projects have played a significant role in altering criminal justice response to violence against women in the home. To illustrate some of the issues and problems associated with the introduction and implementation of change in the justice system, we shall examine three innovative programmes, two of which were LEAA supported.

The San Francisco Family Violence Project

The San Francisco Family Violence Project (FVP) began in March, 1980 with the overall aims of improving the criminal justice response to domestic violence, providing services to victims and their families and educating the community about the serious nature of this violence.[15] Like all LEAA projects on violence in the family, it was justified on the grounds of the severity of this violence, its widespread existence in the community and the general lack of positive and effective responses from the CJS. The basic premise was that 'domestic violence is a very serious crime and often develops into lethal situations if no effective interventions occur'.[16]

Located in the office of the district attorney (prosecutor), the project employed a comprehensive and multifaceted approach to strengthening and co-ordinating all sectors of the justice system (police, district attorney, probation and courts).[17] A broad based community alliance, including the Mayor's sub-committee on domestic violence, city department heads and community experts, was formed in order to intensify the community impact of the project.[18] The areas identified for development included police procedure and training, protocols for prosecutors, and guidelines for diversion and probation of offenders. The focus of this victim-witness scheme was and still is on the woman as a witness and on enhancing successful prosecutions.

Initially, one of the main areas of attention was police procedure. In order to alter existing practice a training programme was introduced for all ranks of officers. In conjunction with the District Attorney, specific materials have been developed to deal with interviewing, incident reports, court order violations, including civil restraining orders and criminal stay-away orders, follow-up procedures and referral.[19] New policies, procedures and orientations for action set out by the Chief of Police formed the corpus of police training.

Innovative police procedures emphasized treating violence in the home like any other form of violence, not using crisis intervention and mediation as a substitute for criminal proceedings, acting only upon the elements of the crime and/or the victim's willingness to make a citizen's arrest without consideration of other factors to do with the personal financial or emotional relationships involved. Warrantless arrest under conditions of reasonable cause were introduced and emphasized.[20] In a subsequent order, domestic violence was explicitly added to the Incident Report Form, and Platoon Commanders were made responsible for seeing that officers recorded incidents of violence. Fulfilling this requirement led to an assessment of the time and resources expended on such cases, facilitating the monitoring and improving of the processing of cases.[21]

While the specific emphasis of the FVP is on law enforcement and prosecution, the overall orientation is towards stopping continued violence and changing traditional legal responses of acceptance or indifference. In this way the FVP departs from programmes primarily aimed at decreasing the workload of the CJS and from those that fail to challenge institutional forms of complicity. In so doing, an alternative has been developed that is directed at meaningful social change both in the CJS and in the wider community. Some of the more innovative features include: Police and District Attorney's participation and initiation of positive directives for change in policy and practice, training of police officers, district attorneys (prosecutors) and judges; strict and delimited guidelines for eligibility and suitability for diversion of violent men out of the system; and the treatment of this form of violence as serious and the responsibility of the criminal justice system. The limitations of the project appear to be problems associated with co-ordination of criminal justice elements with efforts of the voluntary groups in order to deal with the victim and wider community action. This has more to do with the problems of co-ordinating a multi-level agency approach within a large city than with the motivations and efforts of those who operate the Family Violence Project. Despite its limitations, the Project has succeeded in heightening public awareness and altering persistent patterns within criminal justice.

The Duluth Domestic Abuse Intervention Project

Another successful programme is the Domestic Abuse Intervention Project (DAIP), created in Duluth, Minnesota in 1980. Duluth is a small city with a population of about 100,000 and a police department of about 100 uniformed officers. Duluth's size, a background of progessive community support and the efforts of innovative feminist activists have coalesced to produce what many consider to be the most successful justice project in the United States.

Beginning from a base within the shelter movement and building through local financial support, the project works to achieve a multiplicity of goals: to reduce the screening out and diversion of cases of violence in the home; to shift responsibility for the violence away from the victim and on to the state and the assailant; to 'impose and enforce increasingly harsh legal sanctions on the abusers who fail to stop ...'; to create policies and practices that provide specific deterrence for individuals and general deterrence for the wider community; to provide a pro-active response for victims in order to increase support, protection and the victims' use of criminal justice interventions; and to achieve these aims by improving interagency communication and co-operation 'to secure a consistent and uniform response'.[22] A major strategy of the project is to *protect women* by reducing men's violence through an educational programme aimed at convincing assailants to realize they are accountable and responsible for their violent behaviour. The method for achieving this goal is to treat the violence as a crime and ensure effective processing and sanctioning by the justice system.

Initial concern focused on altering police response. Following the programmes' general principle of introducing innovations through a short-term demonstration project, a six-month programme of training coupled with a new pro-arrest policy was used as the means of initiating the programme. Fifty per cent of force officers participated in the training oriented to assisting them to understand better the nature of battering and the woman's position. A significant aspect of the DAIP approach is to engage in continual and systematic forms of consultation at all levels of the CJS and to deal directly with the reservations and requirements of those working within the system. For example, police officers were concerned that new procedures emphasizing arrest would reduce or eliminate discretion and make them vulnerable to suits for false arrest. They objected to the intrusion of 'do-gooders' from outside the police, were cynical about the possibility of meaningful changes and argued that the programme would disappear in a few months. They were also sceptical that arrest would be backed up by meaningful responses from prosecutors and judges. It was pointed out that the DAIP programme would continue, and that other segments of the justice system would be taking a more serious approach to the problem.[23]

In conjunction with the training, police administrators, with the enthusiastic support of the Chief of Police, issued an order emphasizing the existing grounds for arrest under probable cause. Officers participating in the training were required to follow a pro-arrest strategy when dealing with cases of violence in the family. When it became apparent that this policy was not proving effective because officers were continuing to use their discretion, new guidelines were introduced on arrest and '... officers were required to write reports justifying their decisions not to arrest'.[24] After the initial six months of the programme, significant positive results were achieved. More men had been arrested for minor assault and criminal damage to property, and 77 per cent of these men pleaded guilty; 'The most frequent reason given by the men for pleading guilty was that they had been caught'.[25] During the same period, in the eleven cases where no arrest was made and the victim was required to file charges, there were no guilty pleas. In cases of domestic disturbances, there was a reduction in assaults in the home, repeat calls and injuries to police officers. The justice system was not only more effective, it was also more efficient. These patterns have persisted throughout the life of the project: between 1982 and 1984 there was a 47 per cent reduction in repeat calls, and injuries to officers were reduced to zero.[26] Apparently arrest achieved what crisis intervention had not.[27]

A significant element of the DAIP programme is a commitment and ability to monitor the activities of criminal justice. For the purpose of monitoring, initial reluctance to allow the use of police records had to be overcome. Organizers were initially told that the records 'fell under the Data Privacy Act', but an early challenge lead to the State Attorney General ruling that 'arrest data is public data' and the 'police chief does have the authority to allow, in most domestic violence cases, an advocacy programme to receive copies of police reports'.[28] Proposing and introducing new policies and practices is relatively simple compared to the effort needed to translate them into routine procedures. Police organizations present special problems when introducing innovations. Police officers are relatively independent agents within communities, operating with considerable latitude and discretion. Distance from management control and a strong culture emphasizing autonomy make it difficult to implement and monitor routine procedures and practices.[29] Police officers in Duluth demonstrated this independence when, after the six month demonstration period, the new policies and practices were extended to the entire force. Compliance with the new policy of mandatory arrest was high during the initial six months among the officers who had volunteered, but there was a considerable drop in compliance once it was expanded to include all officers.

The Duluth project faced this problem head-on by creating specific techniques to increase compliance. Although training provides a groundwork for new attitudes and behaviour, monitoring of activities is essential. Radio dispatcher incident books were reviewed each week by a Police Inspector to determine if arrest or reports should have been made but were not. In some cases the police or DAIP staff would interview victims about police response. At one point, follow-up telephone interviews were held with all complainants to assess whether or not police action should have been taken. According to Ellen Pence, one of the originators of the programme, 'This somewhat time-consuming monitoring resulted in an increase in arrests and will be repeated whenever rates drop over an extended period of time'.[30] The DAIP staff prepare written follow-up reports on the disposition of cases that are given to arresting officers and provide important reinforcement.

As well as directing efforts at improving police response, DAIP staff work to improve prosecution. At one point, they were able to introduce a policy of not allowing charges to be dropped but it was abandoned because of subsequent reservations about its impact on victims. The current agreed policy is to adopt a case by case approach while continuing to stress prosecution. In order to enhance prosecution the project takes a pro-active approach to engaging the victim. Police records are used to identify victims whether or not there was an arrest, and women are contacted and offered assistance and support, including help should the case be pursued through the courts.

Legal advocates assist victims in their resolve to press charges, help them prepare for court hearings, provide the prosecution with information concerning the case, assist in gathering evidence and accompany victims to court. Work of this nature means advocates gain important knowledge of the case and help increase the efficiency of court processes. This has resulted in a greater use of civil protection orders as well as criminal sanctions. In 1980, the local shelter worked with 260 women, only 45 (17 per cent) of whom were involved in court cases. Three years later, the shelter assisted 719 women, of whom 312 (43 per cent) pursued cases through the courts. The proportion of women filing for orders of protection has tripled over the life of the project.[31]

If convicted, offenders receive one of four possible sentences: (1) jail with no probation, (2) a stayed or deferred jail sentence as part of probation with full participation in a counselling programme for batterers, (3) a jail sentence, partially deferred with probation and the batterers' programme, and (4) straight probation within the batterers' programme. Men are required to attend twelve weeks of counselling sessions followed by twelve weeks of Batterers Anonymous meetings where their attendance is monitored and reported to probation officers. Three unexcused absences and they are returned to court where, depending on the seriousness of behaviour, they may have a jail sentence imposed and/or be mandated to continue in the Batterers Anonymous group. An early obstacle to the success of the programme was the unwillingness of probation officers to revoke probation. With urging from DAIP staff a few revocations were achieved, apparently having a most salutary effect on other offenders on probation.[32]

The Duluth project has made significant progess in shifting the focus of criminal justice intervention from the victim to the assailant, establishing meaningful consequences for violent abusers and reducing the frustrations and dissatisfactions of members of the criminal justice system. Pence maintains that there has been an important shift in perspective.[33] Rather than seeing violence in the family as merely a 'domestic' problem arising from pathological individuals or dysfunctional families, battering is now seen as a criminal offence. The violence is also seen in a more feminist manner, as attempts by men to establish and maintain control in their relationships with women.

184 Women, violence and social change

The Santa Barbara Family Violence Project

Not all innovative programmes have been as successful as the Duluth and San Francisco projects. The best documented example of an innovation that failed to bring about change in criminal justice is the LEAA sponsored programme in Santa Barbara, California. The Santa Barbara Family Violence Project (SB-FVP) began in 1979 with a structure similar to San Francisco, including an umbrella organization to introduce, implement and monitor new responses. In contrast to most other projects, a parallel programme of systematic evaluative research was also conducted.[34] The experiences of Santa Barbara illustrate the importance of support from key individuals in the CJS, the difficulties of using pre-trial diversion, problems of trying to convert into established practice successes based on short-term experimental changes in organizational policy and practice, and the extreme difficulties associated with introducing innovation in the face of persistent, often virulent, opposition.

Four related goals were specified: to encourage police officers to report all cases of violence in the family coming to their attention; to document them properly so that informed prosecution decisions could be made; to increase the number of batterers sanctioned by the criminal justice system; and to use a diversion programme of mandatory counselling as an alternative to fines or imprisonment for the less serious incidents.[35] As with the San Francisco project, considerable effort was devoted to enhancing police and prosecutory cooperation through strategy meetings and training. To this end a special division was created in the district attorney's office to process cases. An assessment of the impact of the first year showed significant progress towards all four goals, especially in bringing more cases into the system. Initial achievements were reversed during the second year.[36] The evaluators concluded, 'virtually all the gains in reporting made during the 1st year of the Family Violence Project were lost during the 2nd year'.[37]

The initial successes and subsequent failures in Santa Barbara highlight many of the salient features associated with social change, factors which can be understood at organizational, cultural and even personal levels. Loss of LEAA funding and the elimination of a team meant to specialize in prosecution reduced the strength of the project. The change from a supportive Chief of Police to one who was disinterested, and the transfer of an enthusiastic criminal investigator were crucial changes with important negative consequences. Frequent transfers and departures of prosecutors and police officers made it difficult to maintain the necessary continuity and supportive atmosphere associated with the initial stages of the project. Departure of key individuals such as the Chief of Police was extremely important because clear and strong support from those in powerful and influential positions within a hierarchical organization encourages the participation of those they command.

Possibly the most important factor was the continuing hostility within the police culture. Initial training was fraught with tension and resistance. There were strong negative reactions to the training film and it mysteriously disappeared during the second year. Police officers expressed their unwillingness to co-operate by not forwarding cases for prosecution and many were 'lost' once received for processing. In such a setting it is not surprising that there was a break-down in relationships between Family Violence Project staff and the police.

The evaluators concluded that the organizational culture in which the project was introduced included very strong orientations towards the notions that the husband is the dominant figure in the household and that wife beating is a private matter in which the CJS could not or should not intervene. A very important factor was the 'occupational prejudice' of many of the police who were 'not prepared to redefine family violence as a law enforcement matter ... were never fully converted by the educational efforts of the FVP and were all too ready to backslide at the first opportunity',[38] an opportunity provided by the change of Police Chief. Likewise, many of the Deputy District Attorneys were either disinterested or opposed to changes in case priorities, and this affected the way judges sanctioned offenders.[39] The project

> faced an uphill struggle from the start and each agency within the criminal justice system experienced strong temptations towards 'business as usual' and away from the treatment of wife battery as a criminal activity, worthy of criminal sanction.[40]

It is useful to compare the success of Duluth with the failure of Santa Barbara. Duluth has an active and persistent shelter group and the financial support of a host of voluntary and commercial organizations which have had a life longer than the LEAA funding in Santa Barbara. The continuous and apparently enthusiastic support of the city's chief of police, members of the judiciary and politicians has been important. This support allowed the project to use consultative forums as vehicles for introducing policy and for monitoring progress. The ability to monitor progress and intervene to alter practice has probably been the most important instrument in the continuing success of the programme. Access to police records has enabled the project to alter practices inconsistent with its aims. Close engagement with criminal justice has also enabled DAIP organizers to deal with the concerns of criminal justice personnel. Pence maintains that the success of DAIP is partially explained by the shelter programme's willingness to adapt 'its advocacy role to the needs of a criminal justice intervention project'.[41] Accommodation has not meant capitulation. Both political and pragmatic successes have been achieved in Duluth through the tireless efforts of activists and the co-operation of management within criminal justice.

NEW LAWS AND CUSTOMARY PRACTICES IN BRITAIN

Civil remedies – injunctions and interdicts

Whatever the successes of innovative local projects, it is also important to consider the impact of the most usual developments and the persistence of customary practices in the majority of locations in the United States and Britain. Despite an apparent emphasis on arrest and prosecution in the United States, the most widespread development in both countries has been the creation and strengthening of civil 'remedies' such as orders of protection, injunctions and interdicts. In Britain, the statutes pertaining to civil law remedies were quickly challenged and clarified through judicial review and mandate. The intent of the new injunctions and interdicts introduced in England, Wales and Scotland was to provide speedier relief and protection for women, to exclude violent, aggressive men from the home and to provide the sanction of arrest when men violated these orders. Despite the existence of two unique criminal justice systems – one for Scotland and the other for England and Wales – judicial interpretations have been remarkably similar.

Provisions of the new Acts were immediately challenged in the courts, first over exculsion orders.[42] Upon appeal, the English courts ruled that the Domestic Violence Act did not alter substantive law and therefore the property rights of a husband should not be restricted by the requirement of safety for women and children. This judgment was quickly overturned by a higher court which ruled that courts did have the right to exclude a violent spouse. The judgment held, however, that there must be evidence of actual, significant molestations amounting to 'serious danger' or 'intolerable conditions'. Importantly, this judgment focused on molestation which could be interpreted in broad terms; as one judge put it, 'any conduct which can properly be regarded as such a degree of harassement to call for the intervention of the court'.[43] Thus, in English and Welsh courts, the spirit of exclusion was upheld and the concept of molestation was given a generous interpretation. Most other provisions of the Acts have not fared so well.

Terms of exclusion orders and the use of arrest have come under considerable scrutiny in both judicial systems. English courts indicated that exclusion was only meant to be a temporary measure. One judge commented, 'I find it difficult to believe that it could ever be fair, save in most exceptional circumstances to keep a man out of HIS flat or house for more than a few months' (our emphasis).[44] A Practice Direction clarified the position, indicating exclusion orders should normally be for a period of three months: presumably the assumption being that a woman should only need a short period of time to find safe alternative accommodation for herself and children. It is also based on the continuing concern about making men homeless and the administrative inconvenience of police having to hold injunctions or interdicts for more than three months. Longer periods are possible, but women must return to court in order to obtain additional exclusion orders. Rulings on the use of arrest have taken a similar direction. The attachment of arrest should not be considered a 'routine measure' and it should not be imposed for more than three months.[45] Clearly, the English courts consider these measures as temporary, 'first aid not intensive care'.

Clarification of the grounds for exclusion has taken two directions in England and Wales. Some judgments have emphasized the protection of children above all other concerns. If children are thought to be at risk then it has been considered 'fair, just and resonable to exclude the husband'.[46] It appears that the protection and support of the woman is considered appropriate primarily or solely in her role as mother. As one authority ruled, 'if there are no children here, if they were two independent adults they *could be left to get on with it* and the court might say it's up to her'.[47] (our emphasis) This position considers the safety of children as the significant feature of the problem. If the mother has custody of the children then she should probably be protected, but as the guardian of children and not in her own right. Although recent rulings have indicated that the interests of children should not necessarily be paramount, one can imagine that judicial thinking will adhere to traditional sentiments.[48]

Those holding the second position focus on the man's conduct. His actions and violence must be weighed against the impact of an exclusion order on his 'lifestyle'. Adherence to this position means a reluctance to issue *ex parte* emergency orders and instead requires the husband to be summoned to court in order to hear his account of the situation. Such a course of action takes time and means that the concept of 'speedy relief' intended in the act is impossible to achieve. Presumably, magistrates and judges attempt to weigh the degree and impact of the violence against the 'hardships' exclusion will inflict.

Scottish courts have proven to be equally reluctant and hesitant about exclusion orders. Although early interpretations were contradictory, an initial, influential opinion condemned exclusion orders as 'harsh' remedies of 'draconian' proportions'.[49] Exclusion of a man from his home should require 'rigid tests' only to be contemplated as a 'last resort'. As one Scottish solicitor observed about the initial reaction of the legal profession, the act 'is maligned by some judges and agents [lawyers] who regard it as excessive'.[50] Scottish judicial opinion recommended non-molestation interdicts as appropriate remedies which would avoid the need for exclusion orders. Judges spoke of exclusion orders as solutions of 'last resort' requiring 'high and severe tests' before being issued. They stressed that women and/or their children should be 'in real and immediate danger of serious injury or irreparable damage before such a drastic remedy is to be applied'.[51]

Evolving standards were far more restrictive than intentions embodied in the legislation. The Matrimonial Homes Act provides for judicial consideration of threatened as well as actual violence and the mental and physical health of a victim and her children. Those who introduced the legislation, the Scottish Law Commission, also made it clear that a 'balance of hardship test' should not be used in reaching a decision on exclusion.[52] Initial court decisions, however, ignored the liberal spirit embodied in the legislation, raising the standard for exclusion to a consideration of the 'immediate' need for protection serious enough to cause 'irreparable' physical harm or damage, and invoking the need for a 'balance of hardship' test.

After these decisions Scottish lawyers were reluctant to apply for exclusion orders; it was considered 'slightly impudent' by certain judges. Consequently very few exclusion orders were granted in the two years after the effective date of the Act in 1981.[53] In many respects the act became nearly irrelevant, incidental to the conduct of the courts.[54] Evidently for a few years, exclusion orders were 'virtually unobtainable,' a dead letter in attempts to protect battered women. The Scottish legal profession was divided with many welcoming and others opposing these interpretations. Subsequent rulings have upheld the spirit of the Act seemingly making it easier for women to obtain exclusion orders.[55] There is little information about how these various and contradictory interpretations are now affecting judgments in Scottish courts.

Despite these limitations, it appears that legal change, and possibly the publicity surrounding the introduction of these acts, has brought about an increase in the use of injunctions. There has been a steady increase in numbers since their introduction. However, the result of contradictory judgments and controversies in both legal systems has been a reluctance to include exclusion orders and the *potential* sanction of arrest. For example, in 1981 a survey conducted by Women's Aid Federation England, found that only 50 per cent of injunctions included an exclusion order. Judges are even less likely to attach the power of arrest to an order. Out of 6,400 injunctions granted in England in 1980, only 24 per cent included provisons for arrest.[56] In the same year a survey of magistrates in Sheffield, Leeds and Manchester revealed that only 57 per cent of injunctions included exclusion orders, and only 27 per cent the power of arrest. There is an increasing tendency for English and Welsh county courts to use injunctions although only a slight increase in willingness to attach the power of arrest. In 1982, 7,474 injunctions were granted in England and Wales with 25 per cent (1,876) including the power of arrest.[57] In 1987, 15,539 injunctions were granted, with 28 per cent (4,903) attaching the power of arrest.[58] Recent evidence indicates considerable regional variation in the use of powers of arrest and exclusion orders. In the Northeast region of England, in 1987, only 12 per cent of injunctions included powers of arrest and 28 per cent of the total involved exclusion orders; whereas in London in the same year, 38 per cent of injunctions were exclusion orders and 37 per cent of injunctions attached a power of arrest.[59]

It would appear that including the power of arrest is only done with 'great caution' and in 'exceptional circumstances' after the husband has consistently ignored an injunction. Imprisonment for the breach of an injunction should only occur, if at all, after '... attempting to alleviate the offending spouse's underlying grievances or after an adjournment to allow tempers to cool ...'.[60] That is, extra-legal or other responses are preferred to 'drastic' action by the court. In some jurisdictions, married women are required to make application for re-housing under the Matrimonial Homes Act before an exclusion order will be considered with the obvious intention of attempting to settle property concerns as a means of solving the problem or as a pre-condition to court action. The outcome of these developments has been the dilution of the intentions of legislation providing civil protection for women assaulted by their partners.

Limitations on the use of exclusion and arrest follow familiar lines, showing a concern for the property rights and lifestyles of men, for male privilege within the home, the priority of motherhood and a concern for children over the protection of women, and a continuing reluctance to attempt to employ the justice system to alleviate the problems of women and/or to sanction male violence. While there was an increase in the use of injunctions in England and Wales, it should be noted that this represents the use of a civil in preference to a criminal response. The judiciary seems reluctant to use criminal justice sanctions. Such a reluctance is even more apparent when we consider the actions of the British police.

Police enforcement

As we have shown the response of the British police to public recognition of the problem of violence against women and the demands of Women's Aid groups have differed remarkably from those in the US. In their evidence to Parliament, the British police rejected the need for changes in their response to the problem and argued that existing provisions were more than adequate. They vehemently resisted changes and were especially opposed to the attachment of powers of arrest for injunctions and interdicts. Such opposition might well produce resistance and avoidance of the intentions associated with the new injunctions and interdicts. Being more optimistic, we might assume that as a consequence of new laws along with continued contact with victims of violence and with Women's Aid, the police would welcome an additional option. With few exceptions, the evidence indicates a continuing reluctance to use direct action.

In 1985, the London Metropolitan Police, one of the most important forces in the country, conducted an internal investigation under the direction of the Force's Working Party into Domestic Violence'.[61] The Working Party acknowledged that violence against women in the home was a 'significant problem that places demands on police resources'. They concluded that existing research, and the evidence presented by various community groups such as Women's Aid, revealed that police response was usually inappropriate and unhelpful. Research by the Working Party also discovered that the Metropolitan's policies and practices fell far short of effective responses.

An important concern of the Working Party was the methods used for dealing with injunctions. Since police use of injunctions depends on officers' knowledge of their existence, the Working Party focused on methods of recording and storing records within police stations. The results indicated 'serious deficiencies' in all but one of the six stations studied. Injunctions were not usually noted in station records and accessibility was severely limited, usually dependent on personal knowledge. Practices such as these illustrate the low priority given to these court documents and to the plight of women. Women with injunctions are poorly served by officers who arrive at their homes with no knowledge of the history of violence and/or the existence of a court order with the power of arrest. It means that women will have to negotiate with the police over the very existence of a court order.

Additional evidence gathered by the Working Party indicates that training for officers of all ranks was nearly non-existent. The Force offered no special training on the use of injunctions or the nature of the problem. The subject of violence in the home appeared only on an *ad hoc* basis or as an incidental in the cursory discussions of 'domestic disturbances'. The Working Party observed, 'However praiseworthy, the input of *ad hoc* sessions such as these is limited being quickly diminished by prevailing practice'. It is, they argued, 'no substitute for inclusion of the topic on the main training programme'. According to the Working Party, 'The training perpetuates current terminology [domestic dispute] which helps to trivialize marital violence rather than treating it as an allegation of crime'.[62]

Investigation of police practices revealed a strong current of animosity or at best indifference to the plight of women. Prevailing patterns demonstrated 'little understanding' and 'lack of empathy' and 'commitment'. Although attitudes of individual officers varied, most viewed the violence as a normal part of family life and preferred informal mediation and peace keeping as the best solutions. They were convinced, contrary to the evidence, 'that almost all women would withdraw their charge'. The preferred solution, if the CJS must be involved, was to tell the victim to apply to a local magistrate under the provisions for common assault. Many officers thought the problem was not a matter for police intervention, and rationalized their views by invoking ideals of domestic privacy. Some officers thought the whole area was a complete waste of time and concluded, 'it was no help whatsoever when applying for posts or promotion':[63] clearly a reflection of their interpretation of the importance accorded the problem within the police hierarchy. Most felt arrest should be used only in 'those cases where death was imminent or likely'. Only one or two of the officers saw their main role as being the protection of the victim. If the problem was to be dealt with at all it should be the primary concern of women police constables.

The report also revealed widespread ignorance about alternative social service and voluntary provisions for assisting women. Police officers were unfamiliar with the addresses, phone numbers and sometimes even the existence of Women's Aid groups. They demonstrated a similar ignorance of most social, personal and health services. Since referral to another agency was not seen as an important option, this information would be of no use to the police. Despite the much vaunted age of community and corporate (interagency) approaches, police have not yet formed a productive part of such a partnership.

Recent studies in other cities in Britain indicate similar patterns. McCann's research on the use of injunctions revealed that the police sometimes failed to serve injunction papers, causing delays and jeopardizing women's safety.[64] In dealing with women the police employed their own language to rationalize non-enforcement of injunctions or failure to arrest. They tell women it is just a 'personal', 'domestic' or 'marital' problem, and they should apply for a divorce. McCann documents numerous cases where women were the victims of serious violence and the police refused to act.

Through interviews with battered women, research conducted by Cleveland Women's Aid and National Women's Aid Federation England reveals in stark detail the failings of criminal justice response to violence against women.[65] Most women interviewed by Homer, Leonard and Taylor in the Cleveland study were unaware of their rights to protection and of the existence of protective injunctions. Those who contacted the police felt belittled and rejected as a result. The majority of women interviewed by Jackie Barron in the NWAF study found the whole process 'very stressful' and 'harrowing' and felt it had little impact on their violent partners. The Domestic Violence Act was not working to protect women. Women reported persistent disregard of injunctions by police even when the power of arrest was attached. When injunctions were granted, they never exceeded three months. For some men the expiry of this period meant a green light to attack their wives, signalling the court's unwillingness to provide further protection. Only a small minority of women found them useful. In some courts, traditional remedies, such as the man's verbal agreement, 'undertakings' not to molest his wife, were still being used.[66] Women judge these responses as particularly useless. They also pointed out that injunctions only come into effect, if at all, '*after a serious assault*'.[67]

The authors of the Cleveland report concluded that the new injunctions have in some ways exacerbated the situation by reinforcing perceptions of the problem as requiring purely personal and civil solutions. Accordingly, women have no right to make demands on the police or the criminal justice system. Unfortunately, in the absence of alternative information, many women come to accept these justifications and rationalizations. They become accepted 'fact'. As a consequence women sometimes even excuse police inaction. As one woman put it,

> I was unhappy at first but then I could see their point of view, it was a domestic affair and they couldn't really get involved and I understood a lot better after that. I think if they'd been allowed to they might have done something but they have to keep out, don't they.[68]

In light of such evidence, the Cleveland researchers have no doubt about the ineffectiveness of the Domestic Violence Act: 'our evidence suggests, [it has] created a situation in which some women are in more danger and live with greater fear than before the act'.[69]

The research conducted by the Cleveland Refuge and by McCann relied on the significant experiences of women. Faragher's work involved systematic observations of police reactions to incidents within the home. He found that the police were 'ineffective in enforcing injunctions, or assisting householders to enforce injunctions'.[70] Officers often had no knowledge of the existence of injunctions. They told women with injunctions, some including the power of arrest, that the violence was a personal matter. Faragher observed women forced to negotiate with the police to press them to act with the burden of responsibility for pressing charges placed on women. They were pressed 'again and again', usually in the presence of the man who assaulted them, about their willingness to charge him and their resolve to follow through on the charge. According to Faragher, police action is not geared to the severity of the violence or the needs of the victim. Instead, 'police evaluate need for intervention by the degree to which the woman appears to be prepared to embark on legal action'.[71] In doing so, police officers demonstrate little understanding or concern for the woman's predicament and the consequences of such a decision for the lives of women and their children. Predictably arrest was a very unlikely outcome of these encounters, only occurring in 20 per cent of 'life-threatening' cases and 15 per cent of those involving 'severe bruising or black eyes'.[72]

By contrast, North American research has shown that civil injunctions can be effective. A study of the use of injunctions in four States revealed that 72 per cent of the 270 women included in the survey found them effective; 42 per cent judging them very effective.[73] Another small-scale, intensive study of a group of Connecticut women also found injunctions could be effective.[74] Women reported that the police responded in a prompt and usually supportive fashion after the issuance of an injunction. Injunctions seem to deter violent men; one woman said, '... the TRO (order of protection) has worked for me – he hasn't dared to visit me or beat me up again'.[75] The authors of a nation-wide investigation on the use of civil remedies concluded, 'Protection orders, when properly drafted and enforced, were considered effective in eliminating or reducing abuse by most of the judges, victim advocates and victims interviewed'.[76] Although the authors note that in some places offenders '... flout civil protection orders with impunity' and there was often a lack of enforcement, they point out that they are most effective when a number of conditions prevail. These conditions include: protection orders with a broad coverage as well as specific directions regarding restrictions on the offender; the use of legal counsel and victim advocates in the preparation and processing of orders; police and judicial training; judicial commitment to enforcement; and a willingness to impose meaningful sanctions when orders are breached.[77]

These studies provide good indication of the utility of civil injunctions, but as the authors stress the implemetation of new laws must be backed up by explicit policy, commitment and training. In Britain police forces have been slow to develop clear policies and training to deal with the problem. In 1986, an *ad hoc* working group of the Women's National Commission, an Advisory Committe to the Government, conducted hearings on the issue of violence against women.[78] Part of their investigations included a survey of police procedures and training. Of the forty-four police forces in England, Wales and Scotland that replied, twenty-six made no comment on domestic violence or indicated considerable satisfaction with their traditional responses; 'a few very firmly indicated that there was no need for action'.[79] Only a few indicated they were pursuing new procedures or training programmes.

West Midlands police were singled out for good practice involving an interagency approach comprising a working group including police, housing, legal professionals, women's organizations, social services and the education authority. Most police departments, however, reported few developments or only *ad hoc* training programmes such as allowing Women's Aid to provide 'input to the constables course'. Progress was defined by one Chief Constable (Chief of Police) as reduced police concern about prosecution and a new emphasis on 'the safety of vulnerable parties and reconciliation where possible'.[80] This declaration of 'progress' underlines the conclusions reached by the Cleveland researchers. The Advisory Working Party concluded, 'domestic violence is not frequently perceived as an area in which police procedures "fall down", or where new measures are feasible and important'.[81] This perception is reinforced by Home Office policy documents.

The Home Office is responsible for recommending policies and practices for all the police forces in England and Wales. Part of their activities include research and the production of policy documents by the Research and Planning Unit. The 1986 report, *Personal Violence*, was 'prepared ... as an aid to the development of policy' in this area. The document was intended to '... summarize what is known about violent crimes against individuals ...' and '... to make a contribution towards a better understanding of such crime and of what are currently felt to be the best ways of tackling it'.[82] In this policy oriented document, the author sympathizes with police reluctance to become involved in violent incidents in the home and endorses the 'general rule to keep the law, the police and the criminal justice system out of domestic matters as far as possible'.[83] On occasion, he observes, the police are *'unavoidably drawn'* into such violent incidents, and, on these occasions they should deal 'sensitively and skilfully' with 'domestic disputes' (our emphasis).[84] It is unclear what this means but one must assume it does not refer to law enforcement. Although the document acknowledges that 'domestic violence is not an insignificant problem ...' no criminal justice solutions are proposed. The preferred approach is education so that couples can 'develop their understanding of relationships and thus avoid or learn to cope with domestic stresses'.[85] It must be assumed that such education would teach women that if they are victimized by a male within their own home they should not expect much assistance from criminal justice.

Until the late 1980s, Home Office policy appeared to reflect similar orientations. In 1985, apparently in response to the concern expressed by the Women's Commission Working Party, the Home Office issued advice to Chief Constables and produced new notes for the guidance of new police recruits. The advisory circular reiterates the issue of reluctant victims and emphasizes that the opportunities for police intervention may be limited. While the circular notes the powers of arrest, ensuring the safety of victims and children is stressed. In pursuing this aim police officers should be aware of potential social service support and offer advice about these services to victims, possibly with a leaflet.[86] Home Office advice of this nature follows a familiar pattern of social service for women victims rather than arrest and prosecution of violent men. Even stronger messages are sent to new police officers. With resounding continuity with the past, they are advised, 'There is usually no criminal offence involved. ... The object of police attendance ... is to restore the peace'.[87]

Pressures brought at local and national level by Women's Aid groups, heightened awareness created by the National Women's Commission, and new thinking among a few in the police have provided a climate for more innovative policies and practices.[88] For example, as a result of the Metropolitian Working Party's report, new guidelines were issued in the London force for dealing with violence in the home, and a number of special units, usually staffed by women officers, have been established.[89] A few other forces, notably West Yorkshire, South Wales and Northumbria, have issued specific force orders emphasizing more assertive action, primarily to provide better support for victims and children by establishing 'domestic violence units', usually staffed by women officers.[90] Of course, translating policy into practice requires continual reinforcement from the police hierarchy, explicit methods for introducing and monitoring new practices and rewards for the efforts of individual officers.

At the national level the British government seems to be increasing its support for a more assertive police response. In 1989, Lorna Smith of the Home Office Research and Planning Unit produced an informed and critical review of research on violence in the home, *Domestic Violence*, which stands as a corrective to the 1986 Home Office report, *Personal Violence*.[91] In 1990, again through Home Office circulars, police forces were urged to establish registers of victims at risk, to create units of specially trained officers and to place greater emphasis on arresting and charging offenders.[92] Since these suggestions are merely advisory, it is far from certain that Chief Constables will create new force orders (policies) to implement them. The evidence suggests that most forces are not committed to more meaningful responses and are particularly reticent to use the powers of arrest. A recent study of the London police, one of the most progressive, found that only 13 per cent of call-outs to violent incidents in the home resulted in a crime report and just over 2 per cent involved arrest and prosecution.[93] On a wider scale, it appears that the creation of a Crown Prosecution Service and legislation making wives compellable witnesses have had little effect on the problem. Primarily negative effects have been observed, when, for example, women are held in contempt of court and imprisoned for not testifying. Violence against women in the home remains on the fringes of criminal justice responsibility, still perceived as a personal problem best dealt with by individual women or by social services. As an Assistant Chief Constable from South Wales observed in 1990, prevailing police policy involves 'minimum involvement and disengagement' and there is 'no sign of a lasting improvement' in police response.[94]

Disengagement has been aptly illustrated by attempts during the 1980s to introduce into Britain procedures for diverting domestic violence away from the criminal justice sytem. In 1983, a few Scottish jurisdictions began concerted programmes of diverting 'trivial' or 'minor' offences away from the full process of justice.[95] Instead of processing cases through the courts they would be directly diverted to social service departments. One of the 'minor' offences to be included was violence in the home. There were no specific guidelines about the type of cases suitable for diversion. For example, should men using persistent and/or severe violence and previous offenders be eligible? Scottish Women's Aid strenuously objected to diversion of cases of violence against women, pointing out that violence was a serious issue which should be reacted to as a significant and not a trivial matter. The use of diversion, they stressed, sent messages to the community, the couple and the justice system: violence against women in the home is not a crime to be punished or controlled by the criminal justice system, and women are not victims worthy of concern within that system. Scottish Women's Aid's campaign has been carried out in the media and at meetings with local procurators fiscal (prosecutors) and social service departments using diversion. Although the campaign continues, it has been quite successful, persuading some authorities to create guidelines for the types of cases that might be diverted, convincing others to withdraw plans for diversion and pressuring some not to introduce it. National and local pressure has had important consequences and Scottish Women's Aid has successfully challenged a practice deemed detrimental to women.

SUCCESSES IN CRIMINAL JUSTICE IN THE USA

Since the introduction of legislation in the early 1980s, persistent efforts have moved American criminal justice towards new policies and practices in the area of family violence. Continued pressure from legal advocates and the movement, and important legal decisions and research results, have all brought about an increasing emphasis on and use of arrest in the United States. Most developments have not been welcomed by law enforcement agencies and criminal justice personnel. Indeed, the impetus for initiatives has often been the result of the continuation of traditional police and court practices and resistance to new approaches.

Following the succesful legal actions in New York and Oakland, many of the most important changes have come about because of lawsuits instigated by battered women pursuing their civil rights.[96] One of the most tragic examples is the case of Tracy Thurman.[97] She had survived persistent assaults from her husband and for months the police had failed to respond to her requests for help even though she had an order of protection. On one occasion, police officers sat in a patrol car outside her house as she was attacked and suffered a broken neck at the hands of her estranged husband. She sued the city of Torrington, Connecticut, under the equal protection clause of the fourteenth amendment, alleging the city was responsible for the permanent injuries she sustained. In a landmark decision, a jury awarded her 2.3 million dollars (subsequently reduced to 1.9 million).

The court ruled that the city police department's unwritten policy of providing less protection to victims of violence in the home than to other victims was tantamount to 'discriminatory administrative' policy. A significant aspect of the Thurman case was the court ruling that once a police department or other municipal agency enters into a 'special relationship' with a victim based on their specific knowledge of danger, through, for example, a restraining order and/or sustained police contact, they are legally liable for subsequent injuries if they fail to respond to calls for help. Responsibility even applies when there are no specific written discriminatory policies; proof of customary discriminatory practice is enough to establish liability.

The ruling in the Thurman case and others like it have had extraordinary implications for the liabilities of municipalities. As Marjory Fields, Chair of New York's Domestic Violence Commission and Judge of the Family Court of the State of New York, indicates: '... local governments may be held liable for the injuries resulting from a single incident when the violation of constitutional rights is shown to be caused by official policy, accepted practice, inadequate training or negligent supervision'.[98] The Thurman case demonstrates the power of legal action. Mandatory arrest legislation was swiftly enacted in the state of Connecticut after the decision in this case. Other provisions of the legislation include providing greater assistance to victims, attachment of criminal sanctions to protection orders, next day arraignment for offenders and provisions for more victim advocates in courts.[99] According to one authoritative observer the new legislation had an immediate impact:

> The positive effect of mandatory arrest has been that many men who batter have been arrested, and are being subjected to criminal proceedings. Victims are no longer required to 'request' the arrest of the abuser, a practice commonly abused by Connecticut police as a way to avoid making an arrest.[100]

Mandatory arrest policies have also resulted in some unintended consequences, with women being arrested as a consequence of these policies. In Connecticut, women have been arrested for 'technical violations' of the law when, for example, they defended themselves or used minimal forms of violence in the process of being attacked. In the first few months after the introduction of mandatory arrest in the state of Washington there were 'wholesale arrests of battered women ... [and] large numbers of double arrests for mutual assault'.[101] One woman was arrested when she revealed, while seeking treatment for injuries sustained from her boyfriend, that she had spat at him. Another woman was arrested for throwing yoghurt at her partner after an attack. In some instances police officers informed victims and assailants that both parties must be arrested under the mandatory arrest laws. Indiscriminate and over-enforcement of mandatory arrest laws has been used by police officers to express their rejection of the law and to protest the loss of their discretion in family violence cases. Their actions are also aimed at convincing those who created these laws that they are inappropriate and ill-founded.[102]

According to legal advocates, there are various methods for overcoming these attempts to undermine the intent of mandatory arrest legislation. In Washington, efforts were directed at clarifying legislation by providing training regarding the intent of the laws. In Connecticut subsequent legal clarification emphasized that arrest should be for a predominance of violence associated with the primary aggressor. Informal discussions and training are directed at convincing police that they should speak separately to the victim and aggressor to determine the nature of the violence and not arrest women who are responding in self-defence. Discussions, persuasion and training are important, but some advocates believe that 'the most powerful tool to [changing] police behavior would be individual and class action lawsuits claiming damages and injunctive relief against false arrest'.[103]

Again, the solution in the United States is reliance on the courts. It might be prudent to ask if all of the efforts expended on altering judicial and criminal justice responses have had meaningful consequences. Most advocates agree that measures such as mandatory arrest, strengthening injunctions through the attachment of powers of arrest, and improved prosecution reduces violence and provides assistance to battered women. Certainly, strengthened criminal justice policies bring more men into the criminal justice system. With the introduction of mandatory arrest in the state of Washington, there was a four fold increase in the number of arrests for assaults and a 300 per cent increase in successful prosecutions.[104] In some Canadian cities there has been a dramatic increase in charges arising from assaults in the family after the Solicitor General's pro-arrest policy directive in 1982.[105] In London, Ontario there were twelve charges of assault arising from 'domestic trouble' calls in 1979, rocketing to 298 by 1983. Arrest is becoming a preferred option in London, Ontario, rising from 2.7 per cent of all 'domestic trouble' calls in 1979 to 67 per cent in 1983. More cases are also being heard in court, increasing from only one out of sixteen arrests in 1979 to three out of four in 1983.[106] Dramatic increases such as these are illustrative of the sort of changes occurring in some North American cities. It should be emphasized that both the State of Washington and the city of London, Ontario have a strong commitment to altering criminal justice response. Innovative policies and procedures introduced in areas resistant to change, as illustrated by the Santa Barbara case, would be very unlikely to produce such dramatic results in practice.

Research findings appear to provide additional support for the efficacy of criminal justice intervention. They indicate that arrest is more effective in reducing violence than other options and that criminal justice intervention is welcomed by most victims. One of the first indicators of the impact of more vigorous criminal justice intervention was the early results of the DAIP in Duluth, Minnesota. An explicit attempt to test the efficacy of arrest was subsequently carried out in Minneapolis, Minnesota.[107] The research used a classic quasi-experimental design involving three options (arresting and detaining, offering advice and removing the man for 'cooling off') applied in a random manner. Follow-up interviews conducted up to six months after the initial assault revealed that arrest appeared to be the most effective action in reducing the risk of subsequent violence. During the six month follow-up period women experienced at least one subsequent assault in 37 per cent of the cases where police offered advice, in 34 per cent of those where the assailant was removed from the home and in only 19 per cent where husbands were arrested and detained.[108] Using data from a California county, Berk and Newton demonstrated that arrest 'did substantially reduce the number of new incidents of wife battery'.[109] Analysis of National Crime Survey data collected from 1978 through 1982 provides additional support for the efficacy of police intervention. The study compared women who contacted police after being assaulted by their partner with those who made no contact. It revealed that 'Calling the police was thus associated with 62 per cent fewer subsequent assaults'.[110]

Unfortunately, these studies do not provide specific information about the full processing of men or explanations about why specific responses appear to have different effects. These studies provide little information on whether the men were charged, prosecuted in court, convicted and sentenced. That is, we do not know if contacting the police and arrest on their own have a deterrent effect on future violence or if other factors such as detention or court appearances and the actions of women, are also important. It may be that the statistical results indicating a reduction in violence are the result of factors other than arrest or telephoning the police, such as the victim ending the violence by leaving or divorcing the violent partner. In the Minnesota study it seems that the much praised benefits of arrest should actually be associated with arrest and detention since all of the arrested men were held in jail overnight. Another important factor in Minnesota may have been that 'arrest and incarceration was a genuine novelty for virtually all offenders' included in the study.[111] The effect of a court appearance is not known since only three of the men arrested in the Minnesota study actually appeared in court.

Whatever the specific factors affecting the outcomes in these US studies, research conducted in London, Ontario supports their general conclusions. A follow-up study of women in London, Ontario who contacted the police, found a 'significant overall reduction' in violence after reporting of an assault to police. Victims were also more satisfied with police response after the introduction of a policy of pro-arrest. Before the introduction of the policy, 56 per cent of victims reported dissatisfaction. After introduction, only 5.5 per cent said they were dissatisfied with police response. The researchers' conclude that police intervention makes an important difference to the level of violence and the predicament of women. As in the US National Crime Survey, they detected no escalation in violent attacks as retaliation for women contacting police. Rather 'Victims were more likely to be faced with new threats and/or assaults when *no charges* were laid'.[112]

Other evidence points to the possibility of significant reductions in homicides in the family as a result of more pro-active criminal justice practices. Considerable research reveals that in many cases of homicide in the home, the police had had previous contact with the family. For example, a study of homicides in Detroit and Kansas City revealed that the police had previously responded to telephone calls at least once in 80 per cent of the cases and five or more times in 50 per cent.[113] Clearly, this finding points to the possibility of more effective action leading to a reduction in homicides. Evidence is beginning to show that this may be the outcome of more meaningful intervention. The city of Newport News had about thirteen domestic homicides per year prior to a pro-arrest policy. In the first six months of 1986, after the introduction of a pro-arrest approach there was only one recorded homicide in the home over a similar period of time.[114] In the State of Oregon a change in the conditions of probable cause arrest in 1977 was associated with a 10 per cent reduction in homicides in the family compared to a 10 per cent increase in homicides in other settings. Before 1977, domestic homicides made up 29 per cent of all homicides; in the four years after the new legislation this proportion had dropped to 19 per cent.[115] These results occurred in spite of only a partial implementation of new legislation.

Assessing the impact of change in institutional policy and practice is a difficult task and in an attempt to validate the results of the widely cited and influential Minneapolis study, the National Institute of Justice is conducting replication studies in six locations: Dade County, Florida; Atlanta, Georgia; Charlotte, North Carolina; Milwaukee, Wisconsin; Colorado Springs, Colorado; and Omaha, Nebraska. Early results from the Omaha study do not show a significant difference between the impact of arrest and other actions.[116] It is quite likely, given the important problems associated with conducting quasi-experimental studies and the differences in the cultural and institutional practices in these cities, that the results from the replications will be equivocal. Arrest is probably an important element in a complement of responses in cities where there is an overarching commitment to effective action in cases of violence against women in the home. Understanding this process will require a sophisticated research programme including both qualitative and quantitative methods. Unfortunately, the NIJ research programme is limited because it is heavily dependent on quantitative methods. In understanding the impact of any particular form of intervention we need to be attuned to the effects they have on the relationship between men and women and to locate these within the context of wider community action.[117] One of the most important findings of the Minnesota study, one which is rarely noted, is that arrest was most effective, 'when police officers established an alliance with the victim (in the eyes of the victim)' whereby '... she could threaten the offender more credibly in the future with a call to the police'.[118]

CRIMINAL JUSTICE AND THE POLITICS OF THE MOVEMENT

In the United States, members of the movement and advocates for battered women have been successful in placing their agendas and new programmes firmly within criminal justice. In cities such as San Francisco and Duluth they have created special divisions within prosecutors' offices and/or been able to monitor and sometimes even direct new policies and procedures within criminal justice. They have sent important symbolic messages about violence against women. They have also created new institutional frameworks and linkages among criminal justice institutions and between criminal justice and community groups. According to one advocate, the successes in the State of Washington have resulted in battered-women's advocates forming useful alliances and 'productive working relationships' with police, prosecutors and courts; links which have 'enhanced the credibility of battered-women's advocates with criminal justice personnel'.[119] These have advanced the agenda of social change and led to the greater democratization of agencies of the State.

At a national level, the movement has seen its concerns represented in policy documents such as the Final Report of the Attorney Generals Task Force on Family Violence. Activists and advocates have even played a part in criminal justice policy formation at the national level. For example, they served as advisors in the preparation of Confronting Domestic Violence: A Guide for Criminal Justice Agencies, a National Institute of Justice publication aimed at upper-level managers in the CJS.[120] Through political struggle and legal action, advocates have impressed themselves on local and national criminal justice organizations.

In Britain, formal, or even informal, links between the justice system and Women's Aid are rare. Criminal justice usually resists the development of links with community groups, remaining aloof and beyond the reach of the influences or concerns of community. To be sure, there have been useful liaisons and developments in some areas,[121] but the persistent orientation is to provide minimal support for victims and to avoid action associated with the offender. The most significant organizational developments have involved the creation of a few specialist teams of women officers to deal with violence against women and children. While these may be important in assisting a few women, they have done little to affect policy directed at changing the traditional perceptions and behaviour of the vast majority of police officers. Importantly, they also perpetuate the perceptions that this is 'merely' a problem for women, to be dealt with by women, while usual practices remain unchallenged.

Central government directives such as Home Office directives on violence in the home and police policies and practices, are usually not available to the public making it difficult to confront and monitor police activity directly. The public has no right to know the content of Home Office directives and police force orders leaving them without one of the main starting points for change employed by the American movement. In this respect this institution of the state is not public, knowable and accountable, but is secret and therefore difficult to change. Community groups have no legal or institutional means of effecting change, and the police seem to change if and when innovations correspond with their own agendas or in response to government mandates. Even then, as in the case of injunctions and interdicts, change in law enforcement has been difficult to achieve.

Why should there be such a difference in the level of change in the two countries? Some might argue that it is because women's groups in North America have struggled harder and more persistently for changes in criminal justice than British Women's Aid groups and simply have not put enough persistent effort into criminal justice revisions. Based on our own observations, the explanation involves important political, social and structural differences in the two countries.

Criminal justice is more susceptible to challenges in the United States. Particularly since the successes of the civil rights movement, legal opinion and judicial challenges can more easily be brought to bear on the procedures and policies of law enforcement. For battered women and the movement, it was possible to bring civil rights and tort damage suits as means of confronting injustice. Early class action cases in New York and Oakland forced changes in traditional policies and practices, and in the Thurman case damages were awarded for police failure to protect. In these cases criminal justice agencies were forced to accede to demands for policy changes because of 'external' legal pressure and the near certainty that failure to change would mean financial costs. Courts have also mandated monitoring in order to maximize compliance.[122] Legal mechanisms such as these do not exist in Britain. The British state has been especially reluctant to create methods for implementing, monitoring and enforcing their rather meagre civil rights legislation. Similarly, Sivanandan has noted that British race relations laws are merely meant to educate but even so they cannot be effective without the 'the power to penalize'.[123] It is impossible to bring class action suits in British courts. Although suits can be brought to redress police action, even if won, they are unlikely to mandate changes in institutional policy and practice. Instead, they apply only to the individual case under consideration.

Another important factor in achieving changes in the United States has been the inherent responsivesness of local criminal justice systems. Judges, public prosecutors, district attorneys, even heads of county and city police departments are often elected officials. Consequently they must be responsive to the local community. This may mean they are only responsive to conservative law-and-order forces demanding more stringent, repressive forms of criminal justice. Alternatively, it may mean a willingness to consider and implement more progressive policies. It is significant that the Duluth Domestic Abuse Intervention Program developed in a reasonably small city where existing criminal justice and social service agencies may be more accessible and responsive to community groups. In Britain, Chief Constables are ultimately responsible to the Secretary of State in England and Wales and the Lord Advocate in Scotland and are relatively immune to local pressure. The concerns of the local community can be construed as 'political pressure', and Chief Constables need attend only to those issues they deem important. Even demands from the government, as we have noted, are only advisory and Chief Constables may or may not implement them.

In the USA, the legacy of LEAA-supported initiatives and the work of the National Institute of Justice cannot be underestimated. At a national level, the Police Executive Research Forum established through LEAA funds and its successor, the National Institute of Justice, produced several important research and policy documents directed at police professionals emphasizing improved response to violence in the home.[124] At the local level, LEAA inspired victim/ witness programmes, emphasizing the CJS agenda of reduced workloads, prosecution and diversion, have also been useful in meeting the needs of women. LEAA programmes might be seen as the Trojan horses which allowed feminist inspired ideas and programmes to enter criminal justice machinery. Such possibilities seem impossible in Britain where no comparable agency exists and criminal justice continues on its own trajectory, usually unaffected by wider community issues. In many respects the movement has been successful in moving criminal justice away from the non-interventionist and 'therapeutic' approaches associated with the earlier LEAA-supported crisis intervention and diversion and towards policies and practices more oriented to crime control and prevention. However, as we will see in the next chapter, the therapeutic approach continues to have an important place in the CJS response, mostly through the continuation of diversion and court mandated counselling.

The increasing proportion of professional women in justice systems must also be considered a significant factor in developments within the United States. In Britain, women are only now beginning to enter criminal justice professions in significant numbers. In the United States women now represent a substantial proportion of professional lawyers and a reasonable percentage of judges, prosecutors and police officers. In 1986, 40 per cent of all law school graduates were women, and women currently comprise approximately 20 per cent of the legal profession; they represented only 2 per cent of the profession in 1970. Of all the State and Federal judges in the country, approximately 7 per cent are women.[125] Many lawyers in the USA, men and women alike, have inherited the progressive legacy of the civil rights era, and some still consider social justice an important aspect of their efforts. From our observations of American courts, it also seems that many innovative programmes are staffed by women. We do not think that all women are 'naturally' or automatically sympathetic to the plight of other women. Class, race and socialization into professional orientations are important intervening factors in gender empathy, but certainly some of these professional women have feminist orientations and others have considerable empathy for abused women. Such women play a role in facilitating the process whereby the state plays a part in enabling women to overcome violence.

CONTRADICTIONS AND LIMITATIONS

Successes in changing the CJS raise important questions about the politics and pragmatics associated with working against and within the justice system. It is possible to identify a number of problematic issues. There are dangers of overestimating the depth and spread of new practices. There are a host of concerns regarding the potential political costs associated with these developments, and the limits of progressive change within what many believe to be a repressive system. We have already highlighted one of the problems associated with a policy of pro-arrest, that of women being arrested for reacting to male violence. An allied problem is women being arrested and prosecuted for failing to appear in court as witnesses under aggressive prosecution practices.

Another potential problem is that new arrest laws and greater police reactions may amplify discriminatory practices within criminal justice by increasing arrests of men from the working-class and ethnic minorities. For example, in Scotland there were some early indications that Sheriffs (judges) were more likely to use exclusion orders against working-class men living in local authority, rented accommodation than owner occupiers, who are more likely to be middle class.[126] In the United States and in Britain, women of colour working within and outside of the movement have articulated the political and personal dilemmas they face concerning the use of the criminal justice system.[127] On a political level, co-operating with the justice system may mean support for racist state repression leaving individual women to choose between continued violence or the risk of racist treatment to themselves and their partners by police and courts. Women of colour are required to carry a heavy additional burden of responsibility and guilt because given such dilemmas many have traditionally been unable to seek assistance. Contradictorily, while men of colour may be discriminated against by more frequent arrest and harsh treatment, women of colour seeking legal protection are discriminated against by failures to assist.[128] The lack of support for women of colour is often associated with patriarchal and racist assumptions about the supposed unique qualities of minority women.[129] Despite these personal and political reservations, many women of colour have sought assistance in the past and will continue to do so in the future.

The problem faced by women of colour should be a problem faced by all, that is, how to provide assistance without reinforcing racist tendencies within criminal justice. In Duluth the pro-arrest strategy minimizing police discretion appears to have reduced discriminatory patterns of arrest. In a twelve month period prior to introducing mandatory arrest when police still used discretion, only twenty-two arrests were made and 32 per cent were of men from minorities. In the twelve month period after the introduction of mandatory arrest, 175 arrests were made and 8.5 per cent of these were of men from minorities.[130] This percentage is very close to the proportion of minorities within the population. On this sort of evidence, we might conclude that new policies limiting police discretion could if carefully monitored reduce prejudicial responses. It must be pointed out, however, that the Domestic Violence Project in Duluth is unique in its ability to monitor and sometimes redirect criminal justice actions. Most local community groups are not able to carry out such intensive forms of monitoring, and most cities are unlikely to monitor or to correct the unintended consequences of new policies and practices.

Business as usual

We have shown how certain cities and states have introduced new policies and practices aimed at increasing arrests and improving responses to victims. Yet, many still practise traditional approaches, and in other areas, new policies have not resulted in significant changes. A survey conducted in 1985 of police departments in 173 cities with populations over 100,000 revealed that police officers' use of discretion to violence in the home was the preferred option in nearly half the departments. Seventeen per cent preferred mediation, 6 per cent were still sending one of the parties out of the house and only a third indicated arrest as the preferred policy.[131] These figures do not indicate an overwhelming preference for a pro-arrest strategy within the United States. Also, a pro-arrest policy does not mean automatic arrest. As we have shown police officers can still subvert 'shall arrest' laws by interpreting the situation as one in which an assault has not occurred, thus returning to the status quo of using discretion not to arrest.

An impressive body of research in Britain and the USA points to the widespread persistence of traditional perceptions and responses.[132] In both countries, dealing with 'domestics' is still considered 'rubbish' work unworthy of aggressive police action.[133] Collective mythologies and prejudices are still widespread. Police officers continue to see victims as fundamentally 'unreliable and capricious', 'inadequate people', who are only worthy of police response when seriously injured.[134] In light of such perceptions it is not surprising that arrest, even in areas with pro-arrest policies, is an unlikely outcome of police contact. Rates of arrest are rarely above 15 per cent and are usually well below this level, with the lowest rates being reported in studies conducted in Britain.[135] Police officers prefer to get in and out quickly, and use non-arrest tactics such as 'cooling-off'.[136] Research also confirms that the police treat violence in the home differently from violence in public places, and are more likely to arrest and pursue cases of violence in public. Observations of police reactions and interviews with officers reveal that they discourage women from filing formal complaints, often give strong advice against arrest, present victims with all the potential 'negative effects of and barriers to pursuing a prosecution' and pressure women not to press charges.[137] In this way the justice system helps create the reality of dropped charges and reluctant witnesses about which it complains. Overall the evidence shows that when responding to public and private violence police action is shaped more by concerns for public order and the maintenance of police authority than enforcement of the law and protection of the victim.

The costs of working with the justice system

We must also consider the potential political costs to the movement of working with criminal justice. In working with the justice system does the social movment become absorbed by it and its concerns? Does this mean that the agenda for social change must be sacrificed for pragmatic changes? Does it mean abandonment of the agenda of social change and the transformation of the identity of the movement? Does successful negotiations at the national level mean adaptation to a less political agenda? On a local level, has the movement been able to transform specific justice programmes and criminal justice in order to meet the needs of women while maintaining the goals of social change. To what extent have they been able to obtain funding from agencies of the state, such as LEAA, without distorting the vision and goals of the movement.[138] Successful implementation of programmes may mean the entry of professionals and the eventual, some would argue inevitable, subversion of challenging agendas as most professionals lack the wider political vision of activists. Activists themselves may forget, ignore or shed ideals required to take the specific programmes of arrest, prosecution and victim assistance beyond the immediate requirements of the justice system to the politics of wider social change.

The politics of the movement in the United States may now be truncated to the immediate concerns of improving criminal justice. Entering criminal justice machinery may mean yielding to the exigencies of that system. Once encapsulated within criminal justice, reform movements must inevitably serve the needs of that system and potentially assist its expansion into more areas of civil society. The CJS may embrace the movement and yet subvert its demands, particularly within a law and order agenda, as a means of gaining greater resources and of widening the net of its response. An absorbent state may be able to incorporate the pragmatic concerns of the movement while ignoring or even rejecting its politics.[139]

Such a process is certainly evident in Federal government documents resulting from consultations with the movement. The early civil rights hearings represent clear feminist interpretations of the inadequacies and limitations of criminal justice. Several years later, and under a different government administration, the Attorney General's Task Force report on 'family violence' represents a very different sort of political perspective.[140] Although recognizing the issue of violence in the family as one of important national concern and accepting the need for criminal justice action, the language in the document is neutralized, stripped of any gender connotations, and the problem is not located within the context of the position of women in the family and society.

Against the use of justice

Problems and contradictions such as these have led some feminists and members of the abolitionist movement to reject any links with existing systems of criminal justice and to question its utility in effecting social change. For abolitionists, all justice developments are repressive and coercive. Criminal justice systems, they observe, are fundamentally flawed and out of control.[141] By their own accounts, they are primarily engaged in a negative, deconstructing enterprise which is the elimination of a repressive system of prisons and, for some, the police and courts as well. What they seek to create are systems of greater discretion proposing 'aggressive nonenforcement', 'informal handling of disputes' and 'reintegration into community'.[142] Hulsman argues that the discourse of crime, criminals, victims and punishment should be replaced with a language emphasizing 'problematic situations' of those 'directly involved'.[143] For abolitionists there are no moral rights or wrongs only problematic situations which, 'cause considerable suffering to those directly involved, quite often affecting both perpetrator and victim. Consider, for example, traffic accidents, and violence within the family.'[144] Abolitionists eschew notions of responsibility and blame. Instead, they urge the creation of new responses based on compensation, conciliation, therapy and education. The vehicle for achieving these goals is community involvement. Crime, they urge, is about conflicts occurring in communities. Since these have been stolen by criminal justice, they must be returned to the community and to the people who experience them.[145] For some, the police would continue to intervene in 'problematic situations' to provide crisis intervention and to keep the peace. For others, the police would have no role.

For abolitionists, the problem of violence against women has generally been ignored or identified as a prime example of the sort of conflict which should be dealt with outside of criminal justice. Ironically, these approaches parallel the traditional responses of criminal justice. Abolitionists propose that community based techniques, such as mediation and crisis intervention, are particularly useful in cases of sexual and domestic violence because they can fulfil 'an emancipating function'.[146] Consequently some abolitionists have spoken out against the women's movement for its attempts to use the criminal justice system to control rapist and batterers.

> Although part of the feminist movement currently advocates turning to the CJS and forcing it to respond, in the long run this will only exacerbate the problem. Patriarchal social institutions are not going to support the emancipation of women.[147]

It is doubtful whether feminists ever thought criminal justice would lead to the 'emancipation of women'. Their pragmatic aims and political goals for criminal justice have always been more modest.

The political and practical agendas of the movement constitute a challenge to the abolitionist position. The movement has not sought to abolish criminal justice, but to try to use it in order to enable women to eliminate the violence used against them and as a tool to help them establish their own autonomy. Unlike abolitionists, most activists see the possibility, albeit flawed and problematic, of obtaining support for women through the redefined and hence more effective intervention of police and courts. Although both activists and abolitionist use community, power and conflict as key concepts, abolitionists have not dealt with them in a concrete manner while activists have. Abolitionists have not considered the operation of power and repression within the family and community because they seem to assume that power and repression are exclusive to the state and its institutions. Abolitionists have not provided an alternative which speaks in a meaningful manner to the needs of women who are victimized and how they would be redressed within the community. The real personal, social and community harm associated with these acts is rarely considered.[148]

The movement does deal with power, intimate domination, conflicts, community, crime and victims in a concrete manner, thus, providing a more penetrating analysis of violence and a clearer focus on responses and outcomes. For the movement, power not only resides in the state, but in all social institutions including the family and community. Furthermore, it is differentially distributed according to class, race and gender. Since power plays a significant role in settling disputes, whether in the community or the courts, there are obvious problems associated with settlements where there are differences of power between the two parties. Gender, race, class and age provide just such differentials in power that would advantage the individual belonging to the dominant group in any 'settlement' that does not effectively redress this imbalance. The 'community' to which abolitionists would return violence against women would, unless radically transformed, simply reinforce and support traditional forms of patriarchal power. The movement seeks both to employ a transformed justice system and to return the problem to a community of active and supportive women dealing with the issues of differentials in power between various groups.

Activists in some locations have been able to employ the justice system while also returning conflicts to the community. In communities with active and persistent women's groups, important advancements have been made. By linking with criminal justice and creating new institutions to monitor and correct developments, they have reduced the violence of individual men, provided substantial protection for women and established a heightened community awareness of violence towards women. This is a process which also works towards democratizing agencies of the state through active participation of the 'community'.

Attempting to employ the law and the justice system to assist abused women is a historically rooted strategy which implicitly or explicitly accepts the enabling aspects of the state as one means of redressing the violent injustices and imbalances of power within the family. While aware of past failures and of the problems considered in this chapter, state intervention remains one of the primary vehicles for attempting to redress injustices in advanced industrial societies. Violence against women in the home is about power, and any form of intervention must be able to confront and redress that power. At present the state allied with the movement is an integral element of this enterprise.

7 The therapeutic society constructs battered women and violent men

In 1979 new categories, 'battered spouse' and 'battered woman', were added to the International Classification of Diseases: Clinical Modification scheme.[1] The classification scheme is compiled by the United States National Center for Health Statistics and lists 'all known diseases and related entities'. It is employed to ensure a common system of classification throughout the United States and is intended to assist clinicians in dealing with patients. Creation of these two new categories was hailed as a breakthrough by many therapeutic practitioners and some activists. Including the 'battered woman syndrome' in the International Classification of Diseases would, it was argued, 'provide impetus for further exploration of the symptoms, treatment and incidence of the problem'.[2] Official recognition by professional therapists and physicians was greeted as 'the first step in formulating appropriate clinical responses'.

In this chapter we explore the background to this development and show how the North American approach to conceiving of most social problems in terms of faulty individual traits and personalities requiring therapy has had an important impact on the conception of the problem of violence against women and the social movement intended to challenge it. While we are critical of the discourses and technologies of change associated with the therapeutic society, we recognize that certain of these approaches can benefit some individuals. Some of the pitfalls of traditional therapeutic work have been avoided by humanistic and feminist inspired approaches that attempt to work with individuals within the wider socio-economic context in which social problems exist. Especially important are efforts emphasizing certain forms of counselling within non-hierarchical group work which recognizes the commensurable relationship between helper and helped. In the initial stages of the recognition of the social problem of violence against women some professionals did stress these forms of intervention and the relationship between the problem and issues of inequality and male domination.[3] This initial conception resulted in the problem being 'transformed from the status of an unfortunate personal pathology to that of a social problem requiring change'.[4] However, professional perceptions of battering as a social and economic problem were shortlived in the USA.[5] Such challenging perspectives have, for the most part, now been superseded by discourses emphasizing the personal pathology of the women who are the victims of violence and of male perpetrators.

THE THERAPEUTIC SOCIETY

Contemporary North American discussions and reactions to the problem are packed with the perceptions and language of psychiatry, psychology and the mental health movement. In the United States, battered women and male abusers are becoming patients and clients of an ever-expanding complement of mental health professionals. The reforming technologies of therapy are deemed beneficial in the struggle to end violence in the home with professionals and some activists arguing that it is possible to go beyond traditional therapies which often blame the victim and reinforce male violence.

Although these approaches are primarily North American, psycho-pathological conceptions of violent men and battered women have sometimes been proffered in Great Britain. As discussed in an earlier chapter, Erin Pizzey and the psychiatrists, Gayford and McKeith, viewed battered women as suffering from serious emotional and mental illnesses requiring long-term therapy within an institutional setting.[6] Subsequently, Pizzey and Shapiro claimed that battered women are 'violence prone' because they are 'addicted to violence' through childhood or embryonic experience.[7] They claim that women obtain sexual excitement from being abused, 'the ultimate orgasm is death,' and propose that this is the basis for understanding why women find it difficult to leave violent men.[8] For them the cure for these women and their children is long-term confinement in a building with an 'unbreachable facade' to protect neighbours '... from accumulated rubbish being thrown out of the windows, mothers and children hanging out of windows or irritating the neighbors by unseemly behavior'.[9] More recently a clinical psychologist working with the British government's Women's National Commission claimed:

Studies of battered wives have shown that they tend to be reserved, easily upset, timid and low in self-esteem.... They tend to be passive, dependent, inhibited and acquiescent in their behaviour which enhances their victimization by dominating and aggressive husbands.... to maintain their subservience, women prefer men who are older or superior to them in various ways.[10]

For the most part, however, the therapeutic outlook characterizes the American rather than the British approach. In the United States, concepts such as the 'battered woman syndrome' and its associated 'cycle of violence' are widely accepted by many inside and outside the movement, and are commonly used in court cases as a defence for women who kill their husbands. Such terms are integral to the standard parlance of public and media discussions about violence against women. In order to understand the differences in approach we must consider the cultural differences between the two countries. Of particular importance is the emphasis in the USA on individualism and the development and acceptance of therapeutic ideals and interventions associated with the mental health movement. We shall examine how these efforts to transform complex social, cultural and political issues into psychological syndromes are predictable in light of the strength of the mental health business in the United States. We shall also consider how, within the movment in the USA, the politics of emotions has had a much greater influence on the conception of the problem than the politics of the body and material conditions[11] – although the politics of the body have been important in both countries.

The psychological and psychiatric professions are now extremely important in the United States and there has been a rapid rise in the number of professionals engaged in delivering therapeutic services.[12] There were only 12,000 clinical psychologists in the United States in 1968, by 1982 there were over 40,000.[13] Today, about one-half of the world's clinical psychologists are working in the United States. Of all the world's registered psychiatrists, one-third are Americans. New York City has more psychoanalysts than any single European country. The number of professional counsellors, psychiatrists, psychologist, clinical social workers and marriage counsellors is mushrooming and is now well over 300,000. Between 1975 and 1985, the number of family therapists in the USA tripled from three to twelve thousand.[14] There are also thousands of para-professional counsellors, therapeutically oriented clergy and other non-professional counsellors offering various forms of therapy and counselling. America it seems 'is the world capital of psychological-mindedness and therapeutic endeavor'.[15]

These burgeoning professional groups are serving an ever-increasing number of people. By 1983, professional and quasi-professional therapists had conducted encounter or sensitivity groups with over 15 million Americans and delivered 'marriage enrichment programs' to over one million.[16] Between 1957 and 1976, the proportion of US citizens who consulted a mental health expert rose from 4 to 14 per cent. The university educated are even more likely to consult a mental health professional; in 1957, 9 per cent sought assistance, whereas in 1976, over 21 per cent consulted a therapeutic professional.[17] These figures demonstrate a rapid expansion of the mental health professions and an increasing use of their services by a considerable proportion of the population.

Why is the United States a therapeutic society in which almost all social, economic and even political problems are seen as 'personal troubles' requiring therapy, and how does this affect movements for social change? Part of the answer to the first question relates to elements of American culture deeply embedded in its distinct history. European observers, notably Tocqueville, commented on the unique character of early Americans. Early in the nineteenth century, he concluded that, in contrast to Europeans, Americans experienced considerable unease and ambivalence about their social position and emphasized the individual over the community.[18] They imagine, he wrote, '... that their whole destiny is in their own hands'.[19] He was one of the first to recognize the potential problems associated with the unfettered and unrestrained individualism of American society: 'Each man is forever thrown back on himself alone, and there is danger that he may be shut up in the solitude of his own heart'.[20] Individualism, he worried, means that each citizen may, '... isolate himself from the mass of his fellows and withdraw into the circle of family and friends; with this little society formed to his taste, he gladly leaves the greater society to look after itself'.[21]

Tocqueville recognized that such developments would have a significant potential for inhibiting and limiting civic and public participation in wider society. The American ideal was the autonomous individual confronting a hostile, though ultimately conquerable world. His observations provide us with two foundations for the therapeutic society. In the United States, like no other country, extreme individualism coupled with a perpetual concern about one's status and position combined with unrestrained ideals of striving and success are powerful forces shaping individual rather than collective solutions.

The rapid expansion during the nineteenth century of institutions of confinement in Europe and the USA provided a significant impetus to the behavioural sciences and the therapeutic professionals associated with them.[22] This was the age of the great confinement and the rise of the carceral or discipline society. In Britain and the United States, the Victorians built prisons, workhouses, reformatories and asylums intended to distinguish the idle from the able poor, the criminal and delinquent from the 'normal', and the insane from the sane. Within these institutions, new technologies of surveillance and discipline were intended to transform the mad, bad and sad into the disciplined and docile workforce required for the purposes of industrial capitalism. From the beginning of this development, therapeutic professionals were there to adjudicate on the level of criminality and insanity and to create and operate the new reforming technologies. First the physicians, then the psychiatrists, psychologists, criminologists and social workers created new categories such as the 'delinquent'. The process of professional assessment and testing legitimized these new categories and the systems of coercion used in mental and penal institutions which they helped operate for the state. This also helped legitimize the new professions and linked them to the operation of the state.

These new professionals played a significant role in another stage in the creation of the therapeutic society. At the close of the nineteenth century and in the early years of the twentieth, a near panic developed over the 'menace' of mental disorder. In Britain and the United States, 'mental health' professionals, especially psychiatrists, played a significant role in fuelling, if not creating, a public panic over the need to regulate and check the mentally inferior and emotionally disturbed.[23] In Britain, the threat of the deviant, often exemplified in the spectre of the tramp and vagabond, was considered a menace to the purity and strength of the English 'race', and, in both countries, a threat to the veracity of nationhood and one that could be spread across generations. The answer to this threat was separation from society through institutionalization, and, for some, sterilization. Whatever the solution, it usually involved institutionalization to be regulated and administered by the new therapeutic professionals. This nineteenth-century approach is very similar to that suggested by Pizzey, Gayford and McKeith for the treatment of battered women and their children.

Institutional solutions were primarily intended for those on the margins of society, criminals, vagabonds and the insane. A significant step in the spread of therapeutic ideals and technologies into wider society was the conceptualization of most people, those usually considered 'normal', as in need of some form of help and intervention.[24] In 1881, George Beard, a New York neurologist, captured public attention with his book *American Nervousness*.[25] Beard described Americans as suffering from fatigue, irrational fears and the inability to concentrate. In Beard's words, Americans were realizing they were 'the most nervous people in all history'.[26] For the first time, a list of feelings and behaviours associated with the everyday life of the majority of the populace were defined as legitimate medical complaints. Beard was one of the first to identify these complaints as amenable to individual forms of intervention. His proposed technologies for change – drugs, injections and electrical stimulation – although used within mental hospitals, were not generally used on the wider population.

The period 1880 to 1920 was a time of rapid change and unease in the United States, associated with the demise of a rural society with its communal moral order and the rise of national and international economies. These changes fuelled an emphasis on self-reliance associated with the emergence of a number of self-improvement movements oriented to mental and physical health. These developments were stimulated by the publication in 1908 of Clifford Beers popular book, *A Mind that Found Itself*, in which, as an ex-mental patient, he argued for the need for community based treatments of the mentally ill.[27] His book gave considerable impetus to the creation of the National Commission for Mental Hygiene. If the nineteenth century was the period for the rapid expansion of institutions and the growth of institutional psychiatry, the twentieth century has been a time when the professionals who created and operated these institutions have found their way into the general community.

About the same time, another group whose early development was solidly grounded in the community and in material responses to social problems began to embrace psychiatric and therapeutic ideals and individualistic solutions. Around the turn of the century social welfare workers in Britain and the United States began to seek professional legitimation by shifting their emphasis from merely helping and aiding the poor within communities, to various forms of casework counselling linked to 'scientific' interventions associated with psychiatry and psychology.[28] Alignment with medical psychiatry gave professional status and legitimacy to the otherwise pragmatic work of social welfare agencies. Psychiatric perspectives played an important role in shifting the focus away from the social and economic conditions which produced the slums and depriving conditions of social work clients, to a focus on the personalities of the poor. Emerging individual perspectives grounded in the embryonic professions of psychiatry and psychology conceived of poverty and crime as primarily linked to individual pathology and inadequacy. This shift had a profound influence on the course of social work in the United States, making it difficult to consider the common bases for most social and economic problems. The focus of social work in the United States, and to a lesser extent in Britain, became the abstracted, atomized individual with a personal problem in need of psychiatric social work intervention.

Linda Gordon shows how these new perceptions affected notions of abused women. Therapeutic discourses transformed a problem which had been seen by Victorian feminist reformers as intricately linked to 'a whole system of male power' to one associated with 'wifely dysfunctions'.[29] By the 1940s standard social work discourses employed gender neutral terms like 'marital discord and marital disharmony' and conceived of the violence as non-attributable; it just 'happens'. If women tried to hold husbands responsible for their violence they were labelled 'infantile'. Conceptions such as these were accelerated by professional retreat away from the homes and neigh-bourhoods of the poor and into the distant and sanitized clinics and offices. As Bush points out, whatever the limitations of early welfare and charity workers their practical work in communities meant they were able better to understand people 'simply because they were constant witnesses to the details of their clients lives'.[30]

The final significant step in the creation of the therapeutic society occurred when professionals began to encompass the failures of everyday life as personal problems requiring therapy. Prior to the late 1950s, professional therapists and social workers primarily treated only those on the margins of society, the mentally ill and criminals. With the advances of the mental health movement, the usual and 'normal' have became a focus for intervention. The objective now appears to be perfection of self through psychotherapy and counselling.[31] Everyday anxieties, failures, frustrations and setbacks are transformed into psychological ailments which need to be cured. A perfect, or at least vastly improved, personality is meant to enable us to recognize problems and rid ourselves of annoyances. These ideas were apparent in the self-help and self-improvement move-ments of the past in which many Americans participated. The power and success of the therapeutic ideology today is evident in its ability to convince vast numbers of Americans that the major route to individual improvement and a reasonable life is through counselling and therapy administered by professionals and para-professionals.

The community health movement provided an institutional framework for the dissemination of such therapeutic ideals and technologies into communities. In 1946, the National Mental Health Act mandated Federal funding for research and community clinics rather than for mental hospitals, and stressed private rather than public agencies.[32] With the unrest and disorder in the 1960s new initiatives were introduced to deal with the problems in communities. Two thousand community health clinics were proposed as a means of bringing inexpensive, meaningful help to communities. They were to be introduced through the co-operative efforts of community groups and therapeutic professionals, but quickly the medical and psychiatric professionals began to dominate the direction and operation of these clinics.[33] While some feminist and radical therapies emerging during this period have challenged mainstream thinking, they have often been subverted by traditional practices. And although recent social work and therapeutic thinking appears to go beyond the individualized approaches of the past, emphasizing, for example, the wider eco-system, it is interpersonal relationships which dominate the focus and not the wider social, cultural and political contexts of social problems.

Despite their apparent differences, social work, therapy and counselling have a number of common features. Whether practising group work or individual forms of intervention, the unit of analysis is the individual with the 'bedrock of insight' located in psychological disorders. Whatever the therapy, the relationship beween client and professional is usually hierarchical, with one-sided forms of communication in which the person seeking help is transformed into the objectified condition of the client. This is done through the technology of constructing the case history of the individual in which certain behaviours and attributes are emphasized and explored while others are ignored. Thereby, complex personal backgrounds and problems are decontextualized into the abstracted 'case' which is seen as the clue to all past and subsequent behaviour. As taught in most therapeutic interventions, the relationship between the therapist and client is crucial to reformation, and the therapist provides a model of the healthy functioning adult. Growth or development is seen as a purely personal matter with little connection to the wider social and especially the political world. If clients are urged to participate in the wider world it is usually to expand or enhance personal development. The social world becomes a hunting ground for instruments of self-growth. The individualized approach of the therapeutic society makes political perceptions and wider social action in public forums unlikely, if not impossible. Given this, all we can know and change is ourselves.

Therapeutic relationships are the antithesis of the visions of activists seeking social change within the movement. Instead of hierarchical dependence, the goal of the movement is one of women engaged in independent action, sometimes involving pragmatic counselling and assisted self-help. Instead of hierarchy between therapist and client, the effort is to create a sense of mutuality between those who live and those who work in shelters. Instead of creating the abstracted case and concentrating on a few supposedly deviant attributes, there is an emphasis on encouraging women's obvious capabilities while recognizing the enormous problems they confront. Instead of normalizing tendencies associated with middle-class conceptions based on the therapist as a model, there is a recognition that success and development must be assessed relative to the circumstances and possibilities associated with the concrete position of women.

CREATING THE BATTERED WOMAN

The term 'battered woman' was first employed by the movement, especially in Britain. It was a powerful phrase. The everyday word 'battered' had been successfully used to describe persistently abused children and was employed by the movement to convey the experience of persistent and severe violence against women. In Britain, the movement has always resisted the use of this term as a pandemic phrase to capture the essence of the problem or those who experience it. The problems associated with violence are primarily seen as contextual, associated with the violent repression of men. Once women escape this predicament, they can build lives of their own free from the violence and its consequences.

Masochism and relationship addiction

A contrasting perspective identifies women experiencing persistent violence as having unique personality disorders requiring specialist therapeutic interventions. The processes associated with this agenda have resulted in the creation of a distinct social-psychological category, the 'battered woman syndrome'. An important aspect of these developments is both an extraordinary continuity with the past and an apparently novel perspective which is merely the old masquerading as the new. An example of the first is Natalie Shainess's book *Sweet Suffering: Woman as Victim.*[34] Although Shainess claims she is breaking with the past in proposing a new conception of female masochism, the threads knitting the past and the present are very strong indeed. Like traditional psychoanalysts, Shainess believes all women suffer from this ailment: '... no woman in our culture escapes masochism altogether; societal attitudes guarantee this. Intelligence, education, career standing, social position – none of these can immunize us.'[35] The entire book is devoted to reinterpreting the common problems created for women living in a patriarchal society into evidence of masochism. Told in a personal, anecdotal style with examples gleaned from clinical practice, and methods such as, 'listening to the news' and 'talking to a friend', the book appears to connect with a popular culture in which women are urged to seek solutions to wider social problems within their own personalities.

Self-punishment, submission and suffering as a way of life are the central features of this 'new' form of masochism. In her examples Shainess translates the strictures of everyday life into evidence of masochism. The presence of a masochistic syndrome makes certain women especially vulnerable to exploitation and violence: '... I do believe that the victims of violent crime may sometimes play a part either in triggering or exacerbating those crimes'.[36] She states that although all women suffer from a degree of masochism, women subjected to persistent violence at the hands of male partners are profoundly afflicted:

> According to those who operate shelters for battered women, they are generally inhibited, passive and helpless.... In anxiety-arousing situations they are unable to act.... They are at a loss to come up with an effective response – in fact, any response at all.[37]

These are reputedly essential attributes of the masochistic woman, who '... exhibits these characteristics in all her life situations, including potentially dangerous ones, and these masochistic qualities increase her vulnerability to violence'.[38] Descriptions such as these may be summarily dismissed by many because they are summated under the term masochism. However, the ideas of most therapeutically oriented observers do not differ much from these conceptions. This is merely a reiteration of the old ideas of masochism and victim blaming. Rather than contradicting the status quo, these ideas represent an agreement with it.

Robin Norwood has proposed that women who find themselves in bad relationships with men suffer from relationship addiction because they 'love too much'.[39] Norwood thinks that women who experience violence in their relationships are especially afflicted with relationship addiction which she suggests is 'A PROGRESSIVE AND ULTI-MATELY FATAL DISEASE PROCESS'.[40] Like Pizzey, Norwood believes women who suffer persistent violence 'CHOOSE DANG-EROUS MEN AND DANGEROUS SITUATIONS' and are 'highly attracted to drama, chaos and excitement ... in order to stir their glands to release adrenaline ...'.[41] Women experiencing violence thus fear abandonment, which 'produces clinging, placating, nagging and pleading'. This in turn provokes a violent response.[42] Furthermore, she claims that a majority (80 per cent) of these women, are 'co-alcoholics' with their husbands, and daughters of 'violent alcoholics' who are sexually addicted to their partners.

The solution is intensive therapy and/or peer assisted group work modelled on Alcoholics Anonymous. Norwood believes the funda-mental route to a cure lies in initiating 'a search for ... an ongoing contact with the healing and guiding spiritual principle within the person who suffers'.[43] Norwood is a maverick therapist who claims to have abandoned the therapeutic agenda because it involves the imposition of power sometimes associated with sexual abuse.[44] Her suggestions for changing the predicament of the individual are often practical and sometimes go beyond the narrow conceptions usually offered by therapists. Still, she has not escaped the extreme reduc-tionist and traditional patriarchal women-blaming conceptions associated with orthodox psychiatry. In this sense, what is being proposed is merely the old, wrapped in new terminology. In Mathiesen's schema, this competes as a candidate for change but is not new and therefore does not contradict the status quo.

Personality, learned helplessness and the battered woman syndrome

Like Shainess, Norwood's speculations are gleaned from clinical observations and letters from those responding to her ideas. Others have subjected women to various psychological tests and objectifying measurements in order to assess their supposed deviant personalities. Once done, she is no longer a whole person with the weaknesses and strengths possessed by all, she is now diminished in our eyes to a case as revealed in a collection of test scores. Not surprisingly, however, most of these efforts are inconclusive or indicate that women who have experienced violence do not differ from other women.[45] Despite these results, almost all therapeutically oriented commentators and researchers locate the problems of women in their aberrant personalities and backgrounds.

Accordingly, women are deemed to suffer from a host of personality problems and altered mental states rendering them susceptible to violence and/or incapable of managing their own affairs and leaving violent men. This range of reputed aliments is extremely diverse, illustrating the theoretical and ideological starting point of the investigator(s). They include: reserve and caution in emotional expression, low ego strength, inability to cope, shyness and difficulty in self-expression, introspection and insecurity, a tendency to withdraw and avoid interpersonal contact,[46] perceptions of loss of control, poor coping skills, manipulativeness, inability to express anger, splitting mind and body, denial and compliance, a willingness to please,[47] self destructiveness, skill deficits, problems communicating with others, poor impulse control,[48] caution in relationships with others, avoidance of confrontations, inability to cope with stress and trauma, retreats into fantasy, dissatisfaction with current status,[49] 'maladjustive attributional system' and poor 'locus of control'.[50] In their relationships with men their psychological make-up supposedly leads them to play the 'escalation game', to expect to be violated and to accept '... physical abuse as inherent in male–female relationships'.[51]

A few of these characterisitcs, such as caution in personal relationships and dissatisfaction with current status, are not particularly remarkable and are rather predictable given the circumstances of women experiencing persistent violence. Others characterize women as very different than the 'normal' female and some, such as the supposed acceptance of violence, feed into the orthodox ideas of victim blaming. The issue here is not whether or not women are affected by their experiences of violence, clearly anyone would be but we must consider the implications and the limitations of the way we conceive of their predicament.

A narrow therapeutic approach leads to very different conceptions and interventions than more contextual and social interpretations. Similiar to activists, a few therapeutic professionals view the problems of abused women as a direct and temporary result of the experience of violence. However, therapeutic accounts usually emphasize the unique backgrounds and permanent personality traits that make women vulnerable to violent relationships and unable to leave them. Furthermore, since these traits are thought to be rooted deeply in women's psychological make-up, they are intractable and require long-term therapeutic intervention. For many therapeutically inclined observers, these various psychological attributes and traits can be seen as a constellation referred to as the 'battered woman syndrome'. The core of these attributes is represented by the label 'learned helplessness'.

The concept of learned helplessness was developed in Seligman's experiments with animals, mostly dogs and rats. These animals were subjected to electric shocks and attempted drowning in order to demonstrate that a continued inability to escape perilous circumstances reputedly leads to passive, helpless behaviour. The experiments were extended to humans and have now been extrapolated to welfare recipients and peasants in third world countries in order to explain why they have not been able to lift themselves from poverty.[52] According to Lenore Walker, the major proponent of the learned helplessness thesis, 'Battered women's behavior ... appears similar to Seligman's dogs, rats and people'.[53]

Learned helplessness is meant to explain why women do not leave their violent partners, though many of its adherents also think it explains why women become victims of violence. Its supporters claim it provides, '... a psychological rationale for why the battered woman becomes a victim, and how the process of victimization further entraps her, resulting in psychological paralysis to leave the relationship'.[54] Like most therapeutically based approaches it identifies the primary roots of victimization in the background of the victim and not in the offender. Rigid sex role socialization, '... a benign, paternalistic, "Dresden doll" kind of upbringing',[55] and early slavish adherence to demands to fulfil the wishes of males, are seen as the characteristics of women who become victims of male violence. Abnormal backgrounds such as these reputedly result in '... a vulnerability pattern that may be established in childhood which makes a woman more likely to develop coping responses, rather than escape responses, in order to survive relationships'.[56] It is not clear from these accounts whether a majority or a small proportion of women who are abused by their male partners suffer from learned helplessness. Most of this literature implies or explicitly states that all battered women, possibly all women, suffer from learned helplessness.[57]

Once the seeds of learned helplessness are planted in childhood, they will apparently take root in women's relationships with men. When a woman with this type of background begins to experience violence she is thought to be unable to act in order to protect herself and to find alternatives. Such women appear to bind themselves to men in a 'symbiotic relationship'.[58] It is argued that this attachment is often observed by those who attempt to help a battered woman. Shelter workers, therapeutic counsellors and the police reputedly all report '... becoming exasperated and angry with battered women' who 'turn down help and return to husbands ...'.[59] The therapeutic explanation for this behaviour does not involve social, cultural or economic factors associated with why many women remain, although these are sometimes considered, nor do they include men's repeated promises of reform and/or threats of further violence should women try to leave. Instead, the supporters of this notion believe that women will not leave violent men because they are bound to them as a result of early conditioning and a 'cycle of violence' resulting in learned helplessness.

A repetitive cycle of violence involving three stages supposedly binds women to physically abusive partners. It is believed that the first two stages, tension building and 'explosions of acute violence', lead inextricably and invariably to a third stage of 'calm, loving respite' and contrition on the part of the man. This cycle is repeated unaltered by time or circumstances, and as a woman participates in this cycle 'she becomes an accomplice to her own battering'. It functions, we are told, to restore equilibrium to the relationship and to reinforce women's willingness to remain. Seemingly the repetition of this third phase is when '... the battered woman's victimization becomes completed', chaining her '... to her batterer just as strongly as "miracle glues" bind inanimate substances'.[60] An additional consequence is for women '... to develop a stereotype routine which meshes with the batterer's stereotyped routine ...'.[61] Once bound to their partner through this stereotyped pattern of behaviour arising from a repetitive cycle, women's help-seeking behaviour is hopelessly distorted.

Women suffering from learned helplessness supposedly appear powerless, unable and unwilling to act or help themselves. Inaction is rooted in distorted belief systems that lead women to '... see the batterer as all powerful' and '... not believe that anything they do can make the batterer stop ...'.[62] Distortions of this nature mean that seeking help from informal sources such as friends and relatives, and from more formal sources such as counsellors, social services and the police, will either not be initiated or they will be 'aborted or halted' because women believe 'they are useless'.[63] Eventually women will '... not accept the helper's assistance because they do not believe it will be effective' and '... cease all attempts to change their situation'.[64]

Based on this literature, it is impossble to tell whether a woman suffering from learned helplessness finds it impossible to seek help or whether she begins to pursue help and then stops because she suffers from this psychological ailment. It can be inferred that the latter is the usual pattern since it is argued that a woman '... discard[s] from consideration any alternatives for which she has no proof of effectiveness'.[65] Presumably the actions or, more accurately, the inaction of agencies have little to do with this assessment; instead, it is faulty thinking that leads women to assess these alternatives as ineffective. We might surmise from this argument that women become hopelessly and perpetually helpless. But no, according to the major adherent of this position,

> It is not that women think they are helpless all of the time, but rather it is the inability to predict when they will succeed and when they will fail which constitutes learned helplessness.[66]

Adherence to this notion seems to be based on the premise that the contingencies and outcomes experienced by abused women are unimportant to their perceptions. Again, it is only, or primarily, faulty reasoning and personality that count. The assumption is that the normal, healthy functioning adult, in contrast to women who experience violence, is able accurately to anticipate the future.

Accordingly, women experiencing learned helplessness binding them to their abusers can best be described as suffering from a 'battered woman syndrome'. Apparently the only way for them to escape these maladies is through 'individual and group therapy' based on the assumption that the 'symbiotic dependency bonds' must be severed, 'new communication skills' learned, and women must 'relearn the response–outcome contingencies by directly experiencing a sense of power and control over those paradigms which are indeed under her voluntary and independent control'.[67] A woman should also learn 'that she is capable of responding in ways that have a positive impact on her life; that is, that outcomes are contingent on her behaviour'.[68] Those who believe in learned helplessness propose that women who have suffered persistent violence should become more assertive, which '... enables the woman effectively to get her needs met, be they from her partner, her employer or her social network'.[69] On the basis of this proposal, it would appear that a woman will no longer be subjected to violence, will be able to leave a violent relationship and to establish a non-violent one or live independently, if she breaks her bond with the man, overcomes her false perceptions and inefficient actions associated with learned helplessness, and becomes more assertive.

In the United States, concepts such as 'learned helplessness' and the 'battered woman syndrome' are firmly embedded in the thinking of therapists and many within the movement. Adherents believe these ideas are sympathetic to abused women because they provide a short-hand for thinking about the problem and a means of absolving women of the responsibility for remaining with a violent man because of psychological traits obtained through faulty upbringing and conditions of daily life. Sympathetic and feminist therapists claim that these new concepts go beyond earlier ideas of masochism and liberate women from negative images and their own culpability.

Learned helplessness and the courts

The most important pragmatic benefit claimed for the concepts of 'learned helplessness' and the 'battered woman syndrome' is their use in American courts, where they have been employed to absolve or diminish the responsibility of women who kill violent husbands. In 1984, the New Jersey Supreme Court was one of the first American courts to rule that expert testimony employing the concept of the 'battered woman syndrome' was permissible in the defence of a woman who killed her husband. For many attorneys, such as those involved in the Women's Self-Defense Law Project, it is considered essential to bring a greater understanding of the predicament of abused women to the judicial process by educating lawyers, judges and jurors. In American courts, one of the standard ways of achieving this is by using expert witnesses, in this case attempting to overcome gender bias by recognizing how '... women's different experiences and circumstances' lead them to kill their violent partners.[70] Initially, lawyers embraced the ideas associated with the 'battered woman syndrome'; but this enthusiasm has been dampened by experience.

It is now recognized that these concepts, and especially their use in courts, have fuelled existing orthodox images of the innate incapacities of women.[71] As Elizabeth Schneider, one of the founders of the Women's Self-Defense Project, says, '... the term "battered woman syndrome" has been heard to communicate an implicit but powerful view that battered women are all the same, that they are suffering from a psychological disability and that this disability prevents them from acting "normally"'.[72] One court employed the term 'handicap' to describe the 'ailments' of a defendant. The 'syndrome' reinforces and confirms the view of women victims as passive, sick, powerless and ruled by emotions, a view firmly implanted in the criminal justice system from at least the nineteenth century. The reasonableness of the act, that is, that any rational person in such a perilous predicament would behave similarly, is denied or ignored. Instead women who kill their partners are portrayed as passive and capable only of responding in an emotional manner. The act is rarely seen as a 'woman's necessary choice to save her own life'.[73] This leads to a judicial focus on an 'excuse' rather than a justification associated with a reasonable act.

Schneider proposes that the concept of reasonableness associated with an act of self-defence highlights the contradictions and inadequacies associated with the use of the syndrome in court. If a woman was so helpless and passive how did she ever manage to kill her husband? Women who are often in most need of a defence but who do not fit the supposed syndrome (a helpless, passive victim who never fought back or sought help) may not benefit from 'judicial solicitude'. What is being created by the use of the syndrome is a unique, rigid classification of female victims, one that neatly fits with the myriad negative perceptions that have preceded it. Feminist legal commentators are now arguing that a defence should be based on the notion of self-defence and constructed on the elaboration of the argument concerning the reasonableness of the act based on a more gender specific understanding of self-defence.[74]

Another significant problem with these concepts and their use in court is that the voice of women is again silenced; their valid accounts and justifications are obscured, redefined or ignored. As Schneider points out, experts 'may not complement women's voices but become substitutes for them'.[75] A narrow therapeutic focus means that the problems of individual women are not seen in the context of male domination, and the social problem of violence against women is reduced to the troubles of unique, deviant women, and not linked to the nature of the wider oppression and experiences of all women. Significantly the bulk of therapeutic discourses pay scant attention to male domination. The approach produces a one-dimensional, static, stereotypical conception of women and men, making it impossible to perceive of the actions of human beings outside of these rigid categories. For example, the conception of a cycle of violence is static rather than dynamic and changing, does not deal with intentionality, and the notion of the third phase as a 'honeymoon' belies the experience of women who indicate that even the process of 'making-up' or reconstructing the relationship is carried out against the background of a personal history of violence and coercion and in the context of few viable alternatives to the violent relationship.[76] The concepts of 'learned helplessness' and the 'battered woman syndrome' may focus our sympathetic tendencies but they have negative implications for public perceptions and actions associated with the problem of violence against women. They are also based on false premises and unsubstantiated evidence regarding the predicament and actions of women experiencing persistent violence.

THE PREDICAMENT OF BATTERED WOMEN

British and North American research on the predicament and reactions of women who endure severe, persistent, usually escalating violence reveals that they do not remain helpless and inactive but rather seek help from a wide variety of individuals and agencies.[77] Although continuous coercion, intimidation and violence can, at some points, create anxiety, distress and depression, and even attempted or actual suicide and murder, it also creates determination, action and bravery.[78] Throughout the process of surviving violent relationships women engage in constant struggles to comprehend the violence and their predicament, and engage in endless activities attempting to mitigate the violence and change or end the relationship. This frequently involves seeking help from several sources.

In considering women's experience across the duration of their relationship, we found in our own research that over time there are considerable changes in the nature of the violence, women's perceptions of the problem and their predicament, and in patterns of help-seeking.[79] This dynamic process contrasts with the static state presented in the model of 'learned helplessness'. After the first episode of violence, women are startled and shocked and usually define it as a unique event that will never be repeated. At this point women do not usually seek to terminate the relationship. Instead, they believe, as anyone might, in the potential for reform and are still committed to the relationship. In the beginning, their partners often reinforce this interpretation by behaving in a contrite manner, but this reduces over time and often disappears as the violence continues. When women first seek to comprehend the violence, some, though certainly not all, look to their own actions for an explanation.[80] This is not surprising in societies which allocate to wives the responsibility for happy husbands and families; women are expected to ask how their own behaviour 'caused' their husband's violence.[81] Women eventually realize that solutions to the man's violence do not reside in a change of their own behaviour. For some this realization comes fairly quickly while others take longer to overcome such culturally constructed notions. Indeed, this is one of the reasons women are susceptible to accepting notions of learned helplessness despite the very obvious facts to the contrary. Throughout this process, most women, rather than remaining completely passive and helpless, actually make contact with others in order to discuss the violence and its meaning and to seek various forms of assistance in effecting a change in the man's behaviour.

Relatives, especially mothers and sisters, are the first to be contacted in the process of seeking help in order to discuss the violence, attempt to discern its meaning, and to try to effect a change in the man's behaviour.[82] Relatives and good friends provide sympathetic listening, advice and support, occasionally they also provide temporary accommodation. Far from helplessly remaining with violent men, women engage in an active process we refer to as 'staying, leaving and returning'.[83] Help-seeking of this nature is not static, either she stays or she leaves, but is a dynamic, evolving process. In this process, women make active and conscious decisions based on their changing circumstances: they leave for short periods in order to escape the violence and to emphasize their disaffection in the hope that this will stop the violence. In the beginning, they are generally not attempting to end the relationship, but are negotiating to re-establish the relationship on a non-violent basis. Women return for a myriad of reasons: because men promise to reform; they are concerned about the welfare of their husband and children; they accept the powerful ideals associated with an intact family; they do not wish to discard their emotional and material investment in the relationship; they have no accommodation and few prospects for meaningful employment; and they fear the violent reprisals of men who are often at their most dangerous when women leave. Relatives and friends have traditionally played a significant role in these deliberations and negotiations, sometimes helping to remove shame and guilt, sometimes blaming the victim, sometimes providing meaningful economic and material support, and sometimes counselling reconciliation.

If the relationship endures and women decide or are forced to stay, they do not stop trying to change the situation. On the contrary, they usually maintain contact with relatives and friends and often expand the network to include more formal sources of help, such as legal, medical and social agencies, persistently trying to effect a change in the man's behaviour.[84] Throughout this process that might be referred to as 'negotiating for a non-violent relationship', women are active, seeking the involvement of a variety of individuals and agencies, and trying numerous tactics. As the process continues, women begin to change their requests. Instead of seeking help in 'negotiating a non-violent relationship', they seek assistance in ending a violent relationship. Research demonstrates that when women seek help, they often do so in a tentative and ambivalent manner, filtered through shame, self-blame, a sense of failure, concerns about exposing the private problems of their families, fear associated with men's threats if contact is made, and concern about the nature of the response they might receive.[85]

Women are right to worry about what might happen; research and experience in both countries reveals that traditional agency response has often been inadequate and sometimes detrimental. In the past and still today, members of the helping professions have often remained 'neutral', offered sympathetic advice and/or concentrated on the needs of children and reconciliation, or offered therapy to the woman. Women have often been blamed for the violence, asked to change their behaviour in order to meet their husband's demands, and had their own concerns and requests deflected or ignored. Consequently, women are often left to negotiate with violent men in isolation from systems of support.

In contrast to therapeutically oriented conceptions of women bound to men in 'symbiotic relationships' in which they suffer 'psychological paralysis' making it unlikely or extremely improbable that they will seek help, evidence on help-seeking shows that women actively seek support and assistance. They do not cease all attempts to obtain assistance because of false beliefs that agencies and friends cannot or will not help them but sometimes alter their actions because they learn through bitter experience that help will not be given or that which is given will not change the problem and help them escape or stop the violence. Women are usually persistent and often tenacious in their attempts to seek help, but pursue such help through channels that prove to be most useful and reject those that have been found to be unhelpful or condemning. For most women, active pursuit of assistance is a continual aspect of their lives, ebbing and flowing with their experiences at the hands of violent men and of the institutions from which they seek assistance.

The reasons for women failing to leave violent relationships have very little to do with some supposed set of unique psychological traits. Instead, an understanding of their patterns of help-seeking must be located in the nature and ferocity of male domination, coercion and violence; a moral order which places responsibilities for family problems on to women; inadequate, even condemning responses of legal, social and medical agencies; a financial and material dependence on men for the support of women and children; a wider social and economic order that makes it nearly impossible for women to leave and live on their own; the bleak prospects (well understood by most women) for single, female headed households; and the lack of effective intervention in the lives of violent men and abused women.[86] Economic problems are, of course, even more profound for minority women who are usually faced with greater obstacles associated with poverty, housing and employment. Factors such as these make a mockery of therapeutic advice that by becoming assertive, women can escape from male violence. This either ignores the social and economic constraints mentioned above or implicitly assumes that these can be redressed through the psychological transformation of the woman. In considering problems associated with therapeutic responses to women who are raped, Michelle Fine criticizes clinical psychology for assuming that women '*can* control the forces which victimize them' stressing that 'Most people are denied the means to assume control over fundamentally changing their lives'.[87]

An explanation of the behaviour of women trapped in violent relationships does not require the specification of unique psychological traits associated with learned helplessness and a battered woman syndrome. Yet these ideas are in the ascendency in the United States, constituting the new orthodoxy even in some feminist oriented programmes assisting abused women. The recent history of these labels is exemplary of the processes associated with the creation of deviant categories in which the diverse problems of individuals are subsumed under a single tag. This label becomes indexical, referring to an entire panoply of stereotypical traits, attributes and behaviours. Such conceptions stereotype women who have experienced violence and place them in rigid, objectified categories. They also have important implications for the futures of abused women and for the responses of those who are meant to provide assistance.

Psychological trait theories categorize people in a rigid manner. People are either healthy and act deliberately and consistently, or they suffer from a malady which makes it impossible for them to do so. People cannot be hesitant, confused and ambivalent. Women either leave or stay. They, like everyone else, cannot engage in diverse, even contradictory action. These approaches lack a dynamic which conceives of human beings as intentional, rational actors able to interpret their social world. They also propose overly deterministic and rigid accounts of the backgrounds of women, seeing them as socialized into passive, acquiescent roles. Females of all ages, according to these accounts, always behave in a submissive and subservient manner towards men, regardless of circumstances and settings. These conceptions, while purporting to be sympathetic to women, see them as the quintessential victim. It is not so much that women are socialized to be helpless, as they are educated to see their roles as highly circumscribed within the family context. Within that context women are given extraordinary responsibility, and, even outside of it, they take on or they are required to assume a variety of social and economic activities. There are other psychological approaches which are more dynamic, conceive of women as more active decision makers, and are more sensitive to the social and economic contexts in which women live.[88]

There are elements within the American movement which embrace this therapeutic conception of women. It might be argued that therapeutic discourses, their associated technologies of change and the professionals who offer them have co-opted much of the movement in the United States, thus transforming ideals and practices. An explanation of these developments must consider the culture of individualism and the emphasis on personal psychology and emotions within American society as a whole and within feminism and the movement.[89] An important contribution of feminism has been to show how 'the personal is political' and to have revealed the importance of intimate personal domination. But this should not mean the collapse of one into the other or lead to equating the political with an exclusive focus on the person, yet this trajectory has at times led to the minimization and neglect of economic and social factors. As Hester Eisenstein has pointed out about feminism in the USA, 'The emphasis on psychology ... may have given many women the impression that in order to transform their situation, it sufficed to change the way they thought about the world'.[90]

Some individuals and groups within the movement were not merely seduced into these conceptions, they were there from the beginning. The movement was susceptible to such a direction and, it seems clear that in some cases these ideas and approaches were introduced from within the movement and not transported from outside. The more the movement adopts this individual, psychological position on abused women the greater likelihood that it will dismiss or ignore the political, social and economic issues surrounding the problem of male violence against women. Through this process, the vision of the movement and the potential for social change associated with making the private public and political are seriously eroded. The more women are seen as clients in need of therapy rather than people in need of alternatives and choices, the less the movement challenges prevailing conceptions of the problem.[91] The processes associated with clienthood strip the relationship between women and activists as well as the movement of a wider political vision. Clients and the professionals who attempt to help them are rarely political actors. Certainly a few therapeutic observers have considered the significance of other factors, arguing, for example, that the most important role of counsellors and therapists may be that of the advocate who can faciliate legal, economic and medical assistance.[92] Yet, such ideas are usually relegated to a secondary importance and in more recent literature, almost completely ignored.[93] One of the most significant limitations of this approach is that it deflects our attention away from the roots of the problem, violent men, and from the social and political structures which support male violence.

THERAPEUTIC ACCOUNTS OF THE VIOLENT MAN

In the nineteenth century men who beat their wives were described as drunken, loutish brutes. In Britain, such men were seen as members of a class apart, throwbacks to an earlier pre-civilized period of human evolution. For many observers they were predominantely Irish immigrants who were distinct from the civilized English males who were the 'natural' inhabitants of Britain.[94] In the United States, violent men were described as brutish, beer drinking immigrants who must be transformed into law abiding, teetotalling, non-wife beating Americans. These conceptions may account for the apparent willingness to employ the lash and whip to transform them into law abiding Americans.

By this century, wife-beaters no longer featured in the infrequent discussions about violence against women. They were rarely identified by criminologists and therapeutic professionals. If the problem of wife-abuse was considered, therapeutic practitioners usually concentrated on the characteristics of women. They were the ones seeking help, and in a tragic though frequent psychoanalytic twist of the usual process of apportioning responsibility, women's personalities became the focus of attention and, in turn, explanation for men's violence. As one psychiatric report explained, 'the victim in spouse assaults can always be assumed to have played a crucial role in the offence, and may have directly or indirectly brought about or precipitated their own victimization'.[95] In these accounts mothers are blamed for the creation of violent men who, it is claimed, grow up within 'domineering, rejecting mother relationships'.[96]

As with all psychoanalytic approaches, those focusing on violent men locate the source of the problem in personality traits usually established through flawed or disrupted childhood development; in this case arising from poor mothering. These sort of men become dependent on their mothers and then 'parentify their wives'. Other accounts reiterated classic masochistic views of the violence. Accordingly, women are locked into some sort of balanced functioning relationship where periodic violence functions to give them 'masochistic gratification ... helping probably to deal with guilt arising from the intense hostility expressed in her controlling, castrating behaviour'.[97] Violent men, it seems, are victims of their past experiences at the hands of women, usually their mothers, and of wives in their current relationships. In these accounts, men and women are seen as abnormal or pathological, distinct from 'normal' men and women who do not experience these problems. Surprisingly, intervention is not aimed at resolving the conflicts of men and thus ending their violence. The focus of intervention is on women who, it is thought, need to change their behaviour as a means of ending the violence of men

Today, there is a growing interest in violent men, and in the United States there is a burgeoning industry associated with the treatment of men who physically abuse their partners. To a large extent this has occurred through the process of defining violence as 'a clinical condition'.[98] The majority of these approaches are based on the assumption that such men have unique traits causing violent behaviour. Some stress the psycho-biological basis of violence, arguing that domestic violence is associated with 'criminogenic encephalosis' characterized '... by temper tantrums, violent outbursts, antisocial behavior and enuresis'.[99] Schauss suggests that all men who use violence should be given a complete physiological screening, blood analysis and urinalysis as these will reveal the biological anomalies associated with violent tendencies. He claims that controlled studies have found '... a consistent pattern of either nutrient intake deficiencies or overconsumption malnutrition in violent men'.[100] Citing Hungerford, he notes , '... that in nearly 75 per cent of the cases she sees involving serious marital discord, particularly wife-beating, the abuser clinically reveals an abnormal blood glucose level ...'.[101] Biologically oriented commentators claim that in over half of 'couples experiencing serious marital discord' at least one of the partners suffers from a 'treatable biochemical imbalance that could later be demonstrated to provoke the negative behavior'.[102] In this approach violence is primarily associated with diseased brains, incontinence, low-blood sugar, poor diets and bio-chemical imbalances.

Biologically based approaches represent a minority of the therapeutic accounts of violent men. The dominant approach is more eclectic, building on traditional psychiatric views and drawing on more recent psychological explanations of human behaviour. Men are described as suffering from inadequate and impaired 'ego functioning' and 'anti-social' and 'pre-morbid' personalities resulting from 'rejection and inadequacy' in childhood.[103] Deschner, for example, thinks that violent men are the youngest sons in families where they have all experienced or witnessed violence: 'The love/hurt/rage reactions that helpless young boys felt towards their abusive, powerful parents ... were replayed by these men in their marriages.'[104] The 'uncontrollable anger' of a violent man emanates from 'unresolved conflicts' with his parents resulting in 'displacement of anger and aggression onto the most convenient targets in his life – his wives and girl friends'.[105] Such men are described as frightened, victimized bullies who experience mood swings, pain and anger. They suffer from a sort of 'atavistic madness',

> ... the primitive rage reactions leading to aggression and battering are unlearned, instinctual patterns. Angry and aggressive responses are 'wired' into every mammalian brain as a vital part of each individual's survival equivalent.[106]

Violent men are not bad; instead, as Deschner thinks, people transgress because they are ignorant of what they are doing, they are stupid, or emotionally disturbed.[107] Since men are not responsible for their acts, Deschner believes women should forgive them.

Women do not escape responsibility in these contemporary reports. As if imitating their precursors these accounts see women as responsible for creating, recognizing and satisfying the unmet needs of men. Unmet needs are created in childhood and express themselves as violence in later life.

> It is the effect of the abusive father shutting off any meaningful affectionate relationship with his son, leaving that son no other alternative than the mother for emotional gratification. That boy eventually comes to develop a general emotional dependence on women.[108]

Violence erupts in marriage because it is '... really a crude attempt to retrieve the same feelings of warmth and security that he originally received from his mother but that his wife may not even be aware he needs'.[109] Violent men are actually dependent and insecure: 'Excessive control of the very women upon whom they are dependent is simply an attempt by these men to shore up their need for security.'[110]

Therapeutic approaches to violent men also emphasize the influences of stress, drug and alcohol dependency, the inability to play, lack of self-control and the 'imbalance of roles brought about by the women's liberation movement'.[111]

One of the most predominant approaches is the Family Systems perspective in which violence is seen as the product of an interacting couple or, more abstractly, the family. The director of counselling at the Tyler [Texas] Family Preservation Project claims, '... many couples have mutual hostility and resentment against the world. They find each other, ... they form a bond or a symbiosis so that it's "Us against the world"'.[112] In such a family system 'likes do attract likes' with each partner bringing the same weaknesses to adult relationships, '... emotional dependence, childlike insecurity, and a generally low self-image'.[113] It is not merely the man who is the product of an inadequate childhood or employs violence as a reaction to stress, it is the entire family: 'The violent family becomes imbalanced and internally competitive in the face of stress.'[114] It seems that the coming together of two people who suffer 'a general emotional immaturity' and 'mutual obliviousness to interpersonal processes' leads inexorably to '... a violence prone system, and once an incident of abuse is consummated, a battering system'.[115] Family systems of this nature are apparently very different from non-violent ones where, '... normal relationship rules are negotiated, each spouse has the prerogative, alternating control occurs and a symmetrical posture develops'.[116]

Treatment within this systems approach predictably involves intervention in the whole family 'system'. As one therapist put it, 'We will never really make progress in resolving family violence if we do not consider the family as the unit to be helped'.[117] Systems counselling conceives of the problem as emerging from sick, weak and violent-prone systems, with violence solely or primarily understood as a result of 'interactional behavior sequences between the partners'.[118] Consequently there are no victims or abusers. In such work, 'neither partner has an exclusive right to either term',[119] and both are seen as 'equally culpable and victimized'.[120] Therapy involves altering interaction by overcoming 'communication problems' and 'skills deficits'. Accordingly, each member of the family must accept responsibility for change, yet therapists may encounter resistance as the '... two parties join in collusion to avoid changes'.[121] In the face of such obstacles some therapists believe that the best route to overcoming resistance may be to 'discuss and expose the system's characteristics' and 'escalate conflict in order to locate the couple's threshold for change'.[122]

Systems perspectives emphasize work with the family because 'Working with several family members, rather than one individual, is more likely to insure an objective and impartial perspective.'[123] It is argued that working with the family can result in a 'change in the environment in which a person lives'.[124] It is clear that the environment under consideration is narrowly conceived of as the closed world of the interacting couple. The family systems perspective presents an empty, usually gender blind, conception of families and individuals, employing a language that grossly reifies and distorts the family and the violence. Adherents talk about 'consort battering', the 'battering couple' and 'the physically maltreating ... [and] abusive family'. Such phrases make little sense unless these therapists are referring to all members of a family maltreating or abusing members of another family. To speak of 'battering families' who 'choose to isolate themselves' makes a nonsense of the reality of family life and of the social processes associated with violence. It assumes that the interests, actions and beliefs of all family members are identical, ignoring the wealth of accumulated evidence demonstrating the different, at times distinct worlds and interests of men, women and children. It ignores the wealth of evidence indicating how women reject violence and conceive of their problems in a radically different manner than men. The approach is deeply conservative. Embedded in its core is the assumption that members of families should be reconciled and re-united regardless of the potential costs to individuals (read: wives). Family systems perspectives have been widely criticized for their gender neutral approach, isolation from research on women, a failure to consider power and the wider social and cultural context, the use of abstract, 'neutral' language, and contradictorily, an overwhelming tendency to blame mothers and idealize fathers.[125]

Despite their apparent diversity, therapeutic approaches to violent men have a number of common elements. Whether they stress biochemical, neurological or physical disorder, transference of aggression, displacement of needs or situational factors such as stress and alcohol abuse, the basic assumption is that the fundamental cause of violence is faulty personality or psychopathology: '... intrafamilial violence is primarily considered a psychological and social disease'.[126] Men, or in many cases families, are propelled into violence because of underdeveloped ego structures rooted in early development or internal stress that causes uncontrollable, irrational eruptions of rage and violence. No individual man is accountable for his violence; the family, faulty backgrounds or situational factors are the causes.

Motivations, values and intentions play no role in these explanations and interventions, nor do notions of guilt and responsibility. Characterizing people in this way means that it is impossible for them to play an active role in transforming their own behaviour. In allocating responsibility for violence against women, men are seen as having no role to play because the explanations of their actions involve the behaviour of women, the family (women) or other factors beyond their control.

If men's accounts of and rationalizations for violence are considered they are explained as psychological transference, not as rooted in social or cultural patterns linked to men's domination, control and aggression. The wider social and cultural context is almost always invisible. Conceptualizing the problem as a disease also means a specific type of relationship can develop between those who are 'sick' and those who offer cures: '... affliction allows us to distance ourselves'.[127] According to the proponents of the illness model, distancing ourselves results in detached, rational observers and helpers. The perfect client–professional relationship.

Whatever the specific features of this illness, it is always compared, usually tacitly, to the hypothetically healthy male or family. The healthy, perhaps 'mythical' male is not aggressive or violent; he comes from a violence free family; he is 'in touch' with his emotions; and he has close relationships with other males. In his relationships with women, this 'normal' male is warm, expressive and not domineering. He shares authority and decision making with his partner.

CHALLENGING VIOLENT MEN

Conceptions such as these are increasingly challenged by alternative perspectives and practices rooted in interpretative and feminist research and in the experience of those working with this abuse.[128] Alternative explanations of violent men, stressing the interpretative and intentional aspects of human action, have played an important role in more recent explanations of men's violence against their partners. They have also been incorporated into innovative reactions to violent males. In the United States a vast array of programmes, at least 200, exist to deal with violent men. Some are extremely orthodox, others build upon traditional explanations and approaches, and a few break new ground in offering pro-feminist programmes to deal with violent men. Pro-feminist men's programmes have been created to challenge men's violence and, consequently, also challenge traditional therapeutic interpretations. Intervention programmes for men, whether traditional or innovative, have generated an enormous amount of political debate and controversy within the movement. Although the movement has sometimes provided impetus for the development of men's programmes, they are still treated with some scepticism and concern.

The movement and programmes for violent men

For the movement men's programmes present a variety of challenges, dilemmas and controversies There is, for example, the relationship between the movement and its adversaries. Are men's programmes an ally in efforts to seek social change or an adversary against the movement and social change? Do they represent a threat to the identity of the movement should it become transformed by embracing this new activity or an opportunity to expand the agenda of change? Do such programmes offer meaningful alternatives to the status quo of accepting and supporting male violence? These and other issues became the topic of concern and debate within the movement and were highlighted in the United States in a series of encounters between the movement and the newly formed men's groups.

In August 1982 a forum on 'working with men who batter' was organized as an immediate follow-up to the national conference of the Coalition held in Milwaulkee. A position paper, 'Men Who Batter/A Woman's Response', outlining the issues surrounding programmes for batterers, was prepared by several activists and presented for consideration by the conference.[129] Some activists argued that there should be no programmes for batterers who were best handled by the justice system. They emphasized the criminal justice system and the '... role of community education, direct action, and demands for housing, jobs and child care services ...' as the most effective means of ending violence against women. Others, while not rejecting the general notion of programmes for batterers, saw several potential dangers for battered women and the movement. There was the possible adoption of psycho-therapeutic orientations and couple counselling which often resulted in ignoring the violence and the oppression of men and sophisticated forms of victim blaming. It was pointed out that efforts directed at individual men would reinforce the view that the violence is only about a 'few' deviant men: 'Any solution which isolates a small fraction of the oppressors' number and attempts to liberate women by changing them leaves the majority of men to continue their oppression.'[130] For the movement, an individ-

ualized approach would not only fail to serve women, it would also
rob the movement of its wider social analysis of the problem and
neutralize the struggle for reform with social and legal agencies.
There was also a fear that a focus on batterers' programmes would
now take over the centre stage of public attention and programme
development in the continued search for the newest or latest social
problem and thus eclipse the victims of violence and the programmes
assisting them.[131] Alarm was also sounded about possible competition
for the scarce funding needed to assist the victims of violence. This
was acute given the propensity of many sources to provide only seed
funding for a limited period of time in order for an organization to get
started, after which they are expected to find permanent funding elsewhere.

The challenges and confrontations generated by activists' criticisms
and the debates at the Forum led to a subsequent conference organized by the Pennsylvania Coalition Against Domestic Violence,
'VISIONS: Work With Men Against Violence Against Women',
which was intended to lead to a dialogue between pro-feminist men
working in men's programmes and women advocates.[132] As might be
expected the conference bristled with conflict and anger. Barbara
Hart pointed out that 'Many pro-feminist men coming to the Forum
did not recognize the critical importance of women's leadership in
anti-violence work'.[133] Activists questioned the legitimacy of the
entire activity, and were sceptical about the motivations and intentions of the men involved. These concerns and objections brought
angry responses from many men and, in turn, women's anger.

Debates over priorities were also heated. Some activists argued
against any form of counselling or education for men because it was
ineffective and reductionist. Others stressed the importance of
accountability to the movement to abused women, and urged pro-
feminist men to direct their energies at confronting institutions in
order to bring about wider social change. A diversity of positions and
directions was identified and pursued with participants reaching a
number of conclusions. Barbara Hart's summary is telling and still
pertinent.

> Some women left the forum convinced that they would never work
> with men to end violence against women. Some left troubled, but
> still firmly committed to working with pro-femininst men and still
> believing that counselling of batterers was a priority for men's
> work. And some went home convinced that the battered-women's
> movement had no choice but to work with men because the work

of men on their own would endanger battered women and jeopardize the movement.[134]

The Visions conference highlights the ongoing political issues surrounding attempts to engage in pro-feminist work with men. These issues are still alive today and have just begun to be debated in Britain.

Pro-feminist programmes for violent men

One of the fundamental differences between pro-feminist programmes and traditional therapeutic ones, as illustrated in the Visions conference, is the attempt to forge links with the movement. Therapeutic efforts usually ignore the achievements and insights of the movement. While some acknowledge the early importance of the movement, they, nonetheless, deny it any continuing role. For example, Shupe, Stacey and Hazelwood claim to identify three phases in family violence work: a victim-oriented phase, a direct treatment of male perpetrator phase and a family systems oriented phase.[135] They think that the current family systems phase is rightly dominated by professionals. For them the 'ideological zeal' of the shelter movement is dangerous, whereas the entry of detached professionals elevates the work to a higher plane. Professionals, they argue, '... erode the ideological zeal of the shelter movement, for professionals are trained to respect, if not pursue, scientific inquiry'. New programmes, they approvingly proclaim, avoid 'a radical feminist mindset' because they are 'no longer under the direct control or influence of women's shelter advocates'.[136]

By contrast, many pro-feminist men's programmes were created because of the insights and encouragement of shelter advocates. EMERGE, the first and one of the best known pro-feminist programmes, was started in 1977 at least partly because of the encouragement of Boston area shelter activists such as Betsy Warrior.[137] Today many of these programmes are linked in various ways with the shelter movement. Some exist as an element of an overall co-ordinated community approach to violence while others, like EMERGE and RAVEN, offer distinct programmes linked through continuous dialogue. Programmes, such as DAIP in Duluth and DAP (the Domestic Abuse Project) in Minneapolis–St Paul, incorporate men's programmes into an overall community effort involving services for women, men's programmes and co-ordination of the efforts of criminal justice and social service agencies. Programmes, with this sort of structure, often dubbed the Duluth model, are usually created and operated by women and men involved in or closely associated with the movement. Another method of linking men's programmes to shelter activists is represented by the programme in Marin County, California. Marin Abused Women's Services encompasses a men's programme, Man Alive, within its overall strategy to end violence against women. MAWS does not, however, attempt to co-ordinate the efforts of other community agencies. Other work with abusers, such as that of Ann Ganley, involves independent efforts but with a distinctly feminist orientation.[138]

The promise of pro-feminist programmes is that they directly challenge men's violence. A fundamental principle is to make men responsible for their violence. Consequently, couple or family systems counselling is rejected as ineffective, even dangerous: 'The potential DANGER ... is significant and should not be minimized ... lest we mirror the attitudes of the men we hope to change.'[139] Family or couple counselling conveys, often unintentionally, the message that the man's violence is a family problem and that all members are equally responsible. Men are not held accountable for their actions and, as such, they are not confronted. This sort of counselling, especially when it is done in the context of conciliation or reconciliation programmes, conveys the message that the couple should stay together, no matter what the costs. Couple counselling may place women in a positon of greater vulnerability. Women who report their husbands to agencies may increase the risk of assault. For women to reveal the nature and extent of the violence in joint sessions and expose their feelings in front of their partners may also increase the man's potential for violence and coercion.

Based on the knowledge and experience of nearly two decades of work in the movement, pro-feminist programmes take a more direct and pragmatic approach, seeking to increase men's insight into their own behaviour and emotions and helping them to end their violent behaviour. Traditional therapeutic technologies are sometimes employed but always within the context of more encompassing forms of reaction and critical femininst interpretations. Confrontational group work is the preferred technology for seeking personal change. According to Ganley, '*Appropriate use of confrontation* is crucial to alter the client's characteristics of minimization, denial and externalization'.[140] Confrontation involves attempts to convince men to acknowledge their violent behaviour and to accept responsibility for actions and for the need to change.

Pro-feminist programmes for men have confirmed the wealth of research on the characteristics of men who are violent towards women. They are men who have very little empathy for others, especially women. They use violence to coerce, control and dominate, while rejecting their own reponsibility. Ganley suggests violent men often deflect responsibility on to women and deny the consequences of their own acts. As Purdy and Nickle put it, they are involved in blaming the victim, justifying the violence, distorting and minimizing, externalizing and omitting and lying.[141] These constitute formidable barriers to personal change. Overcoming denial and creating a sense of responsibility is a vital first step when working with violent men.

Because of the formidable nature of this task some pro-feminist programmes work only with men who have begun to take responsibility for their violence by seeking assistance through their own initiative. Other programmes take the position that most men are incapable of such an initiative and must be required to participate through programmes linked to criminal justice believing that '... the client may benefit from having an external motivator for going through the change process'.[142] In reality, very few men are actually self-referred. The vast majority of voluntary participants are 'socially mandated', entering men's groups because their partners demand it as a condition of continuing and/or returning to the relationship.

In pro-feminist group work the focal point is the violence. Traditional work sometimes ignores and usually slights the violence, preferring to focus on supposed psychological maladies buried deep in the biography of the individual. As David Adams, a founding member of EMERGE, says, some of these approaches collude with batterers '... by not making their violence the primary issue or by implicitly legitimizing men's excuses for violence'.[143] Therapeutic interventions seek to uncover the supposed well-springs of behaviour. It is never made clear, however, how these background characteristics or conditions are explicitly linked to violence and how knowledge or insight into these 'problems' will lead to a change in the problem behaviour.

Pro-feminist programmes deal with the violence in a direct and concrete fashion, first by 'achieving a non-negotiable abstinence from violence' and often by requiring men to re-enact or discuss specific violent events as a means of revealing the sequence of emotions and actions within the overall event. Almost all men can reconstruct their violence, provide accounts of what they said and did, and describe their partner's reactions. This demonstrates that the violence is not the result of uncontrollable 'atavistic' impulses, blind rage or alcoholic induced actions beyond comprehension and control. Reconstructing violent events is also important in increasing men's awareness of their own intentions and motivations.[144] An important feature of these re-enactments is the identification of what some have termed the 'critical moment'.[145] This is the point where a man could have acted differently and chosen a non-violent alternative. Once the critical moment is identified, the incident can be re-created and alternative actions considered, discussed and practised. Locating interventions in actual behaviour is an important means of building and modelling new forms of conflict resolution.

Concrete approaches provide a foundation for discussing other fundamental issues, making it possible, for example, to follow the event through to consider the immediate and long-term impact on women and children. This helps increase empathy. It can also lead to a consideration of the effect violence has on family and friends, showing how it operates to isolate both the man and the woman. Focusing on the violence in the context of a group of men also provides a forum for examining the social, cultural and political issues associated with wife abuse and relating these to individual behaviour. Attempts to link individual actions to wider social processes constitute one of the most important differences between pro-feminist programmes and traditional therapies. Few traditional approaches explore the links between individual behaviour and the wider society; even fewer are sensitive to gender and power.

Pro-feminist programmes see violence as one end of a continuum of male domination. It is seen as an expression of the power and control of men over women, and these interpretations are conveyed to violent men and pinpointed and demonstrated in reconstructions. Andrew McCormick of EMERGE says, 'Our basic premise is that the cause of abuse is the fact that men dominate women both in personal relationships and in social institutions ...'[146] This approach invariably leads to a consideration of other forms of domination, such as intimidation, and psychological coercion. The widely used Power and Control Wheel developed at Duluth which incorporates various forms of control is the most explicit examplar of this concentration on power.[147] The overall goal is the elimination of male dominance within the family and society. Group discussions can also deal with the myths and justifications which are intricately linked to men's violence and domination. This makes it possible for men to recognize their rigid and distorted beliefs and expectations, such as those associated with extreme possessiveness. Recognition of rigid, authoritarian beliefs is the first step in altering them and avoiding many of the confrontations and conflicts associated with violence. A crucial goal is to liberate men from their perceptions that a man is only a man when he is dominating and controlling a woman.

Those who operate pro-feminist programmes for abusive men differ about who can best confront violent men and provide positive direction. Some believe groups must be led by men because it is time men accepted collective responsibility for their violence and because they can best understand batterers and confront their violence. Others argue that men, even pro-feminist men, cannot be trusted with sole responsibility. They point out that it is too easy for men to collude about women's faults and responsibilities for men's violence, and thus support the beliefs and prejudices that generate and excuse men's actions.[148] For them, women should play a central role as programme co-ordinators and group leaders because they are more likely to recognize such problems and redirect the group back to fundamentals. It may also be important for abusive men to see men and women working together as equals. Whatever the mix of group leaders, it is considered crucial that women's groups and abused women provide insight and direction in developing the principles and goals of these programmes. The Duluth programme, for example, developed its power and control model through lengthy discussions with women who had experienced violence.

Programmes for violent men are still in an early stage of development, and pro-feminist programmes as well as a host of others represent a wide spectrum of philosophical aims and pragmatic approaches. Most draw heavily on psychotherapeutic approaches. Some are grafted on to feminist insights, while others have developed with little or no contact or knowledge of the movement, its philosophy and practice. A few stand outside the psychotherapeutic tradition and, instead, use an educational approach. For example, the Duluth programme was partially inspired by the ideas of the radical Brazilian educationalist, Paulo Freire, and the Volunteer Counseling Service offered in New York State is a court-mandated six week educational programme.[149]

Fundamental principles of pro-feminist programmes

Given the diversity of these programmes, it is impossible to cover them all. However, we shall provide a brief account of the major philosophical positions of pro-feminist programmes and consider their implications for relationships with the movement and for social change. In this ideal typical account, we shall accentuate the unique attributes of a pro-feminist approach, recognizing that not all of these features operate in some programmes.

A significant feature of pro-feminist work is an alternative conception of violence and the behaviour of men. Violence is seen as intentional behaviour chosen by men as a tactic or resource associated with attempts to control and dominate women. By contrast, therapeutic discourses usually ignore the violence or see it as an irrational act of emotional ventilation emerging from forces beyond the control or comprehension of violent men: '... violence occurs when a person loses control of himself'.[150] Alternatively, defining violence as intentional leads to a moral discourse identifying men as responsible and accountable for their acts. One of the significant contributions of the movement has been to insert this moral element into the abstract discourses about male violence. Violent behaviour becomes the major and concrete focus in these programmes, not something to be skirted over and ignored. It is a retributive starting point, a continual referent for reminding men of their responsibility and of the harm they have inflicted on their partners and children.[151] The past is continuously linked to the present by communicating disapproval of violence and emphasizing its relation to other individuals and the wider community. Men are not allowed to forget how their acts have affected those around them.

Beginning from this retributive starting point leads more clearly to reparative and reformative goals for personal behaviour. Making amends and remedying wrongs is a fundamental part of the reformative process. These approaches seek to engage men as active participants in their own transformation. Communication is always two-way, involving confrontation, dialogue, persuasion, even argument, with, at its most radical, a sense of commensurability between those who lead groups and those who participate in them. All men, not just those engaged in violent repression, are seen as participating in efforts to control and dominate women.[152] Efforts to promote and intensify feelings of guilt and responsibility are a starting point intended to encourage men to begin a process of self-reflection and censorship. Rebuking and confrontation is direct, never hiding behind a mask of therapeutic neutrality, but intended to be supportive of personal change. Looking backwards is a process which continually links the responsibility for violence with its impact on the victim. Looking forwards encourages personal change.[153] In this way, men might learn new non-violent patterns of behaviour and begin to work on improving their relationships with women.

To the extent that these programmes enter into the arena of social change they will not limit their work to the reform of individual violent men, but also seek to have an effect on the wider community. Community in these programmes is usually characterized in two ways. There is the specific community of women to whom the programmes should be directly responsible and there is a wider community to which efforts of re-education are directed. Efforts must be responsive to the leadership and knowledge of the battered-women's movement and to women who have experienced violence. Mechanisms are established to enhance the responsiveness of men's programmes to the concerns of the movement and to ensure the leadership of women. Programmes sometimes agree to subject themselves to monitoring by shelter groups and not to compete for scarce resources.[154]

Forming links with the community also involves a wider presence in communities. For example, EMERGE and Man Alive, the men's programme of the Marin Abused Women's Service, give talks to professionals, at schools and in all male professional groups. They combine individual reform and community change by urging former batterer's to give talks in the community and to raise the problem with workmates and male friends. According to Hamish Sinclair, of Man Alive:

> The Men's Program strategy is to promote a principled and active awareness among all men in the county to take responsibility wherever they are for a new public community response to dissolve the male role alliance that traditionally turns a blind eye to men's violence against women.[155]

EMERGE believes that talking about the problem in public forums can play a role in 'preventing it' and in reaching men who might not otherwise seek to end their violence. Public exclamation of the links between violence and male domination may also reduce stigma and create 'a climate of admission in the community which permits men to consider getting help without feeling they are sick.'[156] This account constitutes the vision, and sometimes achievements, of pro-feminist programmes for violent men which face extraordinary obstacles in implementing these ideals.

Programmes for men also present several dilemmas. A continual concern is that programmes for men will divert energy, resources and public attention away from the urgent needs of abused women and their children. They may increase risks to women if they inadvertently reinforce violence while seeking to end it and some programmes are not properly attuned to the problem of protecting victims. Group work may offer many competing messages, and men may choose those which appear to reinforce their existing interpretations and actions. There is always the danger that those who run such groups may inadvertently collude with batterers by supporting, or failing to reject, common notions that deny or diminish the violence and/or men's responsiblity, that deflect blame elsewhere and generally shift attention away from the violence and the man. Programmes may also increase the risks to women by giving them false hopes that their partners will be transformed through this work, and thus provide another mechanism for entrapping women in violent relationships. Programmes may even provide men with new techniques and a language for moving from physical to psychological coercion. Many programmes report that men go into counselling for the purely instrumental reason that they want their partners to return, and drop out once this occurs. As with criminal justice innovations, there is always the danger of race- and class-based forms of discrimination by funnelling only working-class and minority men through court mandated programmes.

It is too early to determine the success of the pro-feminist programmes although the limited amount of initial research has shown some success in reducing violence.[157] Whether this means that men acquire new and sustained patterns of non-violent behaviour is not yet known. Nor do we know, and this has not been researched, whether such programmes are making meaningful contributions to social change. It seems clear, however, that if social and personal change is to occur, these efforts should be linked to the movement and the wider community. The ideal of the pro-feminist approach offers a better prospect of moving towards change than traditional therapeutic approaches because it alone addresses the issue of wider social change, and it alone rejects the violence unequivocally and holds the perpetrator responsible for eliminating his violent behaviour.

8 Knowledge and social change

What is the role of research in the context of social movements and social change? What role does research have in shaping public perceptions of the social problems and social issues addressed by social movements? Does research have any relationship to social movements, to social change and to the activities of the state? If so, what is that relationship and what impact does such work have upon the progress of social change? There are those who would say that research has and/or should have no impact on the 'real' world; that researchers are isolated in ivory towers cut off from the rest of society; or, that, at best, research produces knowledge only for others in academia. On the other hand, there are those who maintain that knowledge gained through research can and should shape the policies and practices subsequently designed to guide and direct social life. Among researchers there are differing views about applicability and relevance. One position is that research can and should remain apart from all social and political considerations as an objective, value-free, technical activity uncontaminated by any form of contact with the world in which it is produced. Another position is that research is constructed within and is affected by the context of the world in which it exists, and that it enters into the arena of social and political change. A more extreme position of the latter is that research not only enters into the arena of social change but should, in fact, direct such activity.

Based on studies of the development of science, it is now clear that the entire research process is affected by the historical background and the contemporary arenas in which it is conducted and that research, in turn, affects that social context.[1] Values, beliefs and judgements are an integral aspect of all research affecting choices at every point in the research process.[2] For those who would define research as completely divorced from the social world, one has only to consider, for example, the orientation of the Moynihan Report towards the black family in the USA in the late 1960s, the continuing impact of John Bowlby's work on maternal bonding in Britain in the 1930s, the profound influence of Keynesian economics in the post-war era and, in the same period, the effect of Cyril Burt's work on British educational policy.[3] All of these, along with many others, have had considerable impact on public conceptions of issues of the day and on public policies concerning those issues.

Briefly to cite but one of these examples, the focus and findings of Cyril Burt's researches on inherited 'educable capacity' reflected the class and race orientations and prejudices of their time. Using the Standford–Binet IQ test he supposedly discovered persistent and significant differences in test results for working- and middle-class youngsters. These findings entered into the public arena early in the twentieth century and were subsequently instrumental in the creation of the 'eleven-plus' examination, an important pillar of the English system of selective education in the immediate post-war era. The 'eleven plus' examination was the pivot of a tiered education system effectively excluding from elite schools most working-class children, who were considered to have a limited capacity for learning, and streaming them into separate schools with a restricted range of subjects. It is important to note that Burt's findings were, in fact, falsified, yet they were accepted unchallenged for several decades by the public, policy makers and academics alike, largely because they clearly reflected and supported the dominant prejudices about inherent class difference.[4]

ACADEMIC PERSPECTIVES, DEFINITIONS OF PROBLEMS AND SOLUTIONS

Research is not only affected by the wider social context; more specific factors also make a difference. In approaching any area for study, the researcher usually begins from the vantage point of their academic discipline and often with a view to using a particular method for gathering information. While this may seem to make little difference, it is, in fact, important as it affects how the problem is initially defined. This, in turn, sets a path for the research which includes certain categories of explanation, methods of investigation and solutions, while excluding others. For example, the beginning point for studying an issue such as violence against women may reside in biology, psychology, sociology, economics, theology or history. Each sets parameters within which the investigator operates in defining the problem, shaping theoretical ideas and selecting the methods deemed most appropriate for gathering valid information. For example, socio-economic and historical accounts focus on the specific individual manifestations of a social problem but also place individuals within a wider context. This approach makes it possible to consider the nature of violence as a dynamic process affecting the lives of men and women while locating this process in a wider context. A contextual approach includes an analysis of factors such as the impact of cultural beliefs and values on violent behaviour and the response of victims; the effect of economic factors (particularly women's economic dependence) on the ability of women to leave violent men; and the impact of institutional response on such violence. Historical analysis, important in its own right, also provides an even wider context from which to understand the contemporary manifestations of a problem. Solutions to problems so defined may be located in the motivational and interpretative repertoires of individuals concerned, but also within the wider beliefs and values about men and women and wives as well as institutional responses to violence in marriage. Biological and psychological approaches primarily emphasize the traits and characteristics of individuals, and the topics to be researched are defined accordingly.

Once an issue has been defined in a specific way, the method of investigation and the possible solutions are encapsulated within that original definition. For example, the focus on individuals and their characteristics might lead to research questions such as 'what are the psychological attributes of violent men?' and 'what are the psychological maladies of women who will not leave them?'. We saw in the last chapter how a focus on individuals has led to a stress on research questions focusing on individual traits rather than on social and economic factors, and to questions framed in terms of the characteristics of women who stay with violent men. Since the answer to this particular question has been sought in the backgrounds and personality traits of women, then the solutions to the problem so defined can only reside in these characteristics and behaviour. Thus, it can be seen that such an approach leads to proposed solutions to the problem that reside in women and necessitates change in their behaviour in order that they solve the problem of male violence. The technology for achieving these changes is individual therapy with women.

In both countries, investigations of violence in the home have included a range of issues and used a variety of research methods. In the USA, however, an emphasis on individual characteristics and the social survey have dominated. The survey has been used to investigate the extent of the problem and to try to identify the social and psychological characteristics of those involved. Using the results of surveys, social scientists correlate background characteristics such as age, level of education, race, social class and occupation with incidence of violence in an attempt to discover what kind of people experience it and why. The main thrust of research in the USA has been attempts to correlate background characteristics of individuals with the incidence of violence.

In Britain, the majority of the research has extended beyond individual characteristics and used a broader range of methods for gathering information. Very little British research has tried to describe or explain the problem in terms of the background or psychological characteristics of the individuals involved. Instead, the focus has been on the dynamic processes associated with the problem itself as well as the responses to it. Major government funded research projects have focused on living and working in refuges; detailed accounts of violent events and a violent relationship; the beliefs and reactions of professionals working within social institutions including housing, the justice system and social and medical services.[5] While most of these facets of the issue have also been studied in the USA, they have not enjoyed the attention received in Britain largely because this diversity of issues and approaches has been overshadowed by an emphasis on national surveys exploring the characteristics of individuals. In Britain, the data collection techniques used to study the various facets of the problem include surveys of women experiencing violence and seeking assistance, depth interviews, analysis of official police, court and social work records, historical analysis, ethnographic approaches and participant observation. Again a diversity of methods has been used in the United States, but they are often accorded inferior status to surveys.

Contrasting approaches to research reflect different orientations to the nature of valid knowledge and alternative sources of sponsorship. In the post-war era social science has become increasingly dependent on support from agencies of the state and today the official response to new or emerging social issues almost always includes a call for research, much of which is funded by agencies of the state. Consequently forms of research and the questions asked are, to some extent, a reflection of the orientations of state agencies. In the United States much of the research on violence in the home has been supported by the National Institute of Mental Health (NIMH) and for the criminal justice system, LEAA and later the National Institute of Justice (NIJ).[6] They reflect concern for individual mental health and law enforcement, and each funds research according to their remit.

The NIMH has been especially important in funding research in this area and it has emphasized the use of the social survey. In Britain, funding has come from a range of agencies, including the Home Office, Welsh Office, Scottish Office, the Department of Environment, the Department of Health and the Department of Social Security. Accordingly, they have funded research on the provision of refuge and housing, criminal justice response, and health and social services. British government support for research on violence against women has included considerable funding for projects involving researchers from within or closely aligned with the movement and for a number of collaborative efforts of academic researchers and the movement.[7] As with the public hearings in Parliament and Civil Rights Commission whose proposals for change ultimately reflected the basic focus and resources of existing state agencies and the usual responses to social problems (legal, therapeutic or material), funded research also follows a predictable pattern. While not determining findings *per se*, state funding often determines the focus of research on particular aspects of the problem to be studied (sometimes even the research method) and these, in turn, have an impact on the findings.

THE MOVEMENT AND RESEARCH

From the vantage point of social movements, research and the researchers themselves may be seen as allies or adversaries. Research may assist social movements in identifying social issues and bringing them to public attention. In this way research in both Britain and the USA has been instrumental in establishing that violence against women in the home is both widespread and severe, and in this respect, research has been an ally of the movements.[8] But in terms of debates about the nature of the problem itself and proposals for social change, research has sometimes been an ally, sometimes an adversary. The identity of the movement and of the issue itself, as well as the authority of activists and of their knowledge, are all at stake in their relationship with academic research. To the extent that a social movement has identified the social problem, those who experience it and the movement itself in a particular way, research programmes may sufficiently challenge or change the definition of the problem and those who experience it to such an extent that the movement loses the problem, its own identity and/or its *raison d'être*.

In both countries, the movements raised several issues concerning research. At the Parliamentary hearings in Britain and at the Civil

Rights hearings in the USA, activists asked whether resources should
be spent on research or channelled directly into social services. Activists in the USA were particularly concerned about what they felt
was an overemphasis on research to the detriment of funding for
services. In her presentation before the Civil Rights Commission,
Shelley Fernandez, founder of La Casa de las Madres shelter in San
Francisco, stated:

> We don't want research and demonstration grants, we don't need
> the luxury of research grants. Women are suffering and hurting.
> We know the problems of battered women, we need money to
> establish shelters to work on methods to share our knowledge with
> the thousands of people across the Nation who need to open
> shelters with adequate and ongoing funding.[9]

They particularly objected to vast sums of money being expended on
investigations of the magnitude of the problem, arguing that it was
unnecessary because their work made it clear that the problem was
widespread and significant. Research, they stressed, should focus on
helping the movement, 'understand the problem better and [to] do
something about it'.[10] In Britain, Women's Aid urged 'further
research as soon as possible' and in both countries the principle of
collaborative research was seen as the best method of ensuring the
production of valid and useful knowledge.[11] Lisa Leghorn, an
American activist, urged, 'Any research that is conducted should be
conducted hand in hand with women who have been through the
abuse', a sentiment echoed by Scottish Women's Aid: '... we feel
research should be undertaken *by interested and committed groups
like Women's Aid* and that it is a matter of urgency that *central
government* should make *money* available for this purpose'.[12]

While not altogether antagonistic to research, activists, nonetheless, did not see it as a priority in light of the pragmatic problems they
faced in meeting the immediate crisis of responding to women and
children fleeing from violence. To the extent that research was to be
undertaken, concern was expressed about the level of activists'
participation in the process, whether their insights would be built
upon or ignored, and whether their own source of knowledge
founded on a growing base of direct experience would be used,
ignored, subverted and/or lose its legitimacy in the face of academic
knowledge. There was concern about who was to do the research,
what their orientations might be, and how the privacy, integrity and
safety of abused women would be respected. Would the research be
useful to women and to the agenda of change, or would it be an

abstract enterprise destined for the lecture halls and the library shelves of academia? In the USA, activists initially articulated concerns about research based on experiences of the anti-rape movement in which resources allocated for direct services were diverted to research.[13] In Britain, it was asked whether research funded by the government would or could be of value to abused women, the movement and an agenda of social change.[14]

In the USA in particular, relations between the movement and researchers and among researchers themselves are even more complex and raised very early the spectre of the researcher as ally or adversary. This centred on the notion of 'battered husbands'. From the beginning, in every public forum where the topic of violence against wives was discussed, the question of 'what about battered husbands?' was usually raised but rarely taken too seriously. In the USA, however, this notion has been defined by some researchers as a problem of equal or even greater frequency and severity to that of violence against women. Accordingly, the definition of the problem shifts to beaten men and violent women. The issue of 'beaten husbands' was identified as a contentious issue at the hearings of the Civil Rights Commission where advocates and others objected to the nature of the research conducted and the claims made. Leghorn pointed out that the researchers did not consider the issue of self-defence.

> This represents an inexcusable oversight, since most women who have been violent towards their husbands have done so only as a last resort, in self-defense against long-standing terror and abuse from their husbands.[15]

Thus, early in its history, the American movement was forced to struggle against these notions because, in the words of Leghorn, they have been and '... will continue to be used as an argument against funding shelters for women'.[16] Groups have reported difficulties in obtaining shelter funding because they were not providing services to 'battered husbands'.[17] Activists have expended considerable time and resources attempting to counter this view and to minimize its potentially damaging effects. There is an overtly antagonistic relationship between the movement and some researchers in the US and in 1987 the Activist Research Task Force (ART) was formed as a means of bringing together activists and more sensitive and informed researchers.[18]

The notion of 'battered husbands' and the research which spawned it has been the major focus of debate regarding research within the movement and among researchers. In light of the public and academic attention accorded this notion and the debates surrounding it, it is important to explore the claims and research methods of those who have identified violent women and battered husbands as a problem of equal importance to that of violent men and battered women. In the remainder of this chapter notions and evidence regarding the supposed symmetrical nature of violence in the home – women as equally violent as men – will be contrasted with the evidence and research methods demonstrating the asymmetrical nature of violence in the home. Two main research approaches and the competing evidence they have produced will be considered in this analysis. These two research positions shall be referred to as the family violence approach (FV) and the violence against women approach (VAW).[19] In order to explore the issues surrounding this debate, we shall examine the claims and counter-claims of these two approaches, consider alternative evidence and explanations and analyse the methodological assumptions leading to competing findings. In conducting this analysis we shall demonstrate that the claims of equivalence in violence and its impact are false and that this has come about because of the choice of a narrow, and ultimately, flawed approach to research.

FAMILY VIOLENCE RESEARCH AND THE 'BATTERED HUSBAND SYNDROME'

FV researchers believe that the problem in the United States and elsewhere is not one of violent men or one of violence against women, but is, instead, one of 'spouse abuse', 'violent people' and 'violent couples'. According to these commentators, women and men are equally likely to be aggressors and victims of violence in the family, and they maintain that there are as many beaten and battered husbands as battered women.

In 1974 a member of the FV group claimed his research revealed that wives were almost as violent as husbands.[20] Two national surveys conducted by FV researchers have reinforced these early claims and even found that wives are more violent than husbands. Based on the results of the first survey, FV researchers concluded that in 1974, 11.6 per cent of men were victimized by their wives and 12.1 per cent of women were victimized by their husbands. In 1985, this near equivalence of husbands and wives as victims was found again, except this time men were slightly more likely to be victims (12.1 per cent) than were women (11.3 per cent).[21] When these researchers focused only on what they defined as 'severe violence', they found more male than female victims. 'Severe violence' was inflicted on 4.6 per cent (n=91) of husbands and 3.8 per cent (n=81) of wives in 1975, and 4.4 per cent (n=154) of husbands and 3.0 per cent (n=105) of wives in 1985.[22] Based on these results, FV commentators estimate that in 1985 6.8 million US husbands and 6.25 million US wives were physically victimized by their partner.[23] Following the theme of women as more violent than men, they further estimate that, in a given year, the women in their study perpetrated ten attacks on their husbands while the men committed nine assaults on their wives.[24] FV commentators also claim that women often take the initiative in starting violent quarrels and violence,[25] and are more likely to use or threaten to use weapons than are their male partners.[26] On the basis of these data, FV researchers have concluded that men and women commit the same amount of violence and have similar intentions and motivations:

> Everything we have found points to parallel processes that lead women and men to become violent.... Women may be more likely than men to use kitchen utensils or sewing scissors when they commit assault, but their frustrations, motives and lack of control over these feelings predictably resemble men's.[27]

In the late 1970s, FV researchers proclaimed a 'battered husband syndrome' although no equivalent 'battered woman syndrome' was reported.[28] Extrapolating from the first national survey, it was claimed that 'at least 250,000 American husbands are severely thrashed by their wives [every year]. ... The most unreported crime is not wife beating – it's husband beating.'[29] According to some of these reports, men are more likely to suffer injuries within the family: 'Clearly, violence against men is much more destructive than is violence against women.... Male victims are injured more often and more seriously than are female victims.'[30] Summarizing the results of the two national surveys another FV exponent claimed, 'When all severely violent acts were examined, the data indicated that women as a group were more violent to their male partners, and more men than women were victimized'.[31] In light of evidence and claims such as these, the leading proponent of the FV position proclaimed that 'the marriage license is a "hitting license"', and asserted that

> ... violence between husband and wife is far from a one way street. The old cartoons of the wife chasing the husband with a rolling pin or throwing pots and pans are closer to reality than most (and especially those with feminist sympathies) realize.[32]

These remarkably counter-intuitive claims are primarily based on the results of two national surveys of American couples in which men and women were asked questions from a list of acts included in a scale referred to as the Conflict Tactics Scales (CTS).[33] The CTS presents respondents with a series of questions about how they settle 'disputes' and a list of nineteen 'acts' (eighteen in the original version), ranging from 'discussed an issue calmly' to 'threw something at him/her/you' and 'beat him/her/you up'. These acts are then grouped into three sub-scales: 'Reasoning', 'Verbal Aggression' and 'Physical Aggression' (also called 'Violence'). The 'Violence' scale is then further divided into 'Minor Violence' and 'Severe Violence' based on the assumed *potential* for injury associated with each of the acts. Based on the results of surveys using the CTS, FV researchers believe the 'truth about' domestic violence is that 'women are as violent, if not more so than men'.[34]

To a much lesser extent, FV researchers have attempted to use historical and psychological reports to support claims of equivalence in violence between men and women. Citing experimental psychological studies of aggression, McNeely and Robinson-Simpson claim that this literature shows that women are at least as physically aggressive as men.[35] Although the FV approach is basically ahistorical and representatives of this position do not actually conduct historical research, they, nonetheless, invoke eighteenth-century community chastisements of women accused of violent behaviour towards husbands as indicators of the widespread existence of husband beating in the past.[36] Comic strips from the 1950s depicting domineering and violent women and down trodden men are also used as further support, with FV researchers claiming that such comics were popular 'because they approximated, in a non-serious manner, common family situations...'.[37]

In trying to establish that women are just as violent as men, the FV researchers not only assert symmetry between adult partners but also invoke women's abuse of children and infanticide as evidence of the violent inclinations of women. Without citing any supporting evidence, FV researchers also imply that women who have been abused by male partners are prone to abuse their children, claiming, for example, that 'Almost all shelters for battered women are creating policies to deal with the high rate of child abuse ...' among their residents.[38] They further claim that the violence of mothers is responsible for creating the 'next generation' of abusive males.[39] Significantly, the violence and sexual abuse men direct at children is never or rarely considered in these discussions, leaving the impression that woman are the sole or primary perpetrators of child abuse. In reaching these conclusions, FV researchers first conflate acts such as 'neglect', 'severe physical abuse' and 'spanking', then define them all as child abuse. Having first conflated all of these acts in order to establish the violent nature of women, they then insinuate that women's violence towards children is equivalent to men's violence towards women. They go on to imply that these experiences cancel each other out and make women at least as responsible and guilty of violent behaviour as men, if not more so.[40] As Wardell, Gillespie and Leffler note the implication is '... that a mother's spanking her child, ... is equivalent to a husband's breaking his wife's ribs'.[41]

FV researchers further claim that men subjected to the violence of women '... are reluctant to come forward to seek help ...' and, just like women, are trapped in violent relationships, unable to obtain help from agencies and incapable of leaving.[42] Having claimed for abused men the same entrapment as for abused women, it follows that it is wrong to assume that men would encounter fewer social and economic difficulties in leaving a violent woman. It is a serious fallacy, one FV commentator notes, to assume battered husbands would find it easy to leave.

> This perspective rests on erroneous sexist assumptions. Although males, as a group, have considerably more economic security, if the husband leaves the family, he is still responsible for a certain amount of economic support of the family in addition to the cost of a separate residence for himself.... Interviews with abused men suggest that leaving the family home means leaving ... the comfortable and familiar, that which is not likely to be reconstructed in a small apartment.[43]

It is further asserted that many husbands endure persistent and severe violence at the hands of women, sacrificing their own well-being for the sake of their children: '... men are afraid to leave for fear that further violence would be directed towards the children ... they feel that by staying they are providing some protection for them'.[44] It is also claimed that these actions may lead to the further victimization of a man when, '... he steps in to protect the children and becomes the target of abuse'.[45] The same observer indicates that 'Only when the violence appeared to be affecting the children, rather than affecting the husband's physical safety, did the husband consider leaving'.[46] No substantial evidence is offered in support of either of these contradictory claims.

Seeking public policy for battered husbands

Family violence researchers are not detached, ivory tower academics; rather they seek to affect public perceptions and values concerning violence and to change policies and practices. Two of the main proponents note that they have produced books for the 'general public', had their work '... reported in every major [American] newspaper and on every major TV network', and '... appear on television several times a year'.[47] In these public settings and in their policy oriented statements, special concern is expressed about the failure to deal with the widespread violence against men in the home. Despite persistently reporting equivalence in the incidents of violence between spouses and the reputed existence of a 'battered husband syndrome', FV researchers bemoan the fact that violence against men is not considered a serious problem or accorded a high priority on the national agenda. They claim that denial and the lack of national recognition means that abused men do not receive the services they need: 'Any criminal justice concern for battered husbands was lost amidst the vociferous claims by those concerned with battered women that the issue of battered men was a red herring.'[48] In comparing the results of their two surveys, Straus and Gelles report that violence by wives against husbands has increased because:

> Violence by wives has not been an object of public concern. There has been no publicity, and no funds have been invested in ameliorating this problem because it has not been defined as a problem. Our finding of little change in the rate of assaults by women on their male partners is consistent with the absence of ameliorative program.[49]

Apparently this set of circumstances also operates to deny cadres of violent women '... legitimate access to resources that may reduce the stress and conflict that result from the multiple roles faced by women today, and that may help them develop nonviolent forms of interaction'.[50]

Family Violence researchers criticize activists and other researchers who fail to recognize the validity of the findings about violent women and battered men or who reject the methods used to create these findings:

> Unfortunately, there is a tendency for some feminist writers to deemphasize the importance of women's use of violence, and to attempt to discredit any research that suggests that women may use violence on their spouses.'[51]

They claim that 'There has been an almost conspiratorial silence about discussing women's violence towards men'.[52] Evidence indicating that men are actually more violent than women is discounted by FV researchers because they believe that all methods except their own result in overestimates of men's violence and under-estimates of women's, particularly because men are unwilling to report their wives violence because '... it would be unmanly or unchivalrous to go to the police for protection from a woman'.[53] The unwillingness and inability of women to report husbands is rarely, if ever, discussed by FV researchers.

They believe that national action is needed to correct erroneous conceptions about wife abuse and to deal with the significant and serious problem of 'battered husbands'. Evidence of other researchers which reveals the preponderance of male violence in the family is seen as mischievous, unfortunate, even dangerous: 'The danger of these misconceptions is that social policy, legislation, and the attitudes of officials and the public are being shaped by erroneous information.'[54] Some FV researchers even express concern about the efforts of the women's movement to assist female victims of violence in the home, alleging that supporting female victims has had deleterious consequences for men by creating an atmosphere in which women can 'falsely' accuse men of violence: 'Men increasingly are defenceless when allegations of domestic violence are made.'[55] More broadly,

> The politically charged atmosphere that pervades the broad array of gender-sensitive crimes such as marital rape, sexual abuse of children, and child abuse increasingly provides the means by which women are able to victimize men socially merely by alleging their occurrence.[56]

FV researchers have, by their own accounts, an unfortunate relationship with the movement in the United States primarily because of the claim of symmetry of violence between husbands and wives. The main protagonist of the FV perspective has complained that during the course of his research, '... the fact that wife beating became a feminist issue also created problems because it embroiled us in the politics of the women's movement'.[57] They report feeling besieged by other academics and members of the movement, and accuse them of '... bitter scholarly and personal attacks...'.[58]

VIOLENCE-AGAINST-WOMEN RESEARCH AND THE ABUSED WOMAN

The other body of research in this area, which we shall refer to as Violence Against Women (VAW), predates the discovery of battered wives in the 1970s and encompasses a wide-ranging body of knowledge emerging from a diverse research base. For the purpose of this discussion the main findings of this approach are that violence in the home is asymmetrical (with women the usual victims and men the usual offenders) and that the motivations and intentions of men and women are radically different. It is against this body of evidence that FV research stands as a pronounced and solitary counter-factual. In contrast to FV researchers' primary reliance on two surveys, these researchers use a variety of methods to gather evidence, including: historical, documentary, ethnographic, case-history, intensive interview and the survey. In addition, VAW researchers have gone beyond the narrow questions and restricted methods of the FV traditions to consider the dynamic nature of violence between men and women and to analyse the wider cultural and institutional contexts within which the problem emerged and continues.[59] VAW research has been especially important in documenting the dynamic nature of the violent event, the predicament of victims, and legal, medical and social service responses. Both qualitative and quantitative findings have been used and provide a very different view of violence between marriage partners – one which is often, though not always, informed by a feminist perspective.

Violent men and abused women

Criminal justice statistics show that men are much more likely than women to commit violent crimes whether in public or in private.[60] For assaults in the home, evidence from police and court records also demonstrate that men are disproportionately the perpetrators and women the victims. In the early stages of research in this arena when FVs researchers were first proclaiming the existence of a 'battered husband syndrome', other researchers were producing reviews of existing evidence on homicide, assault and divorce records which revealed a persistent pattern in the direction of violence in the home.[61] In 1975 after an extensive review of existing evidence, Lystad concluded, 'The occurrence of adult violence in the home usually involves males as aggressors towards females'.[62] We reached similar conclusions in our own review of research findings that existed prior to the public recognition of the problem in the 1970s.[63]

Research conducted after the public discovery of the problem of violence against women confirms these early conclusions. Evidence from police and court records and from national victim surveys unequivocally support the finding of asymmetry. A remarkably persistent pattern of male violence directed at female partners emerges from the analysis of police files in Britain and North America. Reports from the United States and Canada indicate that 90–95 per cent of the victims of domestic assaults are women and only 5–10 per cent are men. Investigations of police calls/reports and court records reveal a consistent pattern with violence against women constituting the overwhelming proportion of cases: 96 per cent in Minnesota, 95 per cent in two Canadian studies, 95 per cent in New York study; 94 per cent in San Diego County, 93 per cent in Detriot, 92 per cent in Ohio, 90 per cent in Monroe County, New York.[64] Scottish research employing a more intensive analysis of police and court records found that 99 per cent of assaults between spouses involved men assaulting their partner.[65]

Other evidence of the asymmetrical nature of violence between spouses emerges from national surveys of victims conducted in the United States, Canada and Great Britain. The United States National Crime Survey of victims has been conducted annually since 1972, and has used national probability samples of nearly 60,000 households. As many as seven consecutive intensive interviews have been conducted with members of each household resulting in nearly a million interviews. Gaquin's analysis of National Crime Survey data for the period between 1973 and 1975 reveals that men 'have almost no risk of being assaulted by their wives'.[66] Ninety-seven per cent of all assaults on adults in the family were attacks on wives. Using the National Crime Survey data for the period between 1973 and 1980, McLeod reports that 94 per cent of assaults between adults in the home were wife assaults.[67] Based on a compilation of the National Crime Survey data from 1973–82, Schwartz found only 102 men (4 per cent of incidents) who claimed to be victims of assaults by their spouses in contrast to 1,641 women.[68] For Canada, the 1988 Canadian Urban Victimization Survey of 60,000 respondents and the 1982 General Social Survey of 10,000 show that ... women account for 80–90 per cent of victims in assaults or sexual assaults between spouses or former spouses. In fact, the number of domestic incidents involving male victims was too low in both surveys to provide reliable estimates.[69] Half of the female victims in the Victimization Survey were assaulted more than once during the year of the survey, and 6 per cent of the women were attacked five or more times. Finally, the

1982 and 1984 British Crime Survey revealed that *all* victims of domestic violence were women.[70] Results such as these provide strong evidence from a variety of data sources that women, and not men, are overwhelmingly the victims of violence between spouses. These data stand in direct opposition to the claim that women are just as violent as men.

National Crime Surveys and criminal justice records also demonstrate that women are much more likely than men to suffer injury from assaults. In southern California, research based on police records found that when injuries were used as the criterion, the idea of mutual combat between husbands and wives becomes a myth. Berk, Berk, Loseke and Rauma conclude that '... a marriage license is a hitting license BUT FOR MEN ONLY'.[71] Schwartz's analysis of USA Crime Survey results reveals that the problem of injuries to women is much more serious than for men. He also shows how some commentators have misrepresented evidence of injuries by considering only the rate, which is based on an extraordinarily small number for men and is therefore unreliable. He points out that there are '... more than 13 times as many women [as men] seeking medical care from a private physician for injuries received in a spousal assault'.[72]

FV researchers do not accept this evidence maintaining that official reports are subject to reporting bias and that the results of Crime Surveys are suspect because they explore violence in the context of asking about 'crime'. Their strongest criticism is based on the assumption that men will simply not come forward to report their victimization at the hands of women. Steinmetz maintains that 'husband-beating' is a very camouflaged social problem because men who report their violent partners would face extraordinary stigma. The under-reporting of women is rarely referred to in these discussions. Fortunately there is some evidence regarding women's rate of reporting and a few comparisons of the differentials in reporting by men and women. In our own study, we estimated that of nearly 35,000 violent attacks experienced by women, only 2 per cent were reported to the police.[73] Rouse and colleagues reported that men were more likely than women to call the police after experiencing violence by intimate partners.[74] Kincaid found, in her analysis of 337 cases of violence drawn from 3,125 family court files in Ontario, Canada, that men are more likely than women to press charges against their spouses. She found, '... while there were 17 times as many female as male victims, only 22 per cent of women laid charges while almost 40 per cent of men did so'.[75] Men were also four to five times more likely than women to pursue a complaint, and were less likely to drop charges. Kincaid's intensive investigation also reveals that men bring wives to court not so much because of their violence, but when women attempt to leave or when they are considered quarrelsome and nagging. A male 'victim', she notes, goes to court '... in order to get help in bringing his wife "into line" (his line!)' and many court personnel appeared to collude with these efforts.[76]

Historical evidence

Historical evidence has repeatedly demonstrated that women were the most usual victims of violence in the home in European and American societies.[77] Within the family the use of physical force and violence has traditionally been a prerogative of men who were given the rights and responsibilities over all members of households, including women, children, servants and, in the United States, slaves. This prerogative was supported well into the nineteenth century through religious and legal prescriptions and rulings. Throughout recorded history, men were urged, usually by the Church, to rule over their domestic subjects with kindness and respect; beating them only for serious transgressions against family order. It appears, however, that many men ignored this ministerial advice, preferring to employ coercion, intimidation, violence and terror as a more usual means of control. Men, at least before the nineteenth century, were rarely punished for these offences. It was only when men's conduct became flagrant outrages and/or a public nuisance that they might be subjected to community censure and rebuke.[78]

Despite the claims of FV researchers, VAW researchers have not ignored or denied the violence of women in the past or the present. Indeed, they have conducted the most comprehensive and scholarly historical and anthropological work in this area analysing, for example, the role of women in child abuse, infanticide and other forms of violence.[79] These studies have also been careful to explore the cultural, situational and motivational contexts within which such violence occurs. This provides a foundation for explaining such behaviour which completely undermines the claims of FV researchers. A context based approach demonstrates, for example, that when women do commit acts such as infanticide, these are usually 'acts of desperation ... principally the products of desperate circumstances'.[80] Cross-cultural evidence demonstrates that infanticide sometimes occurs because of cultural beliefs about deformed children but, most commonly because of desperate material circumstances that 'limit the capacity to care for the child', often because men are unwilling to assume responsibility for parental support.[81] Historical evidence for eighteenth- and nineteenth-century Britain and the United States demonstrates that infanticide often occurred after unmarried women were seduced or raped, frequently by masters or sons of the household.[82] Such infanticides occurred in the context of virulent Christian persecution of bastardy in which women could be executed both for concealing a pregnancy out of wedlock and for infanticide. This wider and more careful analysis illustrates quite clearly that these were usually acts of desperation. Although certainly resulting in tragic consequences, they cannot reasonably be equated with acts motivated by base aggression and hostility.

Historical studies of community responses to violence also point to the unusual occurrence of violence against husbands. Scholars have shown how this was an unusual event in the deeply patriarchal societies of the past.[83] Community rituals, such as charivaris and misrules, were sometimes performed against the husband or the wife to censure a violent wife, but these were rare because of the rarity of the behaviour. More common were rituals and physical punishments aimed at censuring the wagging tongues of nagging wives for upsetting the 'natural' patriarchal order.[84] From late medieval times to well into the nineteenth century women could be subjected to symbolic and physical punishments, such as cucking and ducking stools and the branks bridle, as means of restoring domestic tranquillity. Men might also be subjected to community rituals, usually because they were considered guilty of allowing an inversion of the natural, patriarchal order or were judged to be dominated or cuckolded by a wife. It is important to note that such men were not usually punished physically or severely for 'domestic crimes', as were wives, but were, instead, subjected to highly ritualized and symbolic ceremonies such as rough music and the cuckold's court.[85] Cuckold courts and other responses to men so 'abused' by their wives were generally frivolous, mocking affairs, ridiculing and condemning a *monstrous* and *unusual* inversion of the patriarchal order.

The same interpretation applies to twentieth-century comics which were popular because they mocked and ridiculed the unusual inversion of the patriarchal family and not, as FV researchers claim, because they represented 'common family situations'. They are a modern representation of the lessons portrayed in the traditional domestic manuals warning against the evils of 'marriages turned upside down'.[86] Some manuals were solemn while others were satirical, but all expressed misogynist male concerns about controlling domestic order (read: women). Dutch manuals of the seventeenth century often included cartoons representing these concerns depicting wives overturning the domestic order by wearing the breeches, beating husbands and forcing them to do all the domestic chores.[87] Contemporary cartoons are merely perpetuating a centuries long tradition associated with the symbolic support of the domestic order. Mocking community rituals and their modern equivalent in comics are attempts to remind both partners by ridiculing one or the other that a woman is not to 'forget the respect she owes her husband'.[88]

The nature of violence against women

Evidence from police and court records, national crime surveys and historical documentation all confirm the asymmetrical pattern of male violence directed at female partners. In addition to the patterning of violence, it is also important to examine in detail the nature of the violent event, the relationships in which it occurs, the intentions of offenders, the predicament of victims and the responses of agencies. Using depth interviews with women who have experienced violence as well as detailed analysis of official documents from police, court and social service records, VAW researchers have constructed fullsome accounts of the lives of victims, the violent events they experience and their treatment by agencies of the state.

Research has shown that violence experienced by women is most likely to occur in intimate relationships with men. Whether it be sexual assault, rape or physical assault, females are at greater risk from fathers, husbands, boyfriends and acquaintances than from strangers, and there is almost no risk from other women.[89] The onset of systematic and severe violence against women is almost exclusively associated with entering a permanent relationship with a man. Violence against women in the home is a unique phenomenon in the world of violence. Only in a prison or similar total institution would an individual be likely to encounter such persistent abuse, violence and terror.

The intensive study of the violent event makes it possible to provide full 'blow-by-blow' accounts of the whole event including the sequence of events preceding the violence, the various forms of physical and sexual attack composing a single event, the intentions of the attacker, the responses of the victim, a detailed account of resulting injuries, and the immediate responses of the victim and attacker.[90] Examining the violent event as a dynamic process from beginning to end shows that various forms of physical attack are usually employed by men in any single violent episode, and that violent episodes may occur as often as twice a week. Findings from our own research and those of others show that the most common form of attack involves men repeatedly slapping and punching women, often to the floor, followed by kicking.[91] In any single event men usually use a diverse combination of violent acts, including: pushing and pulling (sometimes against injurious objects), hair pulling, punching, kicking, hitting with belts and household objects, biting, banging heads on walls, burning, choking and smothering, and, brandishing and using weapons such as knives and guns.

This research also reveals that women are subjected to another series of acts that are ignored by FV researchers, forced sex and sexual assault. Men often force women to engage in sexual acts against their will as a part of a process of humiliation and domination.[92] Russell's important studies first pointed to the frequent occurrence of sexual assault within marriage and Frieze has recently found that physical violence is often associated with sexual violence, with one-third of the women in her sample reporting being raped by their violent partner.[93] Kelly's intensive interviews with British women provide detailed accounts of the nature of sexual violence within intimate relationships.[94] VAW researchers have also provided much more detailed evidence concerning the nature of injuries received during these violent attacks. This has included elaborate accounts of the consequences of a given violent attack, and shows that the most common injuries women receive are bruising of the face, limbs and body, as well as cuts and abrasions, torn hair, broken teeth, fractured bones, burns, internal injuries and miscarriages.[95]

Even this catalogue of acts and injuries is incomplete, creating only a partial picture of women's experiences. VAW researchers have shown that violent acts involve a wide array of techniques employed in the context of near continuous threats, coercion and intimidation associated with men's attempts to control, dominate and punish women. Women are often captives in their own homes where men seek to isolate them from others including friends, relatives, suspected lovers (milkmen and repairmen), or representatives of official agencies. Given that women as a group are generally under-employed, earning low pay and/or working part-time, they are likely to be economically dependent on a male wage earner or on state benefit. This lack of economic independence means that those who are violently abused have great difficulties in leaving such relationships because they have few viable alternatives.

When women hit back

In studying these facets of the problem, VAW researchers have, unlike FV researchers, actually systematically investigated the responses of women to men's violent acts. The findings show that women sometimes, although not often, respond to men's violence with counter violence, usually in self-defence and occasionally in retaliation for abuse.[96] However, most women attempt to avoid the onset of men's violence by pleading, cajoling and diverting them. Once the violence starts, women continue these efforts while also attempting to protect themselves and/or to escape. Research shows that women rarely respond to men's violent attacks with direct physical force. Fewer than 4% of women in a Scottish study said they sometimes responded with physical force with any frequency.

> There was one time I hit him back. He started to hit me and I really sort of broke. I never used to hit him back when he hit me, but I sort of really cracked. He'd a good drink in him so that he wasn't very sober, and I just took him by the hair and I banged his face on the back of the chair ... And I just screamed at him, and I'm shaking him by the hair, and saying, 'Are you going to hit me again?' And I just kept shouting, 'Are you going to hit me again?'[97]

British and American research reveals that, for the most part, women usually remain physically passive in order, they believe, to avoid a more serious or prolonged attack. Most women believe that attempts at self-protection or retaliation only increase the severity of an attack.[98] Concurring with earlier research, Saunders's study of a group of physically abused women in the United States shows that their violence is typically associated with self-defence, involves a narrow range of acts and is not usually intended to inflict injury.[99]

Violent women and battered husbands?

Findings of VAW researchers based on contemporary and historical studies using intensive and extensive methods persistently reveal a pattern of asymmetrical violence between men and women. Although the predominant pattern is one of male violence directed at a female partner, this does not mean that women absolutely never use violence under any circumstances. When they do, however, it is usually in a context in which they have been repeatedly assaulted by the man and are trying to defend themselves and/or stop his violence.

Although FV researchers persist in claiming that the violence is symmetrical, that women are as violent as men and that men are equally as trapped in relationships thus leading to a 'battered husband syndrome', they offer no systematic, in-depth evidence in support of this claim. Instead, a few anecdotal cases are offered amidst a wholesale conceptual confusion in which non-violent acts are conflated with violent acts.[100] For example, Shupe, Stacey and Hazelwood spend a great deal of time discussing physically violent women terrorizing husbands, yet they present no systematic evidence of this phenomenon. Instead, they become confused and diverted and discuss how women take 'the initiative in starting a violent quarrel with men' and that women file criminal charges against violent men.[101] Starting a *quarrel* whether or not it eventually leads to an event in which a man is violent and *filing charges* against a man who has been violent are not indicators of women's violence. Attempting to file a police charge against a man who has been violent may be an attempt to stop violence, one of seeking help or an expression of anger or retribution, but without a wholesale transformation of definitions, these acts cannot conceivably be defined as violence. While acts such as these do not constitute violence, they are, nonetheless, used by FV researchers as evidence of aggressively violent women. FV observers also fail to recognize that many non-violent tactics used by women trapped in violent relationships are more appropriately understood as defences of the weak. The following example of the responses of the wife of a clergyman who beat her for years appears in a discussion of violent women.

> For years she had purposely misironed her husband's shirts and overcooked or undercooked his meals. She laughed as she revealed that she always made sure she served him food on cracked plates, gave him the bent fork or chipped drinking glass, and even made it a point to break the yokes in his eggs no matter how he wanted them cooked. Her revenge was that he never knew.[102]

Again, where is the violence? Presumably this woman's attempts, through subtle, clever and devious means to preserve some dignity in the face of continuous violence, behaviour often evident in people subjugated by oppressors, are somehow equated with physical violence and used as an indicator of women's aggression rather than being understood as a non-violent response to violence. In light of this sort of analysis, one must seriously ask if this sort of example is intended to provide an illustration of a violent woman or a battered husband. While it is possible to imagine that a few men do exist who have suffered the same sort of continuous violence, intimidation, humiliation and domination at the hands of women in the home as experienced by countless numbers of women at the hands of men, there is no convincing evidence of their existence. Women are not likely to seek to control and dominate their husbands through violence; they are rarely, if ever, equipped with the training, physical stature and cultural supports for carrying-out such an agenda.

Homicides in the home, when women kill

Historical, anthropological and contemporary evidence indicates that the worldwide pattern of homicide is one in which men are over-whelmingly the killers, usually of other men and sometimes of women.[103] The worldwide pattern of domestic homicides, except in the USA, is also one in which men are primarily the killers of wives, fiancés and intimate partners.[104] As victims, men are usually killed by acquaintances and strangers and sometimes by a male or female intimate; by contrast, women are most likely to be killed by male intimates and not usually by strangers. In the United States, of all women killed between 1980 and 1984, approximately 52 per cent were murdered by husbands, boyfriends and male cohabitees.[105] In England and Wales, females are four to nine times more likely than males to be killed by spouses, ex-spouses, cohabitees and ex-cohabitees.[106]

Despite this asymmetrical pattern, some women do employ lethal violence against male partners, and it is important to investigate the nature of these acts and the motivational contexts in which they occur.[107] The evidence indicates that the reasons for domestic homicide are markedly different for men and women. Men often kill women because of sexual proprietariness and possessiveness, and this is especially likely when women attempt to leave. Women do not usually kill men because of jealousy, despite men's more adulterous behaviour. Men, unlike women, commit familicides, killing their partner and children. Men kill women as part of a planned murder or suicide; women rarely do so. Men hunt down and kill ex-partners, sometimes after years of pursuit; women rarely pursue ex-partners and are even less likely to kill them. These are the acts of men and rarely those of women.

When women do kill, the victim is usually an intimate partner and often one from whom they have suffered years of physical abuse.

Women usually kill men in acts of self-preservation when their situation has reached a desperate state, when they believe they are likely to be killed and while defending themselves.[108] Women, unlike men, rarely kill in the context of their own ongoing, coercive, hostile aggression. When women kill men, it is usually in the context of men's aggressive and violent behaviour towards them. It would follow that a reduction in men's violence against women in the home would lead to a reduction in the number of women pressed to the point at which they commit homicide.

'FACTS' OBSCURING REALITY: THE COUNTER FACTUAL AND THE COUNTER INTUITIVE

As this review has demonstrated the asymmetrical pattern of male violence against women in the home is supported by research findings across cultures and across time. Yet, in the United States two contradictory bodies of evidence and analysis compete to represent the reality of assaults between men and women in the home. FV researchers claim to have found symmetry in the nature and occurrence of assaults between men and women in the home. Not only is this claim counter-intuitive to what most members of the public and researchers actually believe, it is also counter-factual and at odds with what the vast body of evidence actually shows. In fact, the vast body of evidence reveals an extraordinary asymmetry in the direction, motivations and acts associated with assaults between intimates. In Britain, Europe, Canada, Australia, Asia, Africa, South and Latin America, and the Soviet Union the problem is believed to be and research findings show it to be violence against women. It is imperative, therefore, that one must ask if there is something peculiar about society in the USA or about its social science. What has created this extraordinarily counter-factual case, resulting in the claim that there are at least as many, and perhaps more, beaten husbands as beaten wives? Could it be that women in the United States are violent viragos? Could it be that men in the United States are unlike men elsewhere? Both seem unlikely. Although the United States has a higher recorded rate of violence than any other industrialized country, this is primarily a result of violence between young adult males in public settings. The reason for the supposed differences in patterns of assaults in the home cannot be situated in the distinct violent behaviour of members of families in the United States, but must reside in the distinct nature of the FV research used to create and support such claims.

Findings reputedly illustrating parity in assaults between husbands and wives are, in fact, an artifact of a narrow and restricted approach to research and an unswerving reliance on a seriously flawed data collection instrument. In order to understand these findings and the debates they have engendered, we need to unravel the methods and overall methodology used to produce these counter-factual results. We begin with an analysis of the specific methods used by FV research as this will help explain how this counter-factual evidence was actually created.

National surveys and the conflict tactics scales

FV researchers have placed an extraordinary confidence in two national surveys employing one scale called the Conflict Tactics Scales. The main proponents of this method have an exceptionally narrow view of valid research. While occasionally suggesting the use of alternative research procedures, their entire agenda represents an unswerving faith in the superiority of this chosen method. Confidence is so high that the proponents of the CTS usually reject, ignore or belittle other research approaches as well as critiques of their own approach. Critics of these methods and the counter-factual results they produce are accused of 'methodological absolutism' and labelled 'feminist', who it is erroneously claimed reject all forms of quantification. Criticism of the methods of FV researcher is equated with the absolute denial of women's violence based on the 'feminist' belief '... that women can do no wrong and anyone who disclosed wrongdoing by women must be using incorrect methods, be a misogynist, or both'.[109] VAW researchers are accused of having a 'distrust of quantitative methodology as a whole' and are chastised for their supposed 'sweeping indictment of quantitative sociology ...'.[110] In these counter-attacks, FV researchers claim that the interpretative, qualitative work of VAW researchers involves the use of 'clinical' samples, when in fact, only a very small proportion of the women studied are receiving treatment, the requisite feature, one would think, for invoking this term.[111]

With these claims, FV researchers attempt to dismiss the critics of their own claims without addressing their substance. Using the term 'clinical' to describe non-probability samples is a political act enabling others to reject such research and its findings. These are powerful political aspersions, as is the use of the term 'feminist'. In North America it is often equated with irrational forms of discourse and qualitative, and thus inadequate, research methods. Although these negative connotations are rarely explicated since there is little need to do so, Shupe, Stacey and Hazelwood have filled in a bit of detail claiming that a 'radical feminist mindset', opposed to 'science and reason', has inhibited the development of work on violence in the family. For most FV researchers, only surveys and scales based on large probability samples (presumably stripped of feminist leanings) can reveal the 'facts' associated with violence in the family.

Counter-evidence from National Crime Surveys, intensive interpretive research with 'clinical' samples and police and court records are usually ignored, disputed or disregarded. Large, preferably national, probability samples, measurement of acts through scales and causal statistical analysis are proffered as the assured route to valid knowledge. Survey research with its emphasis on large probability samples is the bedrock of American social science. It is a powerful tool in investigating relatively straightforward issues which can be probed through short personal or telephone interviews and questionnaires There is, however, a near fetish like commitment to the social survey in the United States.[112] There is a widespread belief that information must be gathered through the use of a survey regardless of the nature of the issue and/or the research question under investigation. Indeed, commitment to the survey shapes researchers' perceptions of social issues and the formulation of research questions. While survey research certainly has its strengths, such as wide coverage, its weaknesses are often overlooked. The survey is particularly poor at investigating complex behaviours, emotions and social processes such as those associated with violence, and its necessary brevity means it can rarely be used to explore the contexts associated with social behaviour. This form of instrumental positivism often means 'Important issues are frequently ignored ... or if studied, they are reduced to trivia by the design of the study', thus radically limiting what we can learn about the social world.[113] Unfortunately, FV researchers have chosen to concentrate their research efforts on this single method, using a short personal interview in the first survey and an even shorter telephone interview in the second. We must ask whether such admittedly superficial one-off, cross-sectional surveys are adequate for investigating problems such as child abuse and violence against women. If these methods are to be employed, panel studies such as the US and Canadian National Crime Surveys would seem to yield more valid results than one-off surveys.

The problems associated with surveys are compounded by FV researchers' use of an inadequate scale to measure violence. The Conflict Tactics Scale (CTS) is hailed by its creator as a 'landmark' instrument in the study of violence. He claims it is a valid and reliable instrument for determining the nature and extent of violence in the family. Many critics disagree and have provided detailed critiques dating back to the inception of the scale. Fundamental criticisms have been raised about the use of a purely behavioural scale to investigate what is a multi-faceted and complex problem involving motivations, intentions, acts and discrete though often overlapping events which occur over extended periods of time. Some interpretative critics note the inherent methodological limitations in the use of scales and argue that only qualitative ethnographic and in-depth methods can truly capture the complex and dynamic processes of violence.

Other critics, while possibly accepting the utility of scales, have nonetheless criticized the internal logic of the CTS and the operational procedures associated with its use. These critics have repeatedly pointed to serious flaws, including the fact that the scale only includes discrete acts and that these acts are confined to a very narrow range. Rape and sexual assault are excluded as are many other forms of physical assault. The immediate and wider contexts associated with violence are ignored. Motivations and intentions of aggressors and the interpretations of victims are not considered. The process and the sequence of events associated with specific attacks are not studied. Acts, motivations and intentions are not linked to the immediate and wider family contexts in which they occur. Items are included which are not mutually exclusive, such as the summary item, 'beating-up'. Minor and severe violence are distinguished solely on the basis of *speculation* that a particular act has the potential for producing injuries rather than knowledge of injuries actually sustained. The labels of minor and severe violence are applied to individuals based on simple additive methods. This means that a respondent who indicates they have slapped their spouse twice is considered the same as one who has twice beaten up their spouse. The CTS also fails to connect outcomes, especially injury, with the acts that produce them.[114]

One of the most significant problems in the use of the CTS is a failure to incorporate theoretical definitions of violence into the scale. Violence, FV researchers assert, '... is defined as an act carried out with the intention, or perceived intention, of causing physical pain or injury to another person'.[115] Very few researchers and observers would disagree with this definition, though many would go further and include the victim's perceptions and the outcome in a wider, more contextually oriented approach.[116] The problem, however, is that intentions are NEVER actually included in the research instruments employed. The CTS only includes acts and this has been rigorously defended by its creator.

Investigating acts and not asking about the intentions associated with them may mean that respondents will answer 'yes' to a question such as 'have you ever slapped or thrown something at your spouse?' even though there is no intention to harm or intimidate. One might, for example, slap a husband or wife on the arm in jest or throw a pillow in order to get their attention. This distinction is not a trivial issue. When Margolin used the CTS followed by depth interviews, she discovered important problems associated with the meanings respondents attached to the items on the scale.[117] One married couple admitted kicking each other. Employing the CTS means we have a case of mutual combat, possibly even 'battered spouses'. In the follow-up depth interviews, Margolin found that this was a playful activity the couple engaged in while in bed. Was this violence? The CTS would indicate it was. The depth interviews revealed it was not. It seems we have a very poor fit between theoretical conceptualization, measurement and reality. By any standards this is a serious threat to the validity of research findings arising from the use of the CTS.

The utility of the CTS is also threatened by failures to substantiate its validity technically. An often employed method of assessing the validity of the scale involves an investigation of the correspondence between the accounts given by husbands and by wives. Attempts to use such concordance as an indicator of the validity of the CTS fail, and reveal instead considerable discordance in the responses of husbands and wives. Straightforwardly, much research and knowledge gained in group work with batterers shows that men systematically underestimate and misrepresent the severity of their violence.[118] Research explicitly directed at determining the correspondence in responses between husbands and wives reveals almost none, especially on the item, 'beat-up'.[119] These studies show that husband/wife agreement is rarely better than what one might predict by chance. Even the creator of the CTS has recently admitted that, '... most of the agreement studies reviewed found large discrepancies between the reports of violence given by husbands and wives'.[120] Such results offer no consolation to those who claim the CTS is a valid instrument for assessing violence between family members.

Another problem with the CTS is the way it is employed to summarize and describe individual experiences of violence. In the FV tradition the application of terms such as 'battered' and 'beaten' are usually connected with the scale score given to each survey respondent. In applying such terms FV researchers do not use or invoke a wider definition, such as 'those individuals defined as "battered" and "beaten" have experienced severe, persistent violence over an extended period of time'. Rather, such terms are employed if an individual is judged to have experienced or used 'severe violence' as assessed solely through their scale score with minimal consideration of duration or persistent severity. This means that individuals could be judged 'battered' or 'beaten' because they experienced one act as recorded through the CTS (e.g. 'hit', 'bit', 'tried to hit', 'beat up' or 'choked'). Is it legitimate to assume that a woman who 'tried to hit' her husband on one occasion can be realistically classified as a violent women and he as a beaten husband (or vice versa)? Is this the same as a woman who has experienced years of violent abuse and intimidation? Using the CTS they would appear to be categorized the same. Again, Margolin's research illustrates this problem. Using the CTS, she discovered a woman who had used violence against her husband during the year of the research. Following the FV tradition her spouse would have been described as a 'battered husband'. In the follow-up interview Margolin found that the woman's single incidence of 'violent self-defence' occurred after years of serious assaults at the hands of her husband. Does this mean he is a battered husband? Is she a battered wife? Are both battered? The two research approaches would answer these questions differently, both using data, but from different research traditions.

In the face of years of mounting criticism and evidence threatening the validity and utility of the CTS, its creator has responded with various reservations about and modifications of the scale. It has, for example, been admitted that even if women were just as violent as men their violence has different consequences because it is less likely to result in injury. Attempting to overcome limitations, a few new items have been added to the scale in an attempt to explore who initiates violence and to assess injuries. However, such changes have done little to deal with the fundamental problems inherent in the scale. For example, in assessing injuries respondents were asked whether or not they experienced violence necessitating medical attention and/or time away from work.[121] Research shows that because of their predicament (threats and entrapment by violent men) the injuries women experience often go unreported and untreated. The economic plight of women and sometimes the demands and threats of men mean that women often find it difficult to take time off work even when injured. Furthermore, since one of the most common injuries is bruising, often massive, the injured do not generally seek medical attention because medicine can be of little assistance. In the

USA, in contrast to Britain, the lack of a national health service and the high cost of medicine also reduces the number of women likely to seek medical attention no matter how badly needed.

Even with these few adjustments the CTS is seriously flawed. Its creator notes there are '... real problems and limitations that are inherent in the instrument as it is currently structured ...'.[122] After years of persistent critiques from other researchers about the flaws and failings of the CTS, most have now been accepted by its creator. The list is substantial. First, the meaningfulness of items in the scale is now questioned, noting that asking someone if they have ever thrown 'something' at their spouse tells you nothing about what was thrown 'a pillow or a brick' and whether it hits its target.[123] Second, it is now accepted that the scale scoring methods misrepresent the nature of violence by treating diverse acts in an equivalent manner. That is, the scale 'combines all forms of violence in a sum index. Consequently, two slaps are counted the same as two knife attacks.'[124] Third, the distinction between defining violence as 'minor' or 'serious' is now acknowledged as problematic because it is '... based on the ASSUMPTION that the latter entail a greater risk of injury and this has never been demonstrated by empirical data'.[125] Fourth, it has finally been accepted that employing perceived risk of injury as the criteria for determining the seriousness of violence '... is not an entirely satisfactory approach'.[126] Fifth, the creator now agrees with critics that the CTS is limited because it only measures discrete acts and '... therefore does not provide information on the specific inter-action sequence that was involved in the use of any of the tactics in the scale'.[127]

The nature and scope of these limitations and faults are so serious that they undermine the validity and utility of the CTS, and, accordingly, any findings based upon it. Having finally acknowledged these flaws, it might be expected that FV researchers would cease to use the CTS in further research or, at the least, to temper claims based on findings arising from its use. This would seem to be particularly important when the results, such as those of symmetry of violence between women and men, are counter-factual and at variance with a wide body of findings arising from other research not based on this problematic scale. It is also important because results emerging from the CTS have been used in the community and in political debates to deny services to abused women. Unfortunately for those who suffer violence, FV researchers continue to defend the CTS as the best possible means of studying the problem and to make strong claims based on its findings.[128]

In continuing to defend the use of the CTS scale, FV researchers reveal their dogged commitment to survey research and to the use of scales as the only, or at least the best, method for studying this and other social issues. They must be used regardless of their limitations and potential distortions. According to the supporters of the CTS, the limited amount of time allocated for each interview makes it impossible to include more than just a 'few acts' of violence, thus restricting '... the amount of data that can be obtained from each subject ...'.[129] Cutting the cloth to fit the 'survey method', the creator of the scale points out, 'The CTS was restricted to relatively few acts of violence because it was developed for use in survey research'.[130]

THEORIES AND EXPLANATIONS

When considered as a whole, the problems associated with the FV research agenda are a consequence of following a positivist and empiricist approach to knowledge. Positivism is now widely discredited in the philosophy of science; as a prominent philosopher of science indicates, 'Positivist philosophy of science has gone into a near total eclipse'.[131] We are now in a post-positivist period in which social scientists are creating new approaches to knowledge. These new approaches are not antithetical to the use of quantitative research and many actively embrace a combination of both quantitative and qualitative methods.[132] Yet FV researchers continue to be guided by the principles of positivism, including an inordinate and misplaced obsession with standardization, measurement, abstract scales and statistical analysis; the compilation of endless lists of purely additive empirical generalizations; and *ad hoc* approaches to explanation. The apparent goal of these researchers is the creation of one grand or single abstract theory of family violence, indeed of all violence, in which the significance of gender is not considered. At present they must content themselves with gathering together, collating and summarizing a seemingly endless array of potentially significant factors (over twenty in one book), empirical generalizations and theories. These are often presented in complex diagrams composed of numerous, usually bewildering, boxes and arrows.[133] The exact relationships among these factors and the specific mechanisms by which they independently and collectively operate to produce violence is never spelled out. In the United States, the roots of this FV orientation are planted in the traditional approach to the sociology of the family.

Family sociologists have traditionally assumed an equivalence in the methods of the natural and social sciences which they think will produce law-like propositions.[134] As one family sociologist claims, '... the goal of theorizing is to acquire laws about nature that can be used to explain and predict more specific phenomena'.[135] In this approach the theories, values and beliefs of researchers do not 'contaminate' empirical research and the technologies, such as the CTS, employed to investigate the social world. As one prominent examplar put it, '... the attitude of science is that of value-free truth-seeking: the method is that of the objective analysis of empirical data and the aim is that of predictive theory'.[136] For these researchers scales such as the CTS can be employed independently of the ideas, values and beliefs associated with its creation and use. Philosophers of science now generally agree that this is impossible – there is no such thing as 'raw data' or 'brute facts'; all observational languages and research procedures reflect the theoretical positions that guide them as well as wider psychological, social and even personal and political contexts.[137]

During the last two decades philosophers of science and social scientists have refuted the 'value-free' stance and positivist approaches, and have developed numerous alternatives. Yet, in the USA sociology of the family has remained relatively untouched. Only recently have a few family sociologists begun to express strong reservations about this outdated approach. Exploring this persistent tradition in family sociology, Thomas and Wilcox have concluded that it leads to an atomization of knowledge and not to systematic explanations.[138] Proposing more critical and realist approaches, they reflect on the rather paradoxical development of family sociology:

> Thus, ... at a time when philosophy of science was turning away from an objectivist view of theory, family theory was moving in a different direction. Philosophy of science was moving to overhaul its basic view of the nature of theory while family theory was building its theoretical foundation on the positivist rubble being discarded by the philosophy of science.[139]

Many VAW researchers are following an alternative agenda seeking to create new forms of critical, disciplined social science. In so doing, they adopt a more holistic approach in which concepts, explanations and empirical evidence are combined into an overall 'interpretive analytic'.[140] The participatory and interactive in-depth interview is the major research tool within this traditon. Some researchers have used highly structured and systematic interviews while others have employed more open-ended and discursive methods. All seek to maximize the mutuality between researcher and those they study, and this has been an especially significant aspect of recent feminist research. In contrast to the narrow linear, inductive approach of FV researchers, VAW researchers seek to explain the problem through a rich mosaic of empirical results and explanations with the aim of achieving a description as well as comprehensive understanding of the problem. In the explanation of violence, the complex explanatory net encompasses a wealth of empirical evidence from contemporary and historical sources, along with wider auxiliary knowledge, explanations and interpretations. In creating these explanations, the centrality of gender based conflicts occurring within the context of male domination is stressed. At the core of this analysis is a concrete analysis of the acts, motives, intentions and interpretations of those who perpetrate and those who experience violence. Close and careful analysis of the violence and the immediate contexts associated with it lead to a link with gender specific cultural beliefs, socialization and practices. These, in turn, are linked to the wider contexts of institutional orientations and actions which, in the past as today, support men's violent repression of women and deny and minimize its impact on them. In this analysis of ever widening contexts, contemporary evidence is linked to the wider historical context as a means of providing a fuller understanding of current patterns. Thus, both the consistency and continuity of the violence can be revealed along with changes in its forms and manifestations in social life. In respect to violence against women, this provides both a glimpse of social change and stern lessons about the difficulties of achieving meaningful change.

In this tradition research and explanatory work is never conducted in a vacuum. For VAW researchers public settings are not merely locations for public pronouncements based on the 'superior knowledges' of academic experts or arenas of annoyances where they must tolerate, though ultimately ignore, critiques or challenging ideas. VAW researchers are keenly aware that 'lively disagreement' and 'public criticism is vital at all stages of research', providing and forcing out 'alternative interpretations'.[141] VAW researchers accept that they are working in a wider political and social world and are often engaged in a fruitful dialogue with activists and women living and working in shelters as well as with representatives of public agencies charged with responding to the problem. Through this process they are able to compare and test their understandings with those who have a rich base of knowledge and experience.[142] Many VAW researchers, especially in Britain, have been directly involved or closely linked to efforts to assist women who have been victims of violence. Contacts such as these have not meant the dilution of scholarship and rigour; quite the opposite, understandings and analyses have been sharpened and enriched. They recognize that detachment from those who have experienced and dealt with the problem, such as that practised by FV researchers, does not lead to the production of better knowledge but to an 'inability to take human beings seriously',[143] and to uninformed research with important negative consequences for the most usual victims of domestic violence, women.

9 Innovation and social change

The movements are in the process of challenging one of the oldest forms of intimate domination and of assisting millions of victims of one of its most brutal manifestations. In the space of little over a decade, coercive male domination and the physical abuse of women in the home have been recognized throughout the world as problems of importance and placed on the agendas of change. The pressure of local and national groups, many inspired by the movements in Britain and the USA, have brought this social problem on to a world stage. From the beginning, the movements faced formidable obstacles in the prevailing public perceptions of the problem itself and of their attempts to create solutions. As one British politician proclaimed in the 1970s,

> ... why should the Government get involved in a family squabble.... Surely they could go to a neighbour or a relative for some time and think things over rather than run to the State to look after them.[1]

Undeterred, activists set about the task of changing such perceptions and the institutional arrangements built upon them. The movements have brought about changes in public and media perceptions and new discourses have now entered public arenas to challenge the ignorance and prejudices of the past. The movement has given us an alternative conception of the private sphere of the family and hope for its transformation. The myth of family unity and bliss has been exploded as the movement made public the unacceptable face of the private by exposing to scrutiny the world of conflict, power and violence which can never again be ignored or denied.

In reflecting on the course of the two movements, we have concentrated on innovations, considering their potential for social change, and the dilemmas and problems faced by the movements. Since the movement is a continuing one, these reflections outline a continuing and evolving social process. Of necessity, this can only be a provisional exploration of paths taken, efforts expended, current directions and possible paths still remaining. Social change must eventually be judged from a greater distance in time, although at this point there can be no dispute about the achievements of this new social movement. An analysis of these achievements not only illustrates many important factors about this particular movement and the changes for which it is struggling, but also about social movements in general and their significance within democratic societies.

Comparing the battered women's movements in two countries helps clarify thinking about the nature of each and illustrates the importance of different social and political contexts to the process of social change. Without cross-national comparisons, it is much easier to overlook issues which have not been recognized as important within one's own nation. Knowledge that something is done differently elsewhere leads to questions about differing contributions to social change. There are, of course, differences in the movements in each country, and an analysis extended to other countries would show still further variation in context and content. The issues that become most salient for particular national movements are often issues that are salient, or at least have a resonance, within the wider society in which activists are thinking about what would constitute change and in which they must work to achieve goals once defined.

In Britain, for example, housing has always constituted a significant social issue and this is reflected in the efforts of the movement. Another example is race and ethnicity. From the beginning, this has been an issue of considerable importance in the movement in the USA, and a great deal of work has been done in this area. In Britain, the issue has not had such prominence even though it has recently become more salient. Reflecting on the wider contexts in which the two movements exist, this difference is, perhaps, not surprising. With the impact of the civil rights movement in the USA has come a more general awareness of the issue of ethnicity and civil rights in all spheres of social life, including within other liberating and democratizing social movements. In Britain, there have been no large-scale or popular movements focusing on race and ethnicity. Even though there are community and government organizations focusing on prejudice and discrimination based on ethnicity, the general level of awareness and of state response is not on the scale reached in the USA. Recently, however, the issue has begun to take on greater importance in Britain, is appearing on political and social agendas.

This can now be seen in work of the Women's Aid Federations and reflected in refuge provision. Thus, the level of awareness about the importance of other groups seeking an enhanced place in society can be seen in the vision and the goals of the battered-women's movement.

A national comparison also provides a framework for examining the negotiations of the movement with agencies of the state. Once again, the context in which activists must operate is affected by the remit and resources of other organizations, by their ideologies and priorities, by their power, and by the willingness to enter into the process of negotiation and change associated with altering policies and practices. While in theory everything might seem possible, the reality is often much more restricting and complex. This realization is critical in reflecting upon the changes obtained from negotiations with the state and on those lost. Without an appreciation of the wider context in which challenges develop and are lost or achieved, it is all to easy simply to consider outcomes alone and to reach simple conclusions about whether the movement has been a success or a failure. Process and context are critical elements in examining the social changes achieved by the social movements. Diverse cultural and institutional approaches and structures within the two national contexts influence and facilitate certain directions and impede others. For example, the US Civil Rights Commission was important not only in putting the issue on the agenda of government concerns but also in facilitating a discourse about the status of women in society. On the other hand, the Parliamentary Select Committee ignored or denied a feminist discourse but praised and supported the pragmatic activities of the movement.

While national comparisons highlight and aid our understandings of some of the differences between the movements in the two countries, they also illustrate persistent similarities that are sustained despite differences in national economies, political order or cultural beliefs. Here we see strong similarities in the identity of the movement, its membership and particularly its pragmatic response to the problem. There are also similarities in the orientation to using the institutions of the state as part of the process of change. Finally, there are similarities in the obstacles faced by the movements as they seek to transform existing orientations, policies and practice.

In assessing the accomplishments of the movement it is important to remember the starting point. The identities of both were firmly rooted in the activism and women's movements of the late 1960s and 1970s and in the feminisms of the past. When the movement began it was based on 'grassroots' membership with women participants coming from diverse backgrounds. Some, like many of those who participated in other new social movements of the period, came from backgrounds in the educational and social services. The concern of feminists to make 'the personal political' moved quickly from the raising of consciousness to that of direct action oriented at specific changes in the economic, political and domestic lives of women. Focusing on the abuse of women and its unacceptability within society is an obvious and important part of the process of seeking change. Activists have entered this process through a variety of routes, some through involvement in other progressive struggles and others with no experience of activism, but all have learned the difficulties of confronting entrenched attitudes and institutionalized patterns of action. The strategies and tactics used in seeking change have at times been ingenious and effective and, at other times, display the inexperience of a new movement up against adversaries with a long and ignoble past.

To the struggle for change, women brought skills, insights and enthusiasms, fuelled by an appropriate anger and passion about the violence used against women. A significant element in social change, perhaps one of the most significant, is the very act of creating new visions and thinking new thoughts. Once a new idea has become established, it is difficult to imagine how it was ever otherwise. But at the moment of launching a new idea, it is difficult to imagine how it could ever be. Thus, it is important to acknowledge that while it may now be generally agreed that it is unacceptable for a man to use physical or sexual violence against his female partner, this is, in fact, an extraordinary departure from thinking of the recent past, a change of considerable magnitude. Once the unthinkable has been thought, it must then be articulated in public settings and initiate the process of transforming the vision of others and overcoming their resistance to the new idea. Finally comes action. In the process of change, it is not sufficient just to think thoughts and articulate new ideas about possible worlds and how things might be. It is necessary to make visions concrete and to act in order to try to create that new world. Such action will, of necessity, involve negotiations and struggles with others who have a different world in mind, usually the retention of the one they already know. Developing a new vision and acting to achieve it is the core of social movements. Forming a vision which truly represents an alternative to the status quo is the core of social change. And struggling for changes which transform the lives of all women is the concrete, constructive core of feminism. All three have come together in the movement for abused women.

The very process of challenging the established order means that large numbers of women have learned the skills and techniques associated with the process of social change. This action provides continuity with and expansion of past struggles and develops models for future action. In these ways challenges are not merely associated with sporadic collective public demonstrations but become a persistent part of everyday culture and of established institutional practices. At the most basic level, the stated preference for more democratic and participatory methods of working within shelters and refuges challenges prevailing patterns and provides an alternative model. The movement's attempts to appreciate and embrace cultural, ethnic and personal diversity represents a challenge to those who would ignore these vital concerns. In linking victims of violence with women working in shelters the movement has simultaneously made concrete the visions of the women's movement and broadened its base of participation.[2]

The refuge itself constitutes the most highly visible and obviously concrete challenge to the legacy of indifference to male violence. By providing a haven for abused women and their children, activists have provided both a practical escape route from violence and a public symbol of the rejection of such violence. Although havens for oppressed women and other groups have existed for centuries, the uniqueness of these refuges and shelters lies in the nature of assistance provided within them and in the wider visions of change beyond them. Within them women find safety and security, but they also find solidarity and an end to their sense of isolation. Shelters are also a location for political thinking and action generated within the context of close contact with those who experience male domination in this direct and brutal form. The vision of working together and in close proxmity to the problem itself corresponds more closely with notions of democratizing relations between women and workers, of renewing the enthusiasm for supporting and assisting women in ways that are meaningful for their lives, and in seeking wider changes that would directly address the problem of male violence. The refuge is, at once, a concrete embodiment of the concern to confront male domination, a site for understanding that domination, and a locus for action. Various strands of feminist thought and action can be seen at work in the refuge. While other orientations, such as the therapeutic, philanthropic and bureaucratic, may also be seen, it is within feminism that the movement was conceived and to which it owes its philosophical allegiance.

The movement has also brought change in the discourse about

violence against women. Silence and a general lack of public discussion has prevailed for over a century. Public chanting and displays of disapproval of men who were brutal beyond the conventions of their time have not been heard since the charavari and misrules of one hundred years ago. Public statements of disapproval are now made by activists throughout the world, and their echoes can be heard in the media, in houses of government and in everyday conversation. The secret and unsharable has been made a topic of public discussion and concern. The discourse is new in that it constructs a vision of the unacceptablity rather than the tolerance of male violence. It departs from previous notions of women by asserting that they occupy a place of value in their own right rather than simply as wives and mothers tending to the needs of others. It leaves behind the image that a 'good wife' is one who remains 'loyal' to her husband by remaining silent about his abuses of her body. It poses a challenge to men who would be violent and to those who would allow their fellows to continue uncensored and unchecked.

Within the movement, the concern about discourse continues to express itself in debates about the terminology and language to be used in naming the movement and in naming the problem and those who experience it. It has been seen as important to name the problem in order that it might be identified as an issue, and to name it in such a way as to increase the possibility of social action and to reduce the possibility of stimatizing the women concerned. The terms used to describe the women who experience persistent abuse have been problematized and scrutinized. 'Victim' has given way to 'survivor', 'battered woman' and 'abused woman' are both in use; words such as 'coalitions' and 'federations' describe organizations, and notions of consensus and co-operation reflect visions about styles of work and relationships. Problematizing the language in relation to a social problem is an important facet of problematizing the problem itself. The discourse evolves as the awareness evolves, and changes accordingly. This is not a straightforward or easy process, and the new discourse is not always elegant or sometimes even as descriptive as the urgency of the problem demands, but it is a necessary process in addressing anew an old problem. In some instances, however, new discourses do not form a part of the agenda of social change.

An emphasis on individual psychology and personal emotions embedded in American culture and feminism has had an important impact on the discourses and directions of the movement in the USA. From the beginning, the movement in the USA exhibited a concern for providing counselling and therapy for women. Much of the counselling appears to be similar to the assisted self-help used in Britain. In this sense, counselling involves recommending, advising and facilitating independent action on the part of the woman. Women who work and live in refuges help new residents, either on an individual basis or within a group setting, by discussing options, providing information about available resources, and assisting in the process of gaining those resources. Through helping one another and discussing their predicament, women move towards overcoming the sense of isolation, stigma and the feeling of being unique, unusual, deviant or sick. This process of counselling or assisted self-help is an invaluable part of the refuge experience and an important part of the process of surviving violence. Therapy is another matter.

Because of an emphasis on the psychology of the individual and a more therapeutic outlook throughout the society, some programmes in the USA have been oriented to creating a different sort of relationship between workers and women, transforming women into clients in need of therapeutic intervention. Through therapy women needing support and assistance in seeking an end to the violence they suffer are transformed into clients with unique, inferior characteristics identified as 'syndromes'. In some cases a condition of receiving 'services' may be subjection to therapeutic assessements and treatment sessions in which women are transformed into objects to be changed by the prevailing regime or into 'willing subjects' meant to transform themselves into the image provided by others. Mutuality – the sense of shared experience and intimacy between individuals – is thus eroded, if not completely destroyed. Therapeutic discourses and their technologies of change threaten the visions and social change potential of the movement. The broad expansive visions and challenging agendas associated with the beginning of the movement may be constricted to attempting to transform individual women through large doses of therapy. Not only does this result in a single finished answer to the problem of violence against women, it also turns the movement inward making it unlikely that it will continue to challenge social injustices, the intimate domination of women, and inequality. While therapeutic discourses may appear to be presenting something new, such solutions are only a rehash of the old, a repackaging that offers no contradictions or challenges to the traditional approach of seeking solutions to male violence within the behaviour of victims.

Therapeutic orientations eliminate wider political visions of social change and move, instead, to discourses associated with individualized medical/psychiatric care. Should this occur on a widespread scale, there will no longer be a social movement and shelters will be utterly transformed into places where women are tested and assessed to determine the depth of their psychological illness and the best treatment or regime to cure them of the various syndromes believed to cause their victimization and their inability to break the 'glue' which binds them to violent men.[3] Such a transformation of the battered-women's movement would be as if the civil rights movement had sought solutions for racist oppression and discrimination in therapy for those who have suffered from it. In moving in these directions the movement will have drifted a long way from its vision, the vision so clearly and succinctly stated by Sharon Vaughan, an important national leader and a founding member of Women's Advocates in St Paul Minnesota:

> A shelter is not a treatment center; residents are not described as clients, battering is not described as a syndrome. Women are not thought of as victims except as victims of a crime requiring redress.[4]

Male domination and female subordination has had some powerful supporters and support systems. Institutional tolerance and indifference have been rife. The movement challenges this legacy as it attempts to change the practices of social, medical and legal institutions. This necessarily involves confrontations and negotiations with institutions of the state as activists seek to provide support and assistance for abused women and to address the continuing problem of male violence. Relations between the movement and the state negate conceptions of the state as a purely coercive or co-opting force seeking to direct and control social movements. While contacts with agencies of the state do demonstrate the potential for engulfment and co-optation, they also point to the possibility of developments that enable and facilitate social change. State orientations and reactions are not monolithic. Instead, they often embody contradictory and conflicting orientations.

It is important to recognize the activities of those working within institutions of the state in facilitating changes. Some have helped facilitate the pragmatic goals of activists. Some have helped make changes in their own organizations. Some have assisted with efforts to provide resources to operate shelters and other services for women. Some have helped secure funding for research by academics and activists seeking to study innovations and changes that challenge the status quo. It is not insignificant that civil servants and representatives of various government agencies have achieved much of this during a period of conservative financial stringency.

By seeking and entering into negotiations with institutions of the state, the movements have made a fundamental statement that the state itself is seen as part of the solution to the problem of male violence in the home. Obversely, this also indicates that the policies and practices of the state have traditionally been part of the problem and are in need of transformation in the process of seeking a solution. At a general level, the very fact that social movements and agencies of the state enter into dialogue about a social problem and into negotiations concerning its solution is itself a process that democratizes the state. Thus the governed enter into the process of government by participating in the process of legislative and policy formation. Simultaneously, the state becomes more democratic and more accessible to civil society as it broadens its base of participation in the process of forming policy.

Through this process some of the proposals for radical change made by the movement have been sponsored by the state. Others have not faired so well or have had unanticipated outcomes, but, nonetheless, the overall process is one in which the state becomes more open to the concerns of the community and to the participation of its citizens in shaping laws and policies that affect their daily lives. Again, at a general level, this process has been one in which the concerns of women have become established as a legitimate part of the concerns of government. It is ironic that in Britain these developments have occurred within a wider context of government attempts to centralize power and to limit access to public information.

The issue of the abuse of women has made it possible for such negotiations to focus on women as such, and not on their social roles as wives or mothers, and thereby move the discourse to one in which it becomes easier and more usual to think and act relative to women in their own right. This has not always been easy nor has it always been successful as attempts have constantly been made to transform the concern about violence against women to a concern about the children who witness it. This is not to imply that the needs of children are not important; indeed the movement has responded to those needs within shelters and refuges, but, rather, to highlight the pressure to transform issues about women that should warrant concern in their own right into issues about others, particularly children. The passage of Federal legislation to fund shelters in the USA illustrates this point. The funding of shelters for abused women was passed only after being attached to a bill focusing on children.

The nature of the state itself has varied across time and has changed during the brief life of this social movement. Of particular importance to women has been its orientation to involvement in the sphere with which women are most closely identified, the private sphere of the family, and, latterly, that of the economy. While in reality, the state has always had some involvement in these spheres of social life, the emphasis within a Liberal state has been to remain apart from issues relating to the family and the economy, thus leaving women traditionally discriminated against within the economy or abused within the family to negotiate on their own with those in power. The orientation within interventionist or welfare states is that of some form of involvement in issues such as health care, housing and the family, thus allowing for some form of provision for issues such as violence against women in the home. Reforming social movements usually emerge within the context of such a state, and, indeed, the battered-women's movement emerged during just such an era.

Interventionist and welfare states provide greater opportunity for reforming social movements in their attempts to effect change within the institutions of the state, changes which either introduce state involvement where once there was none or alter existing policies, practices and legislation deemed detrimental. It is critical that the movements in both countries began at a time when the state was more interventionist and welfare oriented. With the election of the Republican and Conservative governments of Ronald Reagan and Margaret Thatcher in the early 1980s, the orientation moved away from community welfare and to a neo-liberal stance favouring non-involvement. This left the movements in both countries negotiating within a much altered context oriented to a reduction in social provisions and favouring volunteerism and philanthropy. It is, of course, true that government is not monolithic in approach and much of previous activity continues relatively unaltered even with a change of government. Nonetheless, the general climate was altered with respect to social movements seeking the involvement of the state in their efforts to secure social change. Securing resources and negotiating for changes in legislation and policies certainly becomes more difficult during such times. Considerable skill and effort must often be exerted simply to retain the gains achieved under more favourable conditions. Now that the Thatcher and Reagan eras have ended, it remains to be seen if the governments of both countries will again move towards more involvement in issues affecting the community and the welfare of women. Such a change would, of course, affect the climate in which the movements continue to negotiate with agencies of the state for resources and social changes.

The justice system is one arena in which the need for change was first denied and resisted, then grudgingly accepted, and, finally, became the centre of reforming efforts. It has reached a stage where new and meaningful responses have developed in some local areas, yet innovations seem to need constant attention in order to remain a part of established practice. There is now some debate among feminists about the possibility of using law and law enforcement as instruments of social change for women in general or for abused women in particular. Whatever the outcome of this important debate, it is, nonetheless, clear that physically abused women will seek assistance through the law. Possibly because of this, the movement, particularly in the USA, has expended tremendous effort in its attempts to change the justice system. Through this process, they have not only developed and honed their political skills but also engaged in a process that further democratizes the state by expanding the base of those who participate in the process.

From a core of alternative practices rooted in shelter activism, the movements have challenged the justice system. The mere mounting of challenges constitutes an important attainment. Particularly in Britain where the police may more easily ignore or dismiss the challenges of community groups, it must be considered an achievement when the concerns of activists are no longer simply dismissed and are sometimes accorded legitimacy. In engaging the prevailing practices of law and law enforcement the movements have faced a formidable task. Yet those challenges have brought some meaningful changes and had beneficial effects on the lives of some of the large number of women who suffer persistent violence. Changes in law have been reasonably widespread in both countries. Concerning law enforcement, the efforts in Britain have not been as successful in shifting orientations and practices as have those in the USA. The more closed nature of the British system makes it difficult even to know the nature of official policies and practices and, thus, even more difficult to challenge them. As such, changes have often been filtered through government directives and *ad hoc* committees and often implemented through the benevolence of individual Chief Constables. While the movement has greatly influenced the climate in which this occurs, the nature of the system is such that the impact on changes is less direct than that in the USA.

In the USA the levers of change have included the use of the legal system itself to confront the inadequate and dangerous responses of law enforcement. In some areas, individual law suits and class actions against the police have brought swift and often meaningful changes in police response, and this has had an effect on the movement's ability to negotiate for changes in other areas without having to resort to lawsuits. Whatever the gains in changing police response, it is clear that other aspects of the justice system remain relatively unaffected by claims for change. In both countries, for example, prosecutors and judges usually remain relatively unaware of the nature of the problem and of the need to change their own perceptions and practices. Even so, many changes in practices and institutional perceptions have been achieved. Most police forces in both countries now provide improved support and assistance to victims and some are more oriented to enforcing the law against violent men.

In some areas new and novel links have been created between the movement and the justice system. In both countries informal networks have been created between the police and local groups, and these have sometimes been formalized and routinized through the creation of advisory counsultative committees. Particularly, although not exclusively in the USA, inter-organizational approaches now provide significant challenges to past inaction and represent models for meaningful change. One danger in establishing and maintaining these links is that the visions and goals of the movement may become so enmeshed or subsumed under the demands of the justice system that the vision of social change is lost. The lessons of these developments, often involving co-operative work aimed at achieving common goals, should continue to be explored while their consequences remain a topic of critical scrutiny.

Whatever the limitations of institutional change, it is unlikely that the police and others within the justice system can ever again see the problem simply as 'domestic disputes'. Perceptions have been altered, and it is now more fully appreciated that 'domestic disputes' often involve violence against women and are not mere 'family squabbles' of interest to no one except the woman concerned. Activists and legal advocates have had some success in shifting police orientations away from their ideas about the attributes of the victim and on to the violence itself, the abuser and the criminality of the act. Police officers, prosecutors and judges may still want to believe in the nagging, provocative wife and masochistic women, but their actions are less likely to be predicated on such perceptions than on the requirements associated with enforcing the law. In the United States, activists and legal advocates have also challenged the use of diversion, crisis intervention and mediation in cases of violence between intimates. This does not mean that such practices have disappeared;

clearly they have not, but they are being confronted through an emphasis on arrest and prosecution and through direct legal challenges. Several states now have legislation excluding the use of mediation in cases where there is a history of violence.[5] In Britain, where such practices have not been so well established but have recently begun to appear, the efforts of the movement have met with mixed success in ensuring that violence against women is not included in the new schemes meant to divert prior to arrest and prosecution.

The use of arrest has become more prevalent in both countries.[6] We have pointed to some of the unintended negative consequences of these policies, including the arrest of women for acts of self-defence, but there are wider implications, particularly the authoritarian potential associated with policies of mandatory arrest and its extension into other areas. There is a delicate balance between encouraging law enforcement to respond actively to issues in which the justice system has little interest and that of overenforcement which takes racialist or other discriminatory forms. Ironically, discretion is often the key to both. With policies of mandatory arrest, discretion has not been eliminated but has been circumscribed. In general, the purpose has been one of attempting to ensure that the justice system is seen to make a clear and unequivocal statement about the unacceptability of violence against women and to provide a vehicle for holding on to abusers while they go through a process of changing their violent behaviour. For the movement, the concern about the arrest of violent men primarily reflects a concern to provide greater protection for women and their children by controlling violent men and seeking a cessation of their violence. This is also one of the primary goals of the pro-feminist groups for batterers.

There has been a proliferation of programmes for violent men in the USA and Canada, some based on therapeutic orientations and some on a pro-feminist model reflecting the knowledge and lessons learned within the battered-women's movement. They present the movement with a number of dilemmas. Should energy and resources be diverted to work with violent men? Will programmes for men eventually overshadow and overtake the issue of violence against women? Will the knowledge and leadership of the movement be ignored or denied in the rush to deal with men? Will the safety and security of women be threatened through such programmes? And, will they provide an element in changing male domination and the relationship between men and women? These issues have long confronted the movement in the USA, and are only recently becoming a part of the political terrain in Britain. Men's programmes

have been one of the most contentious issues within the British movement generating some of 'the bitterest discussions' during the late
1980s.[7] After much internal debate, Scottish Women's Aid became
one of the initiators of CHANGE, a re-education programme for
violent men linked to criminal justice.[8] The multi-agency programme
includes Women's Aid, social work, probation and others and has
confronted similar controversies to those encountered in the North
America.

In Britain, men, batterers and pro-feminist supporters alike, have
largely been kept at a distance, and the movement has primarily been
embattled with male dominated institutions. This makes even more
problematic the issue of working with men as partners in expanding
the support for abused women through efforts to change batterers
themselves. Men's programmes are beginning to develop quickly. A
few have pro-feminist philosophies and have contact with the movement and/or their local refuge. Years of separation make such
contacts difficult for both sides, and there are few models of how this
might work in practice.[9] The movement cannot stop this development
and now faces the issue of whether to become involved in some way
in order to try to influence the direction of men's programmes or to
remain apart. There are, of course, dangers either way.

The achievements of the battered-women's movement are many.
The goal of social change is an expansive one with implications for
women and men in general as well for those individuals who are
directly concerned. At the very least, their efforts have provided
support for tens of thousands of women throughout the world and
brought this issue into the public arena from which it cannot now be
removed. This has provided a vehicle for change within the institutions of the state as well as within the wider society. Perceptions,
discourse and reactions have all been challenged. The vision of transforming the position of women in society forms the wider goal and
the continuing challenge. The achievement of such a goal may well
involve both the retention of independent action of a single issue
social movement as well as coalitions with other progressive
movements in order to broaden the base of the efforts to achieve
profound change.

Notes

1 VIOLENCE AGAINST WOMEN

1 R.E. Dobash and R.P. Dobash, *Violence Against Wives*, New York, The Free Press, and Macmillan Distributing, Brunel Road, Houndmills, Basingstoke, England, 1979; M. Daly and M. Wilson, *Homicide*, New York, Aldine De Gruyter, 1988.
2 D. Martin, *Battered Wives*, San Francisco, CA, Glide Publications, 1976, pp. 1–2.
3 E. Evason, Hidden Violence, Belfast, Farset Co-operative Press, 1982, p. 27.
4 P. Kincaid, *The Omitted Reality*, Ontario, Canada, Learners Press, 1982, p. 23.
5 R.E. Dobash and R.P. Dobash, 'The nature and antecedents of violent events', *British Journal of Criminology*, vol. 24, no. 3, July, 1984, pp. 269–88.
6 Evason, op. cit., p. 28.
7 L. Kelly, *Surviving Sexual Violence*, Oxford, Polity Press, 1988, p. 130.
8 R.E. Dobash, R.P. Dobash, C. Cavanagh and M. Wilson, 'Wifebeating: The victims speak', *Victimology*, no. 2, vols 3–4, 1977/78, pp. 608–22, p. 612.
9 Evason, op. cit., p. 28.
10 Kelly, op. cit., p. 130.
11 Dobash and Dobash, op. cit., 1984, p. 276.
12 Evanson, op. cit., p. 30.
13 Casey, op. cit., p. 26. See p. 19 for summary of forms of violence recorded in the survey of 127 women in refuges during 1986.
14 Dobash and Dobash, op. cit., 1979, p. 111.
15 M. Casey, *Domestic Violence against Women: The Women's Perspective*, Federation of Women's Refuges and Social and Organisational Psychology Research Unit, UCD, Dublin, 1987–8.
16 Kelly, op. cit., p. 127.
17 Ibid.
18 Kelly, op. cit., p. 130.
19 Dobash, Dobash, Cavanagh and Wilson, op. cit., p. 611.
20 J. Pahl (ed.), *Private Violence and Public Policy: The Needs of Battered Women and the Response of the Public Services*, London, Routledge, 1985, p. 77.

300   *Women, violence and social change*

21 Dobash and Dobash, op. cit., 1979, p. 108.
22 Ibid.
23 Dobash and Dobash, op. cit., 1979, pp. 98–106; Dobash and Dobash, op. cit., 1984, pp. 272–4. See also Kelly, op. cit. p. 131; J. Edelson and Z. Eisikovits, 'Men who batter women: A critical review of the evidence', *Journal of Family Issues*, vol. 6, no. 2, June, 1986, pp. 229–47; M.P. Brygger and J.L. Edleson, 'The domestic abuse project: A multi-systems intervention in woman battering', Unpublished paper, Domestic Abuse Project 2445 Park Ave South, Minneapolis, MN 55404, USA, 1986; Emerge, 'Emerge: A men's counseling service on domestic violence', in Betsy Warrior (ed.), *Battered Women's Directory*, 8th edition, 46 Pleasant St., Cambridge, MA 02139, 1982, pp. 226–42; Raven (Rape and violence end now), 'Men working to end violence against women', in Betsy Warrior (ed.), *Battered Women's Directory*, 8th edition, 46 Pleasant St., Cambridge, MA 02139, 1982, pp. 243–6.
24 P. Langan and C. Innes, 'Preventing domestic violence against women', US Dept of Justice, Bureau of Justice Statistics, Special Report, Washington DC 20531, August, 1986, p. 1.
25 Casey, op. cit., p. 27.
26 Langan and Innes, op. cit., p. 1.
27 Dobash and Dobash, op. cit., 1979, pp. 31–74, 179–222; R.E. Dobash, R.P. Dobash and C. Cavanagh, 'The contact between battered women and social and medical agencies', in Jan Pahl, op. cit., pp. 142–65; M. Homer, A. Leonard and P. Taylor, *Private Violence: Public Shame, A Report on the Circumstances of Women Leaving Domestic Violence in Cleveland*, Middlesbrough, Cleveland Refuge and Aid for Women and Children (CRAWC), c/o Cleveland Council for Voluntary Service, 47 Princes Road, Middlesbrough, Cleveland, England, 1984; M. Maynard, 'The response of social workers to domestic violence', in J. Pahl, op. cit., pp. 125–41; J. Pahl, op. cit., pp. 182–5; T. Faragher, 'The police response to violence against women in the home', in J. Pahl, op. cit., pp. 110–24.
28 M. McGrory, 'A blow to battered wives', *The Boston Globe*, 21 October, 1987.
29 C. Fedders, *Shattered Dreams*, New York, Harper and Row, 1987.
30 B. Campbell, 'The trial of terror' (The case of Joel Steinberg and Hedda Hussbaum), *Guardian*, Monday 2 January, 1989, p. 15.
31 J. Rosen, 'Uproar over conviction in NY child abuse case, *Guardian*, 1 February, 1989.
32 *Guardian*, 18 February, 1989, p. 3.
33 Ibid., *Guardian*, 23 February, 1989, p. 16.
34 A. Jones, *Women Who Kill*, New York, Fawcett Columbine, 1980; A. Browne, *When Battered Women Kill*, New York, The Free Press, 1987; M. Daly and M. Wilson, *Homicide*, op. cit.
35 M. Wolfgang, *Patterns in Criminal Homicide*, New York, Wiley, 1958. Dobash and Dobash, op. cit., 1979, pp. 15–19.
36 N. Cutherbertson and L. Irving, 'Death of a battered women: An examination of the circumstances surrounding the killing of Mary Khelifati by her estranged husband', Scottish Legal Action Group, 1985, p. 148.
37 Homer, Leonard and Taylor, op. cit., p. 4.

38 Daly and Wilson, op. cit., p. 202.
39 M.S. Guttmacher, 'Criminal responsibility in certain homicide cases involving family members', in P.H. Hoch and J. Zubin (eds), *Psychiatry and the Law*, New York, Grune and Stratton, 1955; also cited in Daly and Wilson, op. cit., p. 201.
40 R.C. Showalter, R.J. Bonnie and V. Roddy, 'The spousal-homicide syndrome', *International Journal of Law and Psychiatry*, 3, 1980, pp. 117–41; also cited in Daly and Wilson, op. cit., p. 201.
41 P. Chimbos, *Marital Violence: A Study of Interspouse Homicide*, San Francisco, R&E Research Associates, 4843 Mission St., San Francisco, CA 94112, 1978.
42 Daly and Wilson, op. cit., p. 205.
43 Chimbos, op. cit., p. 67.
44 Ibid., p. 47.
45 Ibid., p. 61.
46 Bernard, Vera and Newman, 1982, cited in Browne, op. cit., 1987, p. 143, no. 1, p. 205.
47 Totman, 1978 cited in A. Browne, and R. Flewelling, 'Women as victims or perpetrators of homicide', Paper presented at the American Society of Criminology Annual Meeting, Atlanta, 29 October–1 Nov., 1986, p. 12.
48 F.E. Zimring, S.K. Mukherjee and B. Van Winkle, 'Intimate violence: A study of intersexual homicide in Chicago', *University of Chicago Law Review*, vol. 50, no. 2, 1983, pp. 910–30, cited in Browne and Flewelling, op. cit., p. 12.
49 Personal correspondence, 1988.
50 Jones, op. cit., Browne, op. cit., Daly and Wilson, op. cit.
51 Jones, ibid., p. 290.
52 Jones, ibid., p. 312.
53 Ibid., p. 298.
54 Ibid.
55 Ibid.
56 Ibid., pp. 298–9.
57 Browne, op. cit.
58 Jones, op. cit., p. 299.
59 R. Kumar, 'Contemporary Indian feminism', *Feminist Review*, no. 33, Autumn, 1989, pp. 28–9.
60 M. Karkal, 'How the other half dies in Bombay', *Economic and Political Weekly*, 24 August, 1985, p. 124.
61 L. Das, 'Hindu family laws and manu's legacy', Paper presented at Women in Interfaith Dialogue Conference organized by World Council of Churches, Toronto, Canada, available from Women's Centre, Bombay, India, B/27 Clifton, Juhu Road, Bombay, India 400 049, June, 1988, p. 5; L. Das, 'Violence against women, An Indian view', in Welsh Women's Aid, *Worldwide Action on Violence Against Women: A Report on the International Women's Conference in Cardiff*, October, 1988, c/o Welsh Women's Aid, 38/42 Crwys Road, Cardiff, Wales, UK, 1988, pp. 8–13, p. 8; Rokhsana Khondker, 'Domestic violence and the law: Case studies from Bangladesh', in Welsh Women's Aid, *Worldwide Action on Violence Against Women: A Report on the International Women's Conference in Cardiff*, October, 1988, c/o Welsh Women's

Aid, 38/42 Crwys Road, Cardiff, Wales, UK, 1988, pp. 8–13, p. 8;
Rokhsana Khondker, 'Domestic violence and the law: Case studies from
Bangladesh', in Welsh Women's Aid, *Worldwide Action on Violence
Against Women: A Report on the International Women's Conference in
Cardiff*, October 1988, c/o Welsh Women's Aid, 38/42 Crwys Road,
Cardiff, Wales, UK, 1988, pp. 35–7; L. Heise, 'Crimes of gender',
World-Watch, vol. 2, no. 2, March/April, 1989, pp. 12–21, pp. 14–15;
Commonwealth Secretariat, *Confronting Violence: A Manual for
Commonwealth Action*, Women and Development Programme, Human
Resource Development Group, Commonwealth Secretariat, Marlbo-
rough House, Pall Mall, London SW1 5HX, 1987, pp. 140–2.
62 S. Maharaja, Women Equal Rights Group, D3, Akashdeep Apartment.
Opp. Telephone Exchange, Ellisbridge, Ahmedabad-380 006, Bombay,
India, 1983, p. 4.
63 Khondker, op. cit., p. 36.
64 Heise, op. cit., pp. 15–16; Women and Law Committee, 'Wife-beating is
a crime', public information leaflet no. 1, Women and Law Committee,
PO Box 3439, Boroko, Papua New Guinea (ND, 1980s); C. Bradley,
'How can we help rural beaten wives? Some suggestions from Papua New
Guinea', in Welsh Women's Aid, op. cit., pp. 43–6.
65 C. Bradley, 'Information and resource materials on domestic violence in
Papua New Guinea', presented to the Welsh Women's Aid International
Conference, October, 1988.
66 Ibid.
67 A, Magezi, 'Violence in Uganda', in Welsh Women's Aid, op. cit.,
pp. 14–17; National Union of Eritrean Women, 'Women's displacement
in Eritrea', Unpublished paper presented at Welsh Women's Aid Conference International Conference, Cardiff, Wales, October, 1988.
68 Heise, op. cit., p. 19.
69 Ibid.
70 Ibid., p. 14.
71 B. Savl, in Welsh Women's Aid, op. cit., pp. 29–31, p. 29.
72 T.P. Halpern, 'Working with battered women in Israel', *ALIYON*,
Spring, 1980, pp. 22–3; Hazelton, 1977, estimates that 20 per cent of
Israeli women are beaten by their partners (cited in Halpern, p. 27).
73 *Guardian*, 1 June, 1988.
74 Women's Aid Organization (WAO), *Battered Women: A Self-help
Guide*, PO Box 493, Jalan Sultan, 46760 Petaling Jaya, Malaya, 1987,
pp. 20–3; C.S. Hong, 'The Malaysian experience', in Welsh Women's
Aid, op. cit., pp. 18–20.
75 S. Scan and C. Novis, 'New home OK'd for the battered', *Jerusalem
Post*, 27 November, 1987, no page.
76 (NCIWR) National Collective of Independent Women's Refuges, 'Home
is where the hurt is', NCIWR, PO Box 6386, Te Aro, Wellington, New
Zealand, 1988, p. 1.
77 Martin, op. cit., p. 202.
78 V. Binney, G. Harkell and J. Nixon, *Leaving Violent Men*, Leeds,
England, WAFE/DERT, 1981, p. 54. See also J. Pahl, *A Refuge for
Battered Women: A Study of the Role of a Women's Centre*, London, Her
Majesty's Stationery Office, 1978; Homer, Leonard and Taylor, op. cit.

79 Binney, Harkell and Nixon, ibid.
80 S. Schechter, *Women and Male Violence: The Visions and Struggles of the Battered Women's Movement*, Boston, South End Press, 1982, p. 60.
81 C. Charlton, 'The first cow on Chiswick High Road', *Spare Rib*, 24, 1972, pp. 24–5; R.E. Dobash, and R.P. Dobash, 'Love, honour and obey: Institutional ideologies and the struggle for battered women', *Contemporary Crisis*, 1, 1977, pp. 403–15, 403–4; Dobash and Dobash, op. cit., *Violence Against Wives*, pp. 223–4; J. Sutton, 'The growth of the British movement for battered women', *Victimology*, vol. 2, nos. 3–4, 1977–8, pp. 576–84; J. Hanmer, 'Community action, Women's Aid and the women's liberation movement', in M. Mayo (ed.), *Women in the Community*, London, Routledge, 1977.
82 B. Warrior, *Battered Women's Directory*, 46 Pleasant St., Cambridge, MA 02139, USA, 1976; Martin, op. cit., pp. 196–231; M. Karl, 'Refuges in Europe', *Victimology*, vol. 2, nos. 3–4, 1977–8, pp. 657–66; no author, 'Resources in the United States and Canada', *Victimology*, vol. 2, nos. 3–4, 1977–8, pp. 666–8; R.E. Dobash, 'Violence against women – A worldwide view', Keynote address, Welsh Women's Aid International Conference, Cardiff, Wales, proceedings published as Report of the International Women's Aid Conference, Cardiff, Wales, Welsh Women's Aid, 38/42 Crwys Road, Cardiff, Wales, UK, 1988, pp. 21–6.
83 Welsh Women's Aid, op. cit., pp. 108–14.
84 Dobash and Dobash, op. cit., *Violence Against Wives*.
85 Schechter, op. cit. For partial discussions of the British movement see, J. Sutton, 'The growth of the British movement for battered women', *Victimology*, vol. 2, nos. 3–4, 1977–8, pp. 576–84; J. Hanmer, 'Violence to women: From private sorrow to public issue', in G. Ashworth and L. Bonnerjea (eds), *The Invisible Decade: UK Women in the United Nations Decade 1976–86*, Aldershot, Hampshire, Gower, 1985, pp. 141–54; R.E. Dobash and R.P. Dobash, 'The response of the British and American women's movements to violence against women', in J. Hanmer and M. Maynard (eds), *Women, Violence and Social Control*, London, Macmillan Press, 1985, pp. 169–79.

2 THE RISE OF THE MOVEMENT: ORIENTATIONS AND ISSUES

1 J. Freeman, *The Politics of Women's Liberation*, New York, Longman, 1975, pp. 44–70; S. Rowbotham, L. Segal and H. Wainwright, *Beyond the Fragments: Feminism and the Making of Socialism*, London, Merlin Press, 1979; D. Dahlerup (ed.), *The New Women's Movement: Feminism and Political Power in Europe and the USA*, London, Sage, 1986; A. Coote and B. Campbell, 2nd ed., *Sweet Freedom: The Struggle for Women's Liberation*, Oxford, Basil Blackwell, 1987, pp. 1–52; *Feminist Review*, no. 31, Spring 1989, special issue on Twenty Years of Feminism; Sheila Rowbotham, *The Past is Before Us: Feminism in Action Since the 1960s*, London, Penguin, 1989.
2 D. Dahlerup, 'Is the new women's movement dead?', in D. Dahlerup

(ed.), *The New Women's Movement: Feminism and Political Power in Europe and the USA*, London, Sage, 1986, p. 3; and citing A. Rossi, *The Feminist Papers: From Adams to de Beauvoir*, New York, Columbia University Press, 1973; E. Wilson, *Only Halfway to Paradise: Women in Postwar Britain: 1945–1968*, London, Tavistock; O. Banks, *Faces of Feminism*, Oxford, Martin Robertson, 1981; J. Rendall, *The Origins of Modern Feminism: Women in Britain, France and the United States, 1780–1860*, London, Macmillan, 1985; N. Cott, *The Grounding of Modern Feminism*, New Haven, CT, Yale University Press, 1987.

3 For examination of earlier ideas see Rendall, ibid., and Banks, ibid., B.S. Anderson and J.P. Zinsser, *A History of Their Own: Women in Europe from Prehistory to the Present*, vols. I and II, London, Penguin, 1988, esp. vol. II., pp. 278–307, 350–406.
4 Anderson and Zinsser, ibid., p. 353.
5 F. Haug, 'Lessons from the women's movement in Europe', *Feminist Review*, no. 31, Spring, special issue on Twenty Years of Feminism, 1989, p. 109.
6 Ibid.
7 J. Freeman, cited in Dahlerup, op. cit., p. 221, Freeman, op. cit., pp. 48–9.
8 Dahlerup, op. cit., p. 221.
9 R.E. Park, *Outline of the Principles of Sociology*, New York, Barnes and Noble, 1939, cited in J.F. Zygmunt, 'Collective behavior as a phase of societal life: Blumer's emergent views and their implications', pp. 25–46 in K. Lang, G.E. Lang and L. Kriesberg, *Research in Social Movements, Conflict and Change*, London JAI Press, vol. 9, 1986, p. 25, no. 45.
10 Zygmunt, ibid., pp. 25–31.
11 J. Gusfield, 'Social structure and moral reform: A study of the Woman's Christian Temperance Union', *American Journal of Sociology*, vol. 61, Nov., 1955, pp. 221–32; S. Messinger, 'Organizational transformation: A case study of a declining social movement', *American Sociological Review*, vol. 20, Feb., 1955, pp. 3–10; D. Sills, *The Volunteers: Means and Ends in a National Organization*, Glencoe, IL, Free Press, 1957; M.N. Zald and P. Denton, 'From evangelism to general service: The transformation of the YMCA', *Administrative Science Quarterly*, vol. 8, Sept., 1963, pp. 214–34, all cited in M.N. Marger, 'Social movement organizations and response to environmental change: The NAACP, 1960–1973', *Social Problems*, vol. 32, no. 1, 1984, pp. 16–30, n., pp. 16, 27–9.
12 C. Tilly, *From Mobilization to Revolution*, Reading, MA, Addison-Wesley, 1978, p. 69 cited in H. Haines, 'Black radicalization and the funding of Civil Rights: 1957–1970', *Social Problems*, vol. 32, no. 1, 1984, pp. 31–43, n., p. 34.
13 J.D. McCarthy and M.N. Zald, 'Resource mobilization and social movements: A partial theory', *American Journal of Sociology*, vol. 82, no. 6, 1977, pp. 1212–41, p. 1220, cited in Haines, ibid., p. 34.
14 A. Oberschall, *Social Conflict and Social Movements*, Englewood Cliffs, NJ, Prentice-Hall, 1973, p. 28 cited in Haines, ibid., p. 34.
15 W.A. Gamson, *The Strategy of Social Protest*, Homewood, IL, Dorsey, 1975; Oberschall, op. cit.; Tilly, op. cit., all cited in Marger, op. cit., p. 16.

16 J.D. McCarthy and M.N. Zald, *The Trend of Social Movements in America: Professionalization and Resource Mobilization*, Morristown, NJ, General Learning Press, 1973, cited in Haines, op. cit., p. 43; C. Perrow, 'The sixties observed', pp. 192–211 in M.N. Zald and J.D. McCarthy (eds), *The Dynamics of Social Movements: Resource Mobilization, Social Control, and Tactics*, Cambridge, MA, Winthrop, 1979, cited in Marger, n., p. 16.

17 Ibid.

18 V. Taylor, 'Social movements continuity: The women's movement in abeyance', *American Sociological Review*, vol. 54, no. 5, 1989, p. 761; V. Taylor, 'The future of feminism: A social movement analysis', in L. Richardson and V. Taylor (eds), *Feminist Frontiers II*, New York, Random House, 1988, pp. 473–90.

19 F. Piven and R. A. Cloward, *Poor People's Movements: Why They Succeed, How They Fail*, New York, Pantheon Books, 1977.

20 Haines, op. cit., illustrates this with the civil rights movement in the USA, comparing the radical Black Panthers with the moderate NAACP (National Association for the Advancement of Colored People).

21 E. Crighton and D.S. Mason, 'Solidarity and the Greens: The rise of new social movements in East and West Europe', in K. Land and G.E. Lang (eds), *Research in Social Movements, Conflicts and Change*, London, JAI Press, 1986, pp. 155–76.

22 This position is particularly strong among some but not all sections of radical feminism.

23 H. Kriesi, 'New social movements and the new class in the Netherlands', *American Journal of Sociology*, vol. 94, no. 5, March, 1989, pp. 1078–116, p. 1079.

24 Crighton and Mason, op. cit., p. 55; Kriesi, op. cit., p. 1079.

25 J. Habermas, 'New social movements', *Telos*, 49, 1981, pp. 33–7, p. 33, cited in Crighton and Mason, op. cit., p. 155.

26 Crighton and Mason, idid., p. 156.

27 See Kriesi, op. cit., p. 1078, for a discussion of the reworking of the 'new class'.

28 A. Touraine, *The Voice and the Eye: An Analysis of Social Movements*, Cambridge, Cambridge University Press, 1981, pp. 77–101.

29 Ibid., p. 80.

30 Ibid., p. 26.

31 Ibid., p. 77.

32 Ibid., p. 80.

33 Ibid., p. 81.

34 Ibid.

35 Ibid., pp. 81–4.

36 P.Y. Martin, 'Rethinking feminist organizations', *Gender and Society*, vol. 4, no. 2, June, 1990, pp. 182–206; C. Olofsson, 'After the working class movement', *Acta Sociologica*, vol. 31, no. 1, 1981; R. Badham, 'The sociology of industrial and post-industrial societies', *Current Sociology*, vol. 32, no. 1, 1984; C. Offe, *Contradictions in the Welfare State*, London, Hutchinson, 1984, p. 247; C. Pierson, 'New theories of state and civil society – Recent developments in post-Marxist analysis of the state', *Sociology*, vol. 18, no. 4, 1984, p. 565; C. Offe, 'New social

movements: Challenging the boundaries of institutional politics', *Social Research*, vol. 52, 1985, pp. 817–68; R. Ingelhart and J.R. Rabier, 'Political realignment in advanced industrial society: From class-based politics to quality-of-life politics', *Government and Opposition*, vol. 21, no. 4, 1986, pp. xxx.

37 For readings on social change, see F.H. Cordoso, 'Problems of social change, again?', *International Sociology*, vol. 2, no. 2, June, 1987, pp. 177–87.

38 T. Mathiesen, *The Politics of Abolition*, London, Martin Robertson, 1974; R.E. Dobash and R.P. Dobash, 'Social science and social action', *Journal of Family Issues*, vol. 2, no. 4, December, 1981, pp. 452–9; and reprinted in K. Yllo and M. Bogard (eds), *Feminist Perspectives on Wife Abuse*, Beverly Hills, Sage, 1988, pp. 61–7.

39 Kriesi, op. cit., p. 1078.

40 Freeman, op. cit., pp. 106–7.

41 Ibid., pp. 106–11; S. Schechter, *Women and Male Violence*, Boston, South End Press, 1982, pp. 29–34.

42 Coote and Campbell, op. cit., p. 9; A. Neustatter, *Hyenas in Petticoats*, London, Penguin, 1990, pp. 3–53; Rowbotham, op. cit., 1989.

43 J. Mitchell, 'The longest revolution', *New Left Review*, Nov.–Dec., 1966; S. Rowbotham, 'Women's liberation and the new politics', Spokesman pamphlet, no. 17, 1969; see Coote and Campbell, op. cit., p. 9.

44 Rendall, op. cit., p. 1; Banks, op. cit., pp. 7–8, 28–47; Schechter, op. cit., p. 45; J. Mitchell, 'Women and equality', in J. Mitchell and A. Oakley (eds), *The Rights and Wrongs of Women*, Harmondsworth, Middlesex, England, Penguin Books, 1976, pp. 379–99.

45 Freeman, op. cit., pp. 71–102; Dahlerup, op. cit., p. 221 refers to The Danish Women's Society, established in 1871, and others in the five Nordic countries which are equal rights organizations, but unlike NOW they did not grow with the rest of the women's movement during the 1960s and 1970s.

46 J. Brenner, 'Feminist political discourses: Radical versus Liberal approaches to the feminization of poverty and comparable worth', *Gender and Society*, vol. 1, no. 4, Dec., 1987, p. 448.

47 G. Lerner, *The Majority Finds its Past. Placing Women in History*, New York, Oxford University Press, 1979; 'Politics and culture in women's history: a symposium', *Feminist Studies*, 6, Spring, 1980, pp. 26–63, cited in Rendall, op. cit., p. 1, note 2, p. 326; J. Mitchell, 'Women and equality', op. cit.

48 D. Dahlerup, 'Is the new women's movement dead?' in D. Dahlerup, op. cit., p. 7.

49 Coote and Campbell, op. cit., p. 19; Schechter, op. cit., p. 46.

50 For discussions of radical feminism, see (GB) Coote and Campbell, op. cit., pp. 18–23; M. Barrett and M. McIntosh, *The Anti-social Family*, London, Verso, 1982; (USA) Schechter, op. cit., p. 46; B. Ryan, 'Ideological purity and feminism: The US women's movement from 1966–1975', *Gender and Society*, vol. 3, no. 2, June, 1989, pp. 239–57. For socialist-feminism see (GB) Coote and Campbell, op. cit., pp. 23–5; Lynne Segal, 'Slow change or no change?: Feminism, Socialism and the problem of men', *Feminist Review*, Special Issue, The Past Before Us,

Twenty Years of Feminism, no. 31, Spring, 1989, pp. 5–21; K. Harriss, 'New alliances: Socialist-feminism in the eighties', in *Feminist Review*, op. cit., pp. 34–54; F. Haug, op. cit., pp. 107–16; (USA) Schechter, op. cit., p. 47; (Europe) Anderson and Zinsser, op. cit., 1990, pp. 371–405.

51 Coote and Campbell, op. cit., p. 9; J.S. Chafetz and A.G. Dworkin, *Female Revolt: Women's Movements in World and Historical Perspective*, Totowa, NH, Rowan and Allanheld, 1986, reviewed in V. Taylor, 'Sisterhood solidarity and modern feminism' – review essay, *Gender and Society*, June, 1989, pp. 283–6.

52 M.M. Feree, 'Political strategies and feminist concerns in the United States and Federal Republic of Germany: Class, race and gender', Paper presented at the XIIth World Congress of Sociology, Madrid, July, 1990; and M.M. Ferree, 'Equality and autonomy: Feminist politics in the United States and West Germany', in M.F. Katzenstein and C.M. Mueller (eds), *The Women's Movements of the United States and Western Europe: Consciousness, Political Opportunity, and Public Policy*, Philadelphia, Temple University Press, 1987, pp. 172–95.

53 Coote and Campbell, op. cit., p. 18; J. Hanmer, 'Violence to women: From private sorrow to public issue', in G. Ashworth and L. Bonnerjea (eds), *The Invisible Decade: UK Women in the United Nations Decade 1976–86*, Aldershot, England, Gower, 1985, pp. 141–54, p. 141.

54 R.E. Dobash and R.P. Dobash, *Violence Against Wives*, New York, The Free Press, and Macmillan Distributing, Brunel Road, Houndmills, Basingstoke, England, 1979, pp. 1–3, 223–5.

55 Ibid., p. 1.

56 Ibid., pp. 223–5; Coote and Campell, op. cit., pp. 36–7; H. Rose, 'In practice supported, in theory denied: An account of an invisible urban movement', *International Journal of Urban and Regional Research*, vol. 2, no. 3, 1978, pp. 521–37, extracted and updated as 'Women's refuges: Creating new forms of welfare?', in Clare Ungerson (ed.), *Women and Social Policy*, London, Macmillan, 1985, pp. 243–59; J. Hanmer, 'Violence and the social control of women', in G. Littlejohn, B. Small, J. Wakeford and N. Yural-Davies (eds), *Power and the State*, London, Croom Helm, 1977.

57 Schechter, op. cit., pp. 53–80; D. Martin, *Battered Wives*, San Francisco, Glide Publications, 1976, pp. 196–216; G. Sullivan, 'The movement against woman abuse', in MCBWSG, Massachusetts Coalition of Battered Women Service Groups, *For Shelter and Beyond*, Boston, MA, c/o Mass. Coalition for Battered Women Service Groups, 1981, pp. 18–19. Although some groups working with male alcoholics had taken in women who had been abused, they cannot be said to have started the movement as their focus was on alcohol abuse and not battering as such.

58 Houseworker's Handbook, 1st ed., Lisa Leghorn and Betsy Warrior, Woman's Center, 1974; B. Warrior, 'Battered lives', in Leghorn and Warrior, ibid., pp. 25–46; B. Warrior, 'Why refuges', in *Working on Wife Abuse* (7th ed.), c/o B. Warrior, 46 Pleasant St., Cambridge, MA.

59 B. Warrior, *Working on Wife Abuse*, 1st ed., c/o B. Warrior, 1976.

60 Dobash and Dobash, *Violence Against Wives*, op. cit., pp. 1–3, 223–9; R.E. Dobash and R.P. Dobash, 'The response of the British and American women's movements to violence against women', in J. Hanmer

308   *Women, violence and social change*

and M. Maynard (eds), *Women, Violence and Social Control,* London, Macmillan Press, 1987, pp. 167–79. *The Theory of Social and Economic Organization,* translated by A.R. Henderson and T. Parsons, New York, Hodge, 1947.

61 See Max Weber for a discussion of authority based on expertise.

62 Freeman, op. cit., pp. 111–14, 120–1.

63 J. Sutton, 'The growth of the British movement for battered women', *Victimology,* 2 (3–4), 1978, pp. 576–84. Rose, op. cit., 1978; Dobash and Dobash, *Violence Against Wives,* op. cit., p. 223; Dobash and Dobash, 'British and American movements', op. cit., p. 175; Schechter, op. cit., p. 154; Coote and Campbell, op. cit., pp. 36–7.

64 Personal correspondence; also cited in Schechter, op. cit., p. 154.

65 Haines, op. cit., p. 31, Freeman, op. cit., p. 106–9; Crighton and Mason, op. cit., p. 169.

66 Cited in A. Mama, *The Hidden Struggle,* London, London Race and Housing Research Unit, 1989, p. 275. For the original wording see J. Sutton, op. cit., 1978; Dobash and Dobash, *Violence Against Wives,* op. cit., pp. 224–5.

67 Sutton, op. cit., Dobash and Dobash, ibid.

68 Mama, op. cit., pp. 276–7.

69 United States Commission on Civil Rights, *Battered Women: Issues of Public Policy,* Washington DC: US Commission on Civil Rights, 1978, p. V; Schechter, op. cit., pp. 133–7.

70 Schechter, op. cit., p. 138.

71 Ibid., pp. 138–9.

72 *Aegis: Magazine on Ending Violence Against Women,* 'National Coalition Against Domestic Violence News', September/October, 1978, p. 15; Schechter, op. cit., p. 140.

73 Mathiesen would refer to the latter as the 'alternative', while Touraine, op. cit., pp. 80–1 defines this as the 'stakes' or totality.

74 L. Kelly, *Surviving Sexual Violence,* Cambridge, Polity Press, 1988, pp. 159–87.

75 Interview with Lisa Leghorn, cited in Schechter, op. cit., p. 126.

76 60 Minutes program; L. Ahrens, 'Battered women's refuges: Feminist Cooperatives vs. social service institutions', *Radical America,* vol. 4, no. 3, May–June, 1980, p. 45.

77 S. Epstein, G. Russell and L. Silvern, *American Journal of Community Psychology,* vol. 16, no. 3, 1988, pp. 345–67, p. 357.

78 A. Sachs and J.H. Wilson, *Sexism and the Law: A Study of Male Beliefs and Judicial Bias,* Oxford, Martin Robertson, 1978; S.S.M. Edwards, *Female Sexuality and the Law,* Oxford, Martin Robertson, 1981; C. Smart, *Feminism and the Power of Law,* London, Routledge, 1989; Dobash and Dobash, *Violence Against Wives,* op. cit., pp. 34–40, 59–64, 207–22.

79 D. Friedman, 'Increased convictions? or lowered expectations?', *Aegis, Magazine on Ending Violence Against Women,* Summer, 1981 pp. 36–8; E. Soler, 'Domestic violence is a crime: A case study – San Francisco Family Violence Project', in D.J. Sonkin (ed.), *Domestic Violence on Trial: Psychological and Legal Dimensions of Family Violence,* New York, Springer, 1987, pp. 21–38; Smart, op. cit., pp. 4–25, 66–89, 138–59.

80 T. Faragher, 'The police response to violence against women in the home', in J. Pahl (ed.), *Private Violence and Public Policy*, London, Routledge, 1985, pp. 110–24; K.J. Ferraro, 'The legal response in the United States', in J. Hanmer, J. Radford and E. Stanko (eds), *Women, Policing and Male Violence*, London, Routledge, 1989, pp. 155–84; Smart, op. cit.

81 S. Schechter *et al.*, 'Men who batter/A woman's response', Unpublished position paper circulated at the NCADV national conference, Milwaukee, Wisconsin, 1982; Schechter, op. cit., pp. 261–7.

82 T. Mathiesen, op. cit., pp. 13–28; Dobash and Dobash, 'Social science and social action'. op. cit.

83 Schechter, op. cit., pp. 241–56.

84 F. Parkin, *Middle Class Radicalism*, Manchester, Manchester University Press, 1968; and discussed in Kriesi, op. cit., p. 1083.

85 Mathiesen, op. cit., pp. 15, 17; Dobash and Dobash, 'Social science and social action', op. cit., pp. 451–9.

86 See M. Foucault, *Discipline and Punish: The Birth of the Prison*, London, Allen and Unwin, 1977; F. Wasoff, R. Emerson Dobash and Dorothy Harcus, 'Simulated clients in natural settings: Constructing a client for study of professional practice', unpublished paper, 1989; M. Bush, *Families in Distress: Public, Private, and Civic Responses*, Berkeley, University of California Press, 1988.

87 D. Friedman, 'Professionalism', *Aegis, Magazine on Ending Violence Against Women*, Summer, 1981, pp. 36–8; S. Schechter, 'Speaking to the battered women's movement', *Aegis*, Winter, 1982, pp. 36–43; P. Roberts and C Lopes, 'Battered women: who will define the solution?', *Aegis*, Winter, 1982, pp. 24–5.

88 Schechter, *Women and Male Violence*, op. cit., p. 283.

89 On this issue and socialist-feminist debates, see Segal, op. cit., pp. 5–21; C. MacKinnon, 'Feminism, Marxism, method, and the state: An agenda for theory', *Signs*, vol. 7, no. 3, 1982, pp. 515–44; H. Hartmann, 'Capitalism, patriarchy, and job segregation by sex', *Signs: Journal of Women in Culture and Society*, vol. 1, no. 3, 1976, pp. 137–69.

90 Cited in Schechter, *Women and Male Violence*, op. cit., p. 279.

91 Ibid., p. 138–49.

92 Ibid., pp. 144–5. On the issue of race and the movement (USA) see Massachusetts Coalition of Battered Women Service Groups (MCBWSG), *For Shelter and Beyond*, op. cit., pp. 49, 53–8; See also *Aegis*, March/April, 1979, special issue on Violence against women and race; Summer, 1981, pp. 14–19, Winter 1982, pp. 16–25; Spring, 1982, pp. 29–38.

93 I.N. Toure, 'Report on the First National Third World Women's Conference on Violence', *Aegis*, Summer/Autumn, 1980, p. 71.

94 Schechter, *Women and Male Violence*, op. cit., pp. 257–86. See Ferree, op. cit., on the importance of race within the women's movement in the USA.

95 Mama, op. cit., p. 285.

96 L. Harvey, unpublished manuscript on Asian women and violence in Glasgow, University of Stirling, Scotland, 1990.

97 Mama, op. cit. On the issue of race and the movement (GB) see K.

Bhavnani and M. Coulson, 'Transforming socialist-feminism: The challenge of racism', *Feminist Review*, no. 23, Summer, 1986, pp. 81–92; A. Mama, 'Violence against black women: Gender, race and state responses', *Feminist Review*, no. 32, Summer, 1989, pp. 30–48; A. Mama, 'A hidden struggle', *Spare Rib*, no. 209, February, 1990, pp. 8–11; Harvey, op. cit.

98 It should be noted that this same form of reasoning has also been used to justify men's use of violence against women.

99 *Social Trends*, 1987. Most of the population live a lifestyle that differs from the 'ideal' nuclear family. The alternatives include the single living alone or with other in non-sexual relationships, cohabitants, adult children living with one or more parents, divorced, widowed, one parent families, couples without children, gay men and lesbians. Only the question of household composition is addressed here. The issue of departure from the ideal of monogamy, either outside the nuclear family with same or opposite sexual partners or inside the family usually in the form of father–daughter incest, is not considered. This would, however, reduce still further the percentage of those living the 'ideal family' lifestyle.

100 On the issue of homophobia and the movement see Schechter, *Women and Male Violence*, op. cit., pp. 267–71; MCBWSG, op. cit., pp. 59–63.

101 Banks, op. cit., p. 5.

102 Piven and Cloward, op. cit., Kriesi, op. cit.

103 On the role of battered women in the movement, see Schechter, *Women and Male Violence*, op. cit., pp. 281–6.

104 Ibid., pp. 300–4.

105 Ibid., p. 302.

106 S. Schechter, 'In honor of the battered women's movement: An appraisal of our work', Unpublished Keynote address, National Coalition Against Domestic Violence, 2nd National Conference, August, 1982; E. Wilson, *What is to be Done About Violence Against Women?*, Harmondsworth, Middlesex, England, 1983, pp. 194–206; Rose, op. cit., 1985, pp. 243–59; Dobash and Dobash, 'The response of the British and American women's movements', op. cit., pp. 169–79.

3 REFUGES AND HOUSING

1 For example, in the eighteenth century magdalen houses were meant to save women forced by poverty into prostitution. Poor houses gave some comfort to the destitute and convents were often places of escape from cruel patriarchs. R.P. Dobash, R.E. Dobash and S. Gutteridge, *The Imprisonment of Women*, Oxford, Basil Blackwell, 1986, p. 37.

2 'Highland clearances and Glasgow rent strikes', in R. Quinalt and J. Stevenson (eds), *Popular Protest and Public Disorder*, London, Basil Blackwell, 1974, pp. 75–114.

3 Christine de Pizan, *The Book of the City of Ladies*, trans. E.J. Richards, New York, Persea Books, 1982, p. 187, cited in B.S. Anderson and J.P. Zinsser (eds), *A History of Their Own*, London, Penguin, 1988, pp. 341–4.

4 Ibid., p. 342.
5 Ibid., p. 343.
6 Ibid., p. 342.
7 Ibid., p. 343.
8 For an early statement about the importance of refuge see Betsy Warrior 'refuges'. *Working on Wife Abuse*, 1976, p. 1.
9 See R.P. Dobash, R.E. Dobash, M. Wilson and M. Daly, 'The myth of the asymmetrical nature of domestic violence', forthcoming.
10 Women's Aid, *Battered Wives: Report by Women's Aid*, June, 1973, p. 3; E. Pizzey, *Scream Quietly or the Neighbours Will Hear*, Harmondsworth, Middlesex, England, Penguin, 1974, pp. 9–10.
11 Ibid., p. 3.
12 Ibid., p. 6.
13 G. Search, 'Notes from abroad. London: Battered wives', *Ms Magazine*, June, 1974, p. 24.
14 Women's Aid, *Battered Wives*, op. cit., pp. 7–8.
15 Search, op. cit., p. 24.
16 D. Martin, *Battered Wives*, San Francisco, Glide Publications, 1976, pp. 197–205; discussion with Sharon Vaughn; Warrior, op. cit., pp. 5, 7.
17 Martin, ibid., p. 198.
18 Personal interview with Fran Wasoff, First National Co-ordinator of Scottish Women's Aid, 1988.
19 K. Kerr, 'In the beginning: The herstory of Women's Aid in Scotland', *Scottish Women's Aid Newsletter (SWAN)*, April, 1985, p. 4; S. Henderson and A. Mackay, *Grit and Diamonds: Women in Scotland Making History, 1980–1990*, Edinburgh, Stramullion, 1990, pp. 78–80, 110–12.
20 M. Whiteland and M. O'Donnell in L. Underwood, 'The herstory of Glasgow Women's Aid: An interview with two founding members', *Scottish Women's Aid Newletter*, Spring, 1987, p. 11.
21 Ibid.
22 M. Butterly, 'Interval House – Glasgow, Scotland', in B. Warrior, *Houseworker's Handbook*, 1974, p. 49.
23 Martin, op. cit., p. 226; *Scottish Women's Aid Newsletter*, April, 1985, pp. 3–5; Scottish Women's Aid, 'The herstory of Women's Aid in Scotland', 1988.
24 V. Binney, G. Harkell and J. Nixon, *Leaving Violent Men: A Study of Refuges and Housing for Battered Women*, Women's Aid Federation England/Department of Environment, printed by King's English Bookprinters Ltd, Leeds, Yorkshire, 1981, p. iii.
25 Ibid., pp. iv–vii.
26 Ibid., p. viii.
27 Ibid., pp. x, 24–7.
28 Ibid., pp. xii, 29–42.
29 Ibid., pp. xiv, xii.
30 Ibid., pp. xii, 44–8.
31 Ibid., p. 48.
32 *Handbook of Federal Resources on Domestic Violence*, Interdepartmental Committee on Domestic Violence, 1980.
33 US Department of Health and Human Services, Office of Human Deve-

312 Women, violence and social change

lopment Services, A Monograph on Services to Battered Women, Washington DC, DHHS no. (OHDS) 79-05708, 1980, pp. 19–77.

34 Ibid., p. 21.
35 Ibid., p. 24.
36 Ibid., p. 19.
37 Ibid., p. 25.
38 Ibid., p. 25.
39 Ibid., p. 23.
40 Ibid., pp. 22–6.
41 K.J. Ferraro, 'The legal response in the United States', in J. Hanmer, J. Radford and E. Stanko (eds), Women, Policing and Male Violence, London, Routledge, 1989, p. 161.
42 SWA Newsletter, Summer/Autumn, 1990, p. 2; Welsh Women's Aid, Annual Report 1989–90, p. 3; personal communication, Women's Aid Federation, England.
43 J. Freeman, The Politics of Women's Liberation, New York and London, Longman, 1975; R. Evans, The Feminists. Women's Emancipation Movements in Europe, America and Australasia, 1840–1920, London, Croom Helm, 1977; O. Banks, Faces of Feminism: A Study of Feminism as a Social Movement, Oxford, Martin Robertson, 1981; A. Coote and B. Campbell, Sweet Freedom, Oxford, Blackwell, 1st ed., 1982, 2nd ed., 1987; J. Rendall, The Origins of Modern Feminism: Women in Britain, France and the United States, 1780–1860, London, Macmillan, 1985; Anderson and Zinsser, op. cit.
44 Ibid. (Anderson and Zinsser), pp. 337–8.
45 M. Wollstonecraft, A Vindication of the Rights of Women, Reprint of 1792, London, Dent, 1955.
46 Anderson and Zinsser, op. cit., pp. 346–9.
47 J.S. Mill, The Subjection of Women, Reprint of 1869, London, Dent, 1955.
48 Anderson and Zinsser, op. cit., p. 338.
49 Ibid., p. 375.
50 Ibid., p. 372.
51 Ibid., pp. 375–6.
52 Ibid., p. 371.
53 Ibid., p. 377.
54 Ibid., p. 338.
55 Ibid., p. 386.
56 Ibid., pp. 368–9.
57 Banks, op. cit., p. 8.
58 Ibid.
59 Ibid., p. 7.
60 Ibid., p. 4.
61 Anderson and Zinsser, op. cit., pp. 397–405; E. Wilson, Halfway to Paradise, London, Tavistock, 1980, pp. 1–40.
62 Anderson and Zinsser, op. cit., p. 339.
63 C.A. MacKinnon, Toward a Feminist Theory of the State, Cambridge, MA, Harvard University Press, 1989, pp. 83–105.
64 Binney, Harkell and Nixon, op. cit., US (OHDS), op. cit., M. Homer, A. Leonard and P. Taylor, Private Violence: Public Shame, CRAWC,

Cleveland Refuge and Aid for Women and Children, Middlesbrough, Cleveland, England, 1984; B. Warrior, *Working on Wife Abuse*, Cambridge, MA, editions from 1976.
65 Some architecture has been oriented to freeing women from traditional divisions of labour that keep them constantly at work in the home. For example, D. Hayden, *The Grand Domestic Revolution*, Cambridge, MA, The MIT Press, 1982, recounts nineteenth-century American experiments in building houses without kitchens and towns designed to reduce housework. Model villages, the co-operative ideal and feminist politics were meant to change domestic and social life using architecture as an important tool in facilitating social change; although with a different focus, Prince Charles has recently caused controversy in Britain with his criticisms of modern architecture and proposals for changes reflecting a more human approach.
66 Information is based on personal visits to the refuges.
67 L. Ahrens, 'Battered women's refuges: Feminist cooperatives vs. social service institutions', *Radical America*, vol. 14, no. 3, May–June, 1980, p. 45.
68 US (OHDS), op.cit., p. 72.
69 Ibid., pp. 73–4.
70 Ibid.
71 Mark Tran in Washington, reported in the *Guardian*, 9 November, 1988.
72 US (OHDS), op. cit., p. 52.
73 Ibid.
74 Ibid., p. 53.
75 Ibid., p. 55.
76 Ibid. These observations are also based on interviews held with staff in 1986.
77 Ibid., p. 69.
78 Ibid., p. 68.
79 Ibid.
80 Ibid., p. 69.
81 Ibid.
82 M.D. Fields and R.M. Kirchner, 'Summary of English and Scottish shelters', Unpublished paper, New York, 1976, p. 24.
83 B. Bowder, 'The wives who ask for it' (interview with Gayford, McKeith and Pizzey), *Community Care*, 1 March, 1979; R.E. Dobash, and R.P. Dobash, 'If you prick me do I not bleed? Replying to "Wives who ask for it"', *Community Care*, 3 May, 1979, pp. 26–8.
84 Fields and Kirchner, op. cit., pp. 24, 27.
85 Bowder, op. cit.; E. Pizzey and J. Shapiro, *Prone to Violence*, Feltha, Middlesex, England, Hamlyn Paperbacks, 1982.
86 *Escape from Violence: The Women of Bradley Angle House*, Portland, Oregon, Bradley-Angle House, 1978, pp. 1–4, 32–3.
87 Ibid., pp. 32, 37.
88 US (OHDS), op. cit., pp. 32–3.
89 Ibid., pp. 33, 37.
90 Fields and Kirchner, op. cit., pp. 22–7.
91 Pahl, *A Refuge for Battered Women*, London, HMSO, 1978.
92 Binney, Harkell and Nixon, op. cit.

93 Homer, Leonard and Taylor, op. cit.; M. Homer, A. Leonard and P. Taylor, 'Refuges and housing for battered women', in J. Pahl (ed.), *Private Violence and Public Policy: The Needs of Battered Women and the Response of the Public Services*, London, Routledge, 1985, pp. 166–78.

94 Homer, Leonard and Taylor, op. cit., p. 47.

95 Ibid., p. 48.

96 Ibid.

97 Ibid.

98 Homer, Leonard and Taylor, *Private Violence, Public Shame*, op. cit.; Binney, Harkell and Nixon, op. cit.; Pahl, op. cit., E. Evanson, *Hidden Violence*, Belfast, Farset Press, 1982; R.E. Dobash and R.P. Dobash, *Violence Against Wives*, New York, The Free Press, and Macmillan Distributing, Brunel Road, Houndmills, Basingstoke, England, 1979.

99 Homer, Leonard and Taylor, *Private Violence, Public Shame*, ibid., pp. 50–1.

100 Ibid., p. 53.

101 Binney, Harkell and Nixon, op. cit., pp. 60–1.

102 Ibid., p. 51.

103 N.M. Rodriguez, 'Transcending bureaucracy: Feminist politics at a shelter for battered women', *Gender and Society*, vol. 2, no. 2, June, 1988, pp. 214–27. This 1988 study of the workings of the Family Crisis Shelter in Hawaii illustrates how this type of egalitarian refuge has learned the lesson of early innovation and continues to deal with creative forms of organization and issues of authority while seeking to fulfil the general goals of empowerment and liberation of women using the principles of self-help and self-reliance. It examines how this form of organization and working philosophy has addressed many of the issues raised during a decade of working for social change within such a framework.

104 T. Mathiesen, *The Politics of Abolition*, London, Martin Robertson, 1974, p. 17.

105 M. Bush, *Families in Distress. Public, Private and Civic Responses*, Berkeley, University of California Press, 1988.

106 Scottish Homeless Group, *Homelessness: Your Rights, a Scottish Guide to the Housing (Homeless Persons) Act*, c/o Scottish Homeless Group, 1986; Report of the Metropolitan Police (London) Working Party into Domestic Violence, 1986, p. 50; Scottish Women's Aid (SWA), 'Battered women and homelessness: An outline of the Code of Guidance to the Housing (Scotland) Act (1987)', 1989; Women's National Commission, An Advisory Committee to Her Majesty's Government, *What Chance of a Home? A Study of Homelessness Particularly as it Affects Women*, Report of an ad-hoc Working Group, c/o WNC, Government Offices, Horse Guards Road, London, 1990.

107 Binney, Harkell and Nixon in Pahl, op. cit., p. 176.

108 Ibid., p. 177.

109 Report of the Metropolitan Police (London) Working Party into Domestic Violence, pp. 36, 37–8, 40.

110 R. Maxwell, 'A place of safety: Meeting the housing needs of battered women in Scotland', unpublished dissertation, Department of Sociology

and Social Policy, University of Stirling, Stirling, Scotland, 1987, p. 44; Scottish Women's Aid, 'Battered women and homelessness', op. cit.

111 Maxwell, ibid., p. 37; H. Rose, 'Women's refuges: Creating new forms of welfare?', in C. Ungerson (ed.), *Women and Social Policy*, London, Macmillan, 1985, pp. 246–8.

112 Rose, ibid.

113 Watchman and Robson, 1983, p. 27 cited in Maxwell, op. cit., p. 38.

114 Maxwell, op. cit., pp. 39–42.

115 Watchman and Robson, op. cit., p. 31, cited in Maxwell, op. cit., p. 38.

116 Maxwell, ibid., p. 49 citing A. Wilson, 1986, p. 23 unpub. dissertation, University of Edinburgh.

117 This law came into force on 7 January, 1987.

118 Maxwell, op. cit., p. 46, no. 19; SWA, 1989, op. cit.

119 See US Commission on Civil Rights, *The Federal Response to Domestic Violence*, Washington DC, 1982 for housing. J. Zorza, 'Federal domestic abuse legislation', *The Women's Advocate*, vol. XI, no. 5, Sept., 1990, p. 1 (Bill, HR 2951).

120 Welsh Women's Aid, 'Housing', in Tenth Annual Report, Welsh Women's Aid, Cardiff, Wales, 1988, pp. 3, 8–9.

121 Maxwell, op. cit., p. 78.

122 Maxwell, op. cit., p. 84; Scottish Women's Aid, *Annual Report*, 1987/88, p. 9.

4 THE STATE, PUBLIC POLICY AND SOCIAL CHANGE

1 An example of such an evaluation was made by Tierney in an article in which she declared that the battered women's movement had not been a success because, after a decade of work, it had not eliminated male violence. K. Tierney, 'The battered women's movement and the creation of the wife beating problem', *Social Problems*, vol. 29, no. 3, February, 1982.

2 S. Hall, 'The state in question', in G. McLennan, D. Held and S. Hall (eds), *The Idea of the Modern State*, Milton Keynes, Open University Press, 1984, pp. 1–28, p. 1.

3 Ibid., p. 1–9.

4 Ibid., p. 15. Whether the terms 'government' and 'state' are interchangeable is the subject of debate. Hall maintains that they are not, saying that the state is more complex and cannot be reduced simply to the technical and administrative functions of government operation, ibid., pp. 19–20. While the focus of our attention in the next few chapters shall be concentrated more explicitly upon the operations of legislation, government, public policy and criminal justice, these should be conceived of as only part of the state as a whole.

5 Ibid., p. 15.

6 Ibid., pp. 18–19.

7 Ibid., p. 20; See also D. Held, 'Central perspectives on the modern state', in McLennan, Held and Hall (eds), op. cit., pp. 29–79, p. 31.

8 Hall, ibid., p. 20.

9 See P. Aries, *Centuries of Childhood: A Social History of Family Life*,

New York, Random House, Vintage Books, 1962, pp. 351, 356; M. Foucault, *Madness and Civilization: A History of Insanity in the Age of Reason*, London, Social Science Paperback, 1967; G.J. Schochet, 'Patriarchalism, politics and mass attitudes in Stuart England', *The Historical Journal*, vol. 12, no. 3, 1969, pp. 413–41; L. Stone, 'The rise of the nuclear family in early modern England: The patriarchal stage', in C.E. Rosenberg (ed.), *The Family in History*, Philadelphia, University of Pennsylvania Press, 1975, p. 54; R.E. Dobash and R.P. Dobash, *Violence Against Wives*, New York, The Free Press, 1979, pp. 48–50; C. MacKinnon, 'Feminism, Marxism, method, and the state: An agenda for theory', *Signs*, vol. 7, no. 3, 1982, pp. 515–44; Hall, op. cit., p. 20.

10 J. Donzelot, *The Policing of Families*, translated by Robert Hurley, New York, Pantheon Books, 1979.

11 *The Shorter Oxford English Dictionary*, Oxford, Clarendon Press, 1973, p. 1205.

12 Hall, op. cit., p. 10; Held, op. cit., pp. 31–2; Stone, op. cit.

13 Hall, ibid., p. 10; Held, ibid., p. 31, 71; D. Held, 'Beyond liberalism and Marxism?', in McLennan, Held and Hall, op. cit., p. 225.

14 Hall, op. cit., pp. 10–11, 25.

15 Ibid., p. 11.

16 Ibid., p. 13.

17 D. Held and J. Krieger, 'Theories of the state: Some competing claims', in S. Bornstein, D. Held and J. Krieger (eds), *The State in Capitalist Europe: A Casebook*, London, George Allen and Unwin, 1984, pp. 1–21, p. 4; B. Jessop, *The Capitalist State: Marxist Theories and Methods*, Oxford, Basil Blackwell, 1982, pp. 1–31.

18 Jessop, op. cit., p. 27.

19 J.B. Elshtain, *Public Man, Private Woman: Women in Social and Political Thought*, Oxford, Martin Robertson, 1981.

20 See, for example, the exchange with Schechter about violence against women. J.B. Elshtain, 'Politics and the battered woman: A provocative study of a major social problem', *Dissent*, Winter, 1985, pp. 55–61; S. Schechter, 'Politics and the battered woman' (response to Elshtain), *Dissent*, Summer, 1985, pp. 332–4; J. B. Elshtain, 'Jean Bethke Elshtain replies' (to Susan Schechter), *Dissent*, Summer, 1985, pp. 334–6.

21 H. Bianchi and R. van Swaaningen (eds), *Abolitionism: Towards a Non-repressive Approach to Crime*, Amsterdam, Free University Press, 1986; J.R. Blad, H. van Mastrigt and N.A. Uildriks (eds), *The Criminal Justice System as a Social Problem: An Abolitionist Perspective*, Rotterdam, Erasmus Universiteit, 1987.

22 S. Schechter, *Women and Male Violence*, Boston, South End Press, 1982, pp. 177–8; L. Lerman, 'Mediation of wife abuse cases: The adverse impact of informal dispute resolution on women', *Harvard Women's Law Journal*, vol. 7, no. 1, 1984, pp. 57–113; also see discussion in Chapter 6.

23 M. Foucault, *The History of Sexuality*, vol. 1, trans. by Robert Hurley, London, Allen Lane, 1976; Donzelot, op. cit.

24 E. Wilson, *Women and the Welfare State*, London, Tavistock, 1977; E. Wilson, *Only Halfway to Paradise*, London, Tavistock, 1980, pp. 88–103, 207–9; E. Wilson, *What's to be Done About Violence Against*

Women, Harmondsworth, Penguin, 1983, p. 478; see also 51–2, 82–3, 87–96.

25 M. McIntosh, 'The state and the oppression of women', in A. Kuhn and A.M. Wolpe (eds), *Feminism and Materialism*, London, Routledge, 1978, pp. 254–89.

26 M. McIntosh and M. Barrett, *The Anti-social Family*, London, Verso, 1982.

27 C. Smart, *The Ties That Bind*, London, Routledge, 1984, pp. 129–46; H. Land, 'Changing women's claims to maintenance', in M. Freeman (ed.), *State, Law, and the Family*, London, Tavistock, 1984, pp. 25–35; C. Ungerson (ed.), *Women and Social Policy*, London, Macmillan, 1985; J. Dale and P. Foster, *Feminists and State Welfare*, London, Routledge, 1986, pp. 3–20; J. Millar and C. Glendinning, 'Invisible women, invisible poverty', in C. Glendinning and J. Millar (eds), *Women and Poverty in Britain*, Brighton, Eng., Wheatsheaf, 1987, pp. 3–27; J. Pahl, *Money and Marriage*, London, Macmillan, 1989, pp. 153–67.

28 On the enabling state, see C. Pierson, *A New Political Economy of the Welfare State*, Oxford, Polity Press, 1991.

29 Held, 'Beyond liberalism', op. cit., p. 234.

30 Ibid., p. 235.

31 Ibid., citing Held and Leftwich, 1984, p. 144.

32 Ibid., pp. 235, 237.

33 Ibid., p. 236.

34 Ibid.

35 Ibid., p. 237.

36 C. Offe, *Contradictions in the Welfare State*, London, Hutchinson, 1984, p. 247; C. Pierson, 'New theories of state and civil society – Recent developments in post-Marxist analysis of the state', *Sociology*, vol. 18, no. 4, 1984, p. 565.

37 Parliament, Report from the Select Committee on Violence in Marriage, Together with the Proceedings of the Committee, vol. 1, Report, London, HMSO, H.C.553-i, 1974–75a; Parliament, Report from the Select Committee on Violence in Marriage, Together with the Proceedings of the Committee, vol. 2 (also including vol. 1), Report, Minutes of Evidence and Appendices, London, HMSO, H.C.553-II, 1974–75b.

38 Parliament, op. cit., vol. 2, p. v.

39 For an analysis of the discourse of the media in covering the women's peace movement at Greenham Common, see A. Young, *Femininity in Dissent*, London, Routledge, 1990.

40 E. Stark and A. Flitcraft, 'Social knowledge, social policy and the abuse of women: The case against patriarchal benevolence', in David Finkelhor *et al.* (eds), *The Dark Side of Families: Current Family Violence Research*, Beverly Hills, Sage, 1983, pp. 337–8; D. Marsden, 'Sociological perspectives on family violence', in J.M. Martin (ed.), *Violence and the Family*, New York, John Wiley, 1978.

41 Parliament, op. cit., vol. 2, p. 3.

42 Ibid., pp. 1–43, 84–91; J.J. Gayford, 'Ten types of battered wives', *Welfare Officer*, vol. 1, Jan., 1976, pp. 5–9; B. Bowder, 'The wives who ask for it' (interview with Gayford, McKeith and Pizzey), 1 March, 1979; R.E. Dobash and R.P. Dobash, 'If you prick me do I not bleed?

Replying to "Wives who ask for it"', *Community Care*, 3 May, 1979, pp. 26–8.
43 Parliament, op. cit., vol. 2, p. 89.
44 Ibid., p. 37.
45 Ibid., vol. 2, op. cit., p. 6.
46 Ibid., p. 29.
47 Ibid., p. 6.
48 Ibid., p. 42.
49 Ibid.
50 Ibid., p. 6.
51 Ibid., pp. 12–13.
52 Ibid., p. 7.
53 Ibid., p. 10.
54 Ibid., p. 15. Gayford indicated that 148 questionnaires were administered but 48 'had to be discarded' for reasons undisclosed – see J.J. Gayford, 'Wife battering: A preliminary survey of 100 cases', *British Medical Journal*, 25 January, 1975, p. 194, and reprinted in Parliamentary Select Committee Memorandum, vol. 2, op. cit., p. 32; E. Wilson 'Research into battered women: Why we need research and why what exists is potentially dangerous: A reply to Dr. Jasper Gayford', available from the National Women's Aid Federation (Now Women's Aid Federation England), 1976; Stark and Flitcraft, op. cit., pp. 333, 337–8, 344–5.
55 Parliament, Gayford, op. cit., vol. 2, p. 88.
56 Bowder, op. cit.
57 Parliament, op. cit., vol. 2, pp. 59–63, 66–83, 155–75, 220–6, 253–66, 270–95, 302–18, 491.
58 Ibid., p. 59.
59 Ibid.
60 Ibid.
61 Ibid., p. 61.
62 Ibid., p. 91.
63 Ibid., pp. 305–6, 311.
64 Ibid., p. 311.
65 Ibid., pp. 84–5, 295, 309–12, 335–6, 340. Note that the memorandum stating the research findings upon which MPs based their questioning was not published even though this was the common practice for those giving evidence.
66 Ibid., pp. xxix–xxxi.
67 Ibid., pp. 462–9, The Lord Advocate, pp. 441–8.
68 Ibid., pp. 469–82.
69 Ibid., p. vi.
70 Ibid., pp. xxix–xxxi.
71 Ibid., pp. 1–53.
72 Ibid., pp. v–xxvii; also reproduced in the introduction to vol. 2.
73 See also H. Rose, 'In practice supported in theory denied: An account of an invisible urban movement', *International Journal of Urban and Regional Research*, vol. 2, no. 3, 1978.
74 Parliament, vol. 2, op. cit., p. 287, para. 1329; p. 306, para. 1380.
75 Parliament, vols 1 & 2, op. cit., p. xiii, para. 29; see also para. 21.

76 Ibid., p. xiii, para. 31.
77 Ibid., p. xiv, para. 33.
78 Ibid., p. xiv, para. 32.
79 Ibid., p. xiv, para. 36.
80 Ibid., p. xiv, para. 34.
81 Ibid., p. xxv, para. 61.
82 Ibid., p. 67, para. 319.
83 Ibid., p. xxvi, Recommendations pp. 6–8, 11–12.
84 Ibid., p. xii, para. 26, Rec. 9, pp. xxvi, 2.
85 Ibid., pp. xii–xiii, para. 28, Rec. 10, pp. xxvi, 3.
86 Ibid., p. xix, para. 49, Rec. 18, p. xxvii.
87 V. Binney, G. Harkell and J. Nixon, 'Refuges and housing for battered women', in J. Pahl (ed.), *Private Violence and Public Policy*, London, Routledge, 1985, pp. 176–7; S. Parker, 'The legal background', in J. Pahl, ibid., pp. 100–8; T. Farragher, 'The police response to violence against women in the home', in J. Pahl, ibid., pp. 110–11.
88 Binney, Harkell and Nixon, op. cit., pp. 166, 174–6; Parker, op. cit., p. 108. The Matrimonial Homes Act 1967 had previously made interim exclusion orders virtually unobtainable in England. A. Solicitor (anon.), 'The Matrimonial Homes Act/working at last', *SCOLAG, The Bulletin of the Scottish Legal Action Group*, October, 1983, pp. 152–7. Also see Parker, op. cit., pp. 104–5 on the use of the exclusion order.
89 Parker, op. cit., pp. 105–6; Farragher, op. cit., pp. 110–11.
90 Cited in Solicitor, op. cit., p. 154.
91 Solicitor, op. cit., p. 154.
92 J. Barron, *Not Worth the Paper?: The Effectiveness of Legal Protection for Women and Children Experiencing Domestic Violence*, Bristol, Women's Aid Federation England, 1990, pp. 18–20.
93 Parliament, vols 1 & 2, op. cit., p. xxv, para. 44, Recommendations pp. 15–16, pp. xxvi–xxvii.
94 Dobash and Dobash, *Violence Against Wives*, op. cit., p. 222.
95 Parliament, vols 1 & 2, op. cit., p. xvii, para. 43, p. 284, paras 1305.
96 Ibid., p. xvii, para. 44.
97 Ibid., p. viii.
98 Ibid., p. ix.
99 Ibid., p. ix.
100 Ibid., p. xvi, Finer Report, Cmnd. 4629, July 1974.
101 Ibid., pp. xxi, xxiii. Although not mentioned by name, this was our own research which was funded by the Scottish Home and Health Department.
102 Ibid., pp. xxiv, xxvii.
103 Ibid., pp. xxiv–xxv.
104 Ibid., p. xxv.
105 Ibid., pp. x–xv, paras 19–40, Recommendations 4, 5, 13.
106 Ibid., pp. xv–xvi, para. 40; Recommendation 13, xxvi.
107 Ibid., p. ix, para. 18, p. xv, para. 37; p. xxvi, Recommendation 4.
108 Ibid., p. xxv.
109 PEP (Political and Economic Planning), *Advisory Committees in British Government*, London, Allen and Unwin, 1960; R.E. Wraith and G.B. Lamb, *Public Inquiries as an Instrument of Government*, London, Allen and Unwin, 1971; R. Chapman, 'Commissions in policy-making', in R.

Chapman (ed.), *The Role of Commissions in Policy Making*, London, Allen and Unwin, 1973, pp. 174–88; G. Rhodes, *Committees of Inquiry*, London, Allen and Unwin, 1975; M. Bulmer (ed.), *Social Research and Royal Commissions*, London, Allen and Unwin, 1980.
110 Schechter, op. cit., 1982, p. 136.
111 United States Commission on Civil Rights (USCCR), Washington DC, *Battered Women: Issues of Public Policy*, 1978, pp. 532–3. The Domestic Violence Prevention and Treatment Act of 1977 (H.R. 7927) was introduced on 21 June, 1977 by Rep. Newton Steers and Rep. Lindy Boggs. Rep. Mikulski introduced another bill and continued to do so in each session until 1983. See Schechter, op. cit., 1982, pp. 140–3; L. Melling, 'Federal legislation for abuse victims', *Response*, March/April, 1984, p. 5.
112 USCCR, op. cit., p. I.
113 Ibid.
114 Ibid., p. III.
115 Ibid., p. IV.
116 Ibid., p. V.
117 Ibid., p. 97.
118 Ibid., p. 3–18.
119 Ibid., pp. 3–4.
120 Ibid., pp. 5–6.
121 Ibid., pp. 7, 9.
122 Ibid., p. 14.
123 Ibid., p. 15.
124 Ibid.
125 Ibid., p. 18.
126 Ibid., pp. 49–97, 176–8, for criticism see pp. 66–8, 81–2.
127 Ibid., pp. 20–2.
128 Ibid., p. 30.
129 Ibid., Flitcraft, pp. 113–14; Lisa Leghorn, pp. 138–9, 449; Hilberman, p. 531.
130 Ibid., p. 138. See also pp. 449–50, Bako, p. 362.
131 Ibid., p. 119. See also pp. 120–2, 362; proposed legislation is analysed by Valle Jones, Feminist Alliance Against Rape, Nov/Dec, 1977.
132 Ibid., pp. 103, 139, 450–2.
133 Ibid., Lisa Leghorn, pp. 139, 450–3; Murray Straus, pp. 169–70, 468; Elaine Hilberman, pp. 157, 527–9.
134 Ibid., p. 144.
135 Ibid., p. 167. See also Judge Richette, pp. 143–4, 150, Commissioner Freeman, M. Straus, L. Walker and E. Hilberman, pp. 166–7.
136 Ibid., p. 144.
137 Ibid., p. 146.
138 Ibid., pp. 171–3, AFDC, Section 406 of the Social Security Act.
139 Ibid., p. 175.
140 Ibid., pp. 79–80.
141 Ibid., pp. 81–2; see also Fields, pp. 20–7.
142 Ibid., p. 183.
143 Ibid., Schechter, op. cit., 1982, pp. 137–8; See US Commission on Civil Rights, *The Federal Response to Domestic Violence*, Washington DC,

1982 for subsequent reports and recommendations.
144 Ibid., pp. IV–V; Schechter, op. cit., 1982, pp. 138–9.
145 Ibid., p. 202.
146 House of Representatives bill (HR 7927), and Senate bill (S 1728).
147 USCCR, op. cit., 1978, pp. 197–203, 532–4, 661; Schechter, op. cit., 1982, pp. 140–3.
148 House of Representatives bill (HR 8948). For the text of the various bills, see USCCR, op. cit., pp. 661–703. For discussions of content see USCCR, op. cit., pp. 197–203, 362, 661; Schechter, op. cit., 1982, p. 140, ref. 21, p. 335; Jones, op. cit.
149 Schechter, op. cit., 1982, pp. 140–1 citing Mikulski's legislative assistant, Note 22, p. 225; USCCR, ibid., pp. 197–203.
150 House of Representatives bill (HR 12299). USCCR, op. cit., pp. 661, 690–703. See also Schechter, op. cit., 1982, p. 141.
151 Senate bill (S 2759), USCCR, op. cit., pp. 661–89.
152 Schechter, op. cit., 1982, p. 141.
153 Melling, op. cit., p. 5.
154 House of Representatives bill (HR 2977).
155 B. Hart, cited in Schechter, op. cit., 1982, p. 142; note 26, p. 335.
156 Schechter, op. cit., 1982, p. 142.
157 Held, op. cit., 1984b, p. 237.
158 Schechter, op. cit., 1982, p. 143.
159 Ibid., p. 147.
160 Melling, op. cit., p. 5.
161 Ibid.
162 V. Sapiro, 'The women's movement, politics and policy in the Reagan era', in D. Dahlerup (ed.), *The New Women's Movement: Feminism and Political Power in Europe and the USA*, Beverly Hills, Sage, 1986, pp. 135, 137–8.
163 Melling, op. cit., p. 5; *Response*, Nov/Dec, 1983.
164 Melling, op. cit.
165 *Response*, Fall, 1984; J. Moore, 'Federal funding for family violence programs, *Response*, Summer, 1985, p. 24; *SANEnews*, Sept. 1987, p. 7; K.J. Ferraro, 'The legal response in the United States', in J. Hanmer, J. Radford and E. Stanko (eds), *Women, Policing and Male Violence*, London, Routledge, 1989, pp. 155–84, p. 159.
166 Ferraro, op. cit., p. 159.
167 J. Zorza, 'Federal domestic abuse legislation', *The Women's Advocate, Newsletter of the National Center on Women and Family Law*, vol. 11,. no. 5, 1990, pp. 1, 4.

5 CHALLENGING THE JUSTICE SYSTEM

1 T. Stang Dahl, *Women's Law: An Introduction to Feminist Jurisprudence*, Oxford, Oxford University Press, 1987.
2 C. Gilligan, *In A Different Voice*, Harvard University Press, Harvard, 1982.
3 Ibid.
4 M. K. Harris, 'Moving into the new millennium: Toward a feminist vision

of justice', *The Prison Journal*, vol. 67, 1987, pp. 27–38, p. 32.
5 Ibid., p. 35.
6 For a critical analysis of these ideas see K. Daly, 'Criminal justice ideologies and practices in different voices: Some feminist questions about justice', *International Journal of Sociology of Law*, vol. 17, no. 1, 1989, pp. 1–18.
7 C. Smart, *Feminism and the Power of Law*, London, Routledge, 1990.
8 Ibid., p. 138.
9 Ibid., pp. 160, 89.
10 Parliament, Select Committee on Violence in the Family, *Report from the Select Committee on Violence in Marriage, Vol. II, Report, Minutes of Evidence and Appendices*, 1975, pp. 79 and 81.
11 US Commission on Civil Rights (USCCR), *Battered Women: Issues of Public Policy*, Washington DC, Civil Rights Commission, 1978, p. III.
12 Ibid., pp. 20–6.
13 Parliament, op. cit., p. 363.
14 Ibid., p. 366.
15 Ibid., p. 374, p. 261.
16 Ibid., p. 369.
17 Ibid., pp. 384, 378.
18 Ibid., p. 378.
19 Ibid., p. 368.
20 Ibid., p. 369.
21 Ibid., p. 377.
22 Ibid., p. 334.
23 USCCR, op. cit., p. 13.
24 J. Garner and E. Clemmer, *Danger to Police in Domestic Disturbances – A New Look*, Washington DC, National Institute of Justice, November, 1986; C.D. Emerson, 'Family violence: A study by the Los Angeles County Sheriff's Department', *Police Chief*, vol. 45, pp. 48–45.
25 USCCR, op. cit., pp. 14, 20–1, 249–56.
26 US Commission on Civil Rights, *Under the Rule of Thumb: Battered Women and the Administration Justice*, Washington DC, USCCR, 1982, p. 14.
27 Ibid., p. 18.
28 USCCR, op. cit., 1978, p. 87.
29 USCCR, op. cit., 1978, pp. 177–8.
30 E.P. Thompson, 'The moral economy of the English crowd in the eighteenth century', *Past and Present*, vol. 50, 1971, pp. 76–136; J.M. Beattie, 'The criminality of women in eighteenth-century England', *Journal of Social History*, 1975, pp. 80–116; R.P. Dobash, R.E. Dobash and S. Gutteridge, *The Imprisonment of Women*, Oxford, Basil Blackwell, 1986, esp. Chap. 2; S. Schama, *Citizens*, London, Penguin, 1989.
31 E. Richards, 'Patterns of Highland discontent, 1790–1860', in R. Quinault and J. Stevenson (eds), *Popular Protest and Public Disorder*, London, Basil Blackwell, 1974, pp. 75–114.
32 Dobash, Dobash and Gutteridge, op. cit.; N.Z. Davis, 'The reasons of misrule: Youth groups and charivaris in sixteenth-century France', *Past and Present*, vol. 51, 1971; pp. 51–71; E.P. Thompson, 'Rough music: Le Charivari Anglais', *Annales*, vol. 27, 1972, pp. 285–312; R.P.

Dobash and R.E. Dobash, 'Community response to violence against wives: Charivari, abstract justice and patriarchy', *Social Problems*, vol. 28, no. 5, 1981, pp. 563–81.

33 Dobash and Dobash, ibid.

34 E. Turinger, 'Marital violence: The legal solutions', *Hastings Law Journal*, 1971, vol. 23, no. 1, pp. 259–76.

35 See, for example, Dobash, Dobash and Gutteridge, op. cit.; W.R. Miller, *Cops and Bobbies: Police Authority in New York and London*, Chicago, Chicago University Press, 1977; M. Ignatieff, *A Just Measure of Pain: The Penitentiary in the Industrial Revolution, 1750–1850*, London, Macmillan, 1978; N.H. Rafter, *Partial Justice: State Prisons and Their Inmates, 1800–1935*, Boston, Northeastern University Press, 1985.

36 Dobash, Dobash and Gutteridge, op. cit.; F.K. Prochaska, *Women and Philanthropy in Nineteenth Century England*, Oxford, Clarendon.

37 For reviews see R.P. Dobash and R.E. Dobash, *Violence Against Wives*, New York, Free Press, 1979; A. Sachs and J. Hoff Wilson, *Sexism and the Law. A Study of Male Beliefs and Judicial Bias*, Oxford, Martin Robertson, 1978; S.S.M. Edwards, *Female Sexuality and the Law*, Oxford, Martin Robertson, 1981.

38 B. Eherenirch and D. English, *For Her Own Good*, London, Pluto, 1979; L. Davidoff, J. L'Esperance and H. Newby, 'Landscape with figures: Home and community in English society', in J. Mitchell and A. Oakley (eds), *The Rights and Wrongs of Women*, Harmondsworth, England, Penguin, 1976, pp. 139–75; L. Davidoff and C. Hall, *Family Fortunes: Men and Women of the English Middle Class, 1780–1850*, Chicago, University of Chicago Press, 1987.

39 Edwards, op. cit.

40 Dobash and Dobash, op. cit., 1981.

41 E. Cox, *The Principles of Punishment*, London, Law Times Office, 1877.

42 Ibid., p. 130.

43 F. Power Cobbe, 'Wife torture in England', *Contemporary Review*, vol. 33, 1879, pp. 55–87. For discussions of these developments see Dobash and Dobash, op. cit., 1979, 1981; E. Pleck, *Domestic Tyranny*, Oxford, Oxford University Press, 1987.

44 Dobash and Dobash, op. cit., 1979. Pleck, op. cit.

45 J. Davis, 'The London garotting panic of 1862', in V.A.C. Gatrell, B. Lenman and G. Parker (eds), *Crime and Law*, London, Europa, 1980; G. Pearson, *Hooligan: A History of Respectable Fears*, London, Macmillan, 1983, pp. 143–53.

46 Dobash and Dobash, op. cit., 1979; Pleck, op. cit.

47 Pleck, op. cit., Chap. 6.

48 Ibid.

49 Ibid.

50 Cobbe, op. cit., p. 61.

51 D. Klein, 'The etiology of female crime: A review of the literature', *Issues in Criminology*, vol. 8, no. 2, 1973, pp. 3–30; C. Smart, *Women, Crime and Criminology: A Feminist Critique*, London, Routledge, 1977; N.H. Rafter, 'Too dumb to know better: Cacogenci family studies and the criminology of women', *Criminology*, vol. 18, no. 1, 1980, pp. 3–25; S.S.M. Edwards, 'Neither bad nor mad: The female violent offender re-

assessed', *Women's Studies International Forum*, vol. 9, no. 1, 1981, pp. 79–87. Dobash, Dobash and Gutteridge, op. cit.

52 Klein, op. cit.; Rafter, op. cit.; Dobash, Dobash and Gutteridge, op. cit.

53 Edwards, op. cit., 1981, Pleck, op. cit.; L. Gordon, *Heroes of Their Own Lives, The Politics and History of Family Violence*, New York, Viking, 1988.

54 J.M. Masson, *The Assault on Truth: Freud's Suppression of the Seduction Theory*, New York, Farrar, Straus and Giroux, 1984.

55 Gordon, op. cit.

56 A. Platt, *The Child-Savers: The Invention of Deliquency*, Chicago, Chicago University Press, 1969. R.I. Parnas, 'Judicial response to intra-family violence', *Minnesota Law Review*, vol. 54, 1970, pp. 539–65. Pleck, op. cit.; Gordon, op. cit.

57 Parnas, op. cit.; Gordon, op. cit.

58 Parnas, op. cit.; Pleck, op. cit.

59 Quoted in Pleck, op. cit., p. 137.

60 Parnas, op. cit.; Dobash and Dobash, op. cit., 1981; Gordon, op. cit.

61 Parnas, op. cit.

62 Ibid.

63 Like so many ideas gone wrong, the ideal of crisis intervention had a noble beginning. It emerged during WWII as a consequence of the aftermath of a fire which destroyed the Coconut Grove nightclub in Boston. Developing out of the tragedy, crisis intervention was intended as a method of dealing with a 'pathogenic situation affecting the whole community rather than with an individual disorder'. R. Castel, F. Castel and A. Lovell, *The Psychiatric Society*, trans. by A. Lovell, New York, Columbia University Press, 1982, pp. 124–5.

64 H.A. Barocas, 'Urban policemen: Crisis mediators or crisis creators?', *American Journal of Orthopsychiatry*, vol. 43, no. 4, 1973, pp. 632–9, p. 636.

65 M. Bard and H. Connolly, 'The police and family violence: Practice and policy', in US Commission on Civil Rights, op. cit., 1978, pp. 304–26.

66 Barocas, op. cit., p. 636.

67 See, for example, M. Bard, 'Family intervention police teams as a community mental health resource', *The Journal of Criminal Law, Criminology and Police Science*, vol. 60, no. 2, 1969, pp. 247–50; G.L. Arthur, P.J. Sisson and C.E. McClung, *Journal of Police Science and Administration*, vol. 5, no. 4, 1977, pp. 421–9; Bard and Connolly, op. cit.

68 Bard and Connolly, op. cit.

69 Arthur, Sisson and McClung, op. cit.

70 Barocas, op. cit., p. 368.

71 For a recent example of this abstract approach, see D.R. Buchanan and P. Chasnoff, 'Family crisis programs: What works and what doesn't', *Journal of Police Science and Administration*, vol. 14, no. 2, 1986, pp. 161–7.

72 M. Bard, *The Function of the Police in Crisis Intervention and Conflict Management: A Training Guide*, Washington DC, US Department of Justice, 1975.

73 See, for example, M. Bard, 'Alternatives to traditional law enforcement',

Police, November–December, 1970, pp. 20–3; Bard and Connolly, op. cit.

74 Bard, op. cit., 1970; M. Bard and B. Berkowitz, 'Training police as specialists in family crisis intervention', *Community Mental Health Journal*, Winter, 1971, pp. 315–17.

75 Bard and Connolly, op. cit., p. 316.

76 P.B. Wylie, L.F. Basinger, C.L. Heinecke and J.A. Reuckert, 'Approach to evaluating a police program of family crisis interventions in six demonstration cities' (Abstract), Washington DC: National Criminal Justice Reference Service, cited in L.W. Sherman and R.A. Berk, 'The specific deterrent effects of arrest for domestic assault', *American Sociological Review*, vol. 49, pp. 261–72.

77 J. Driscoll, R. Meyer and C. Schanie, 'Training police in family crisis intervention'. *Journal of Applied Behavioral Science*, vol. 9, 1973, pp. 62–82, p. 65.

78 Bard and Connolly, op. cit., p. 317.

79 Arthur, Sisson and McClung, op. cit.

80 Bard and Connolly, op. cit., p. 317. It should be noted that these results may reflect an increase in the number of arrests for other crimes which would be reflected in a proportional decrease in the representation of assaults within the family.

81 M. Fields, 'Wife beating: Government intervention, policies and practices', transcript of verbal evidence, in Civil Rights Commission, op. cit., 1978, pp. 20–7.

82 Ibid., pp. 228–87, pp. 240–1.

83 N. Oppenlander, 'Coping or copping out', *Criminology*, vol. 20, nos. 3, 4, 1982, pp. 449–65, p. 461.

84 Ibid.

85 Cited in L. G. Lerman, 'Mediation of wife abuse cases: The adverse impact of informal dispute resolution on women', *Harvard Women's Law Journal*, vol. 7, no. 1, 1984, pp. 57–113, p. 71.

86 Ibid.

87 Ibid.

88 Ibid., p. 70.

89 Ibid., p. 60.

90 In the United States, telephone screening was another official means of limiting the response of the CJS. Telephone screening is the practice of ignoring or deflecting requests for police assistance which are defined as unworthy of response. One type of incident to be screened is a domestic dispute, Dobash and Dobash, op. cit., 1979.

91 Fields, Civil Rights Commission, op. cit., 1978.

92 Ibid., pp. 236–7.

93 *Response*, vol. 3, no. 6, 1980, p. 6.

94 Bruno vs McGuire, Docket Report (1978–9), New York, Center for Constitutional Rights, 1979, p. 12.

95 S. Schechter, *Women and Male Violence, The Visions and Struggles of the Battered Women's Movement*, Boston, South End Press, 1987.

96 Bruno vs McGuire, Docket Report, op. cit.

97 Ibid., p. 12.

98 Commission on Civil Rights, op. cit., 1982, pp. 30–40; see also L.G. Lerman, 'A model State act, remedies for domestic abuse', *Harvard*

Journal on Legislation, vol. 21, no. 1, 1984, pp. 61–143.

 99 Commission on Civil Rights, op. cit., 1982.
100 P. Finn and S. Colson, *Civil Protection Orders: Legislation, Current Court Practice, and Enforcement*, Washington DC, National Institute of Justice, US Department of Justice, 1990.
101 Civil Rights Commission, Thumb 1982, op. cit.; Finn and Colson, op. cit.
102 Finn and Colson, op. cit., p. 42.
103 Civil Rights Commission, Thumb, 1982, op. cit.
104 Finn and Colson, op. cit., p. 27.
105 Civil Rights Commission, Thumb, op. cit., 1982, p. 9.
106 Ibid.
107 Finn and Colson, op. cit., p. 1.
108 Lerman, op. cit., 1984, pp. 129–30, G.A. Goolkasin, *Confronting Domestic Violence: A Guide for Criminal Justice Agencies*, Washington DC, US Department of Justice, National Institute of Justice, 1986; The Women's Advocate, 'Report finds both good and bad results of Wisconsin's mandatory arrest law', *The Women's Advocate, Newsletter of the National Center on Women and Family Law*, vol. 11, no. 4, July, 1990, pp. 2, 4.
109 Lerman, 'A model', op. cit.
110 Finn and Colson, op. cit.
111 Civil Rights Commission, 'Thumb', 1982, p. 10.
112 IACAP Training Key, pp. 245–6, quoted in Commission on Civil Rights, op. cit., 1982.
113 For useful summaries of this legislation see K. McCann, 'Battered women and the law: The limits of legislation', in J. Brophy and C. Smart (eds), *Women-in-Law*, London, Routledge, 1985, pp. 71–96; T. Parker, 'The legal background', in J. Pahl (ed.), *Private Violence and Public Policy*, London, Routledge, pp. 97–109; J. Barron, *Not Worth the Paper ...?*, Bristol, England, Women's Aid Federation England, 1990.
114 A. Solicitor (anon.), 'The Matrimonial Homes Act – working at last', *SCOLAG: The Bulletin of the Scottish Legal Action Group*, vol. 85, October, 1983, pp. 152–7.
115 S.S.M. Edwards, *Policing 'Domestic' Violence*, London, Sage, 1989.
116 Ibid.
117 Parliament, op. cit., p. xvi.
118 McCann, op. cit.; Parker, op. cit.; Solicitor, op. cit.
119 Barron, op. cit., p. 18.

6 NEW LAWS AND NEW REACTIONS

1 For an orthodox left view of these developments see S. Cohen, *Visions of Social Control*, Oxford: Polity Press, 1985.
2 For Britain see J. Boyle, *A Sense of Freedom*, Canongate Press, 1977; for the US see J. Irwin, *Prisons in Turmoil*, Boston, Little Brown, 1980.
3 M.A. Young, 'Victim assistance in the United States: The End of the Beginning', *International Review of Victimology*, vol. 1, 1990, pp. 181–99.
4 S. Cohen, *Folk Devils and Moral Panics*, London, Paladin, 1972; S. Hall,

C. Critcher, T. Jefferson, J. Clarke and B. Roberts, *Policing the Crisis*, London, Macmillan, 1978.

5 Cohen, op. cit., 1985.

6 J. Stein, *Better Services for Victims*, Washington DC, Blackstone Institute, 1977, cited in P. Rock, *A View From the Shadows*, Oxford, Clarendon Press, 1986, p. 86; see Rock pp. 71–100 for an excellent summary of the role of LEAA in the victims movement.

7 US Commission on Civil Rights, *Battered Women: Issues of Public Policy*, Civil Rights Commission, 1978; Interdepartmental Committee on Domestic Violence, *Handbook of Federal Resources on Domestic Violence*, Rockville, Maryland, National Clearinghouse on Domestic Violence, 1980.

8 Commission on Civil Rights, op. cit.; Interdepartmental Committee, op. cit.

9 Commission on Civil Rights, op. cit.

10 Commission on Civil Rights, op. cit.; Interdepartmental Committee, op. cit., p. 219.

11 Interdepartmental Committee, op. cit., p. 220.

12 Ibid.

13 The national centre and newsletter were similar to the network set up in 1972 by Betsy Warrior, an early activist in the movement, and the government was criticized by the movement for failing to recognize and support existing expertise within the movement; S. Schechter, *Women and Male Violence: The Visions and Struggles of the Battered Women's Movement*, Boston, South End Press, 1982, p. 185.

14 L.G. Lerman, *Prosecution of Spouse Abuse: Innovations in Criminal Justice Response*, Washington DC, Center for Women Policy Studies.

15 San Francisco Family Violence Project, *Domestic Violence is a Crime*, San Francisco, Family Violence Project, 1982 (revised in 1985); E. Soler, 'Domestic violence is a crime: A case study – San Francisco Family Violence Project', in D.J. Sonkin, *Domestic Violence on Trial*, New York, Springer, 1987, pp. 21–35.

16 San Francisco Family Violence Project, op. cit., section 11, p. 2.

17 Ibid.

18 Ibid., p. 2.

19 Ibid.

20 Ibid., Section D, pp. 1–2.

21 Ibid., Section D, p. 7.

22 E. Pence, 'The Duluth Domestic Abuse Intervention Project', *Hamline Law Review*, vol. 6, no. 2, 1983, pp. 247–75; E. Pence and M. Paymar, *Power and Control: Tactics of Men Who Batter*, Duluth, MN, Domestic Abuse Intervention Project, 1985; E. Pence and M. Shepard, 'Integrating feminist theory and practice: The challenge of the battered women's movement', in K. Yllo and M. Bograd (eds), *Feminist Perspectives on Wife Abuse*, Newbury Park, CA, Sage, 1988; E. Pence (with M. Duprey, M. Paymar and C. McDonnell), *Criminal Justice Response to Domestic Assault Cases: A Guide for Policy Development* (revised), Duluth, MN, Domestic Abuse Intervention Project, 1989.

23 Pence, op. cit., 1983.

24 Ibid.

25 Ibid.
26 S.M. Buel, 'Mandatory arrest for domestic violence', *Harvard Women's Law Journal,* vol. 11, nos. 2–3, 1988, pp. 213–26.
27 Pence, op. cit., 1983.
28 Pence, op. cit., 1989, pp. 94, 54.
29 E.A. Stanko, 'Missing the mark? Policing battering', in J. Hanmer, J. Radford and E.A. Stanko, *Policing and Male Violence: International Perspectives,* London, Routledge, 1989, pp. 46–69. This paper provides an excellent overview of the cultural and organizational obstacles to introducing innovations into the police.
30 Pence, op. cit., 1983, p. 253.
31 Pence, op. cit., 1989.
32 Pence, op. cit., 1983
33 Pence, op. cit., 1989.
34 R.A. Berk, D.R. Loseke, S. Fenstermaker Berk and D. Rauma, 'Bringing the cops back in: A study to make the criminal justice system more responsive to incidents of family violence'. *Social Science Research,* vol. 9, 1980, pp. 193–215; R.A. Berk, D. Rauma, D.R. Loseke and S.F. Berk, 'Throwing the cops back out: The decline of a local program to make the criminal justice system more responsive to incidents of domestic violence', *Social Science Research,* vol. 11, 1982, pp. 245–79.
35 Berk et al., op. cit., 1982, pp. 245–6.
36 Ibid.
37 Ibid., p. 262.
38 Ibid., p. 277.
39 Ibid.
40 Ibid., pp. 277–8.
41 Pence, op. cit., 1989, p. 53.
42 K. McCann, 'Battered women and the law: The limits of legislation', in J. Brophy and C. Smart (eds), *Women-in-Law,* London: Routledge, 1985, pp. 71–96; T. Parker, 'The legal background', in J. Pahl (ed.), *Private Violence and Public Policy,* London, Routledge, pp. 97–109; S. Maidment, 'Domestic violence and the law: The 1976 Act and its aftermath', in N. Johnson (ed.), *Marital Violence,* London, Routledge, pp. 4–25. J. Barron, *Not Worth the Paper?,* London, WAFE, 1990.
43 Parker, op. cit., p. 11.
44 Quoted in McCann, op. cit., p. 80, our emphasis.
45 Barron, op. cit., p. 28.
46 Quoted in McCann, op. cit., p. 80.
47 Quoted in ibid., p. 81.
48 Barron, op. cit.
49 A Solicitor (anon.), 'The Matrimonial Homes Act – working at last', *SCOLAG: The Bulletin of the Scottish Legal Action Group,* vol. 85, October, 1983, pp. 152–9, p. 153; M. Robertson and P. Robson, 'Operating the Matrimonial Homes Act, the first six months', unpublished paper, The Law School, University of Strathclyde, 1983.
50 Solicitor, op. cit., p. 153.
51 Ibid.
52 Ibid.
53 Robertson and Robson, op. cit.

54 Solicitor, p. cit., p. 153.
55 Solicitor, op. cit.
56 Parker, op. cit.
57 S.S.M. Edwards, 'Male violence against women: Excusatory and explanatory ideologies in law and society', in S.S.M. Edwards (ed.), *Gender, Sex and the Law*, Beckenham, England, Croom Helm, 1985, pp. 183–213.
58 S.S.M. Edwards, *Policing Domestic Violence: Women, the Law and the State*, London, Sage, 1989, p. 62.
59 Ibid.
60 Quoted in McCann, op. cit., p. 83.
61 Metropolitan Police, *Report of the Metropolitan Police Working Party into Domestic Violence*, London, January, 1986.
62 Ibid., p. 23.
63 Ibid., p. 40.
64 McCann, op. cit.
65 M. Homer, A. Leonard and P. Taylor, *Private Violence: Public Shame*, Cleveland, England, Cleveland Refuge and Aid for Women and Children, 1984; Barron, op. cit.
66 Barron, op. cit., pp. 56–9.
67 Homer, Leonard and Taylor, op. cit., p. 65.
68 Ibid., p. 66.
69 Ibid.
70 T. Faragher, 'The police response to violence against women in the home', in J. Pahl (ed.), *Private Violence and Public Policy*, London, Routledge, 1985, pp. 110–24.
71 Ibid., p. 117.
72 Ibid.
73 J. Grau, J. Fagan and S. Wexler, 'Restraining orders for battered women: Issues of access and efficacy', *Women and Politics*, vol. 4, no. 3, 1984, pp. 13–28.
74 M. Chadhuri and K. Daly, 'Do restraining orders help? Battered women's experience with male violence and the legal process', unpublished paper, March, 1990.
75 Ibid., p. 16.
76 P. Finn and S. Colson, *Civil Protection Orders: Legislation, Current Court Practice, and Enforcement*, Washington DC, National Institute of Justice, US Department of Justice, 1990, p. 1.
77 Ibid.
78 Women's National Commission, *Violence Against Women, Report of an Ad Hoc Working Group*, London, Cabinet Office, 1986.
79 Ibid., p. 50.
80 Ibid., p. 56.
81 Ibid., p. 55.
82 R. Walmsley, *Personal Violence*, Home Office Research Study 89, London, HMSO, 1986, p. iii.
83 Ibid., p. 29.
84 Ibid., p. 48.
85 Ibid.
86 A. Bourlet, *Police Intervention in Marital Violence*, Milton Keynes, England and Philadelphia: Open University Press, 1990, p. 67.

87 Quoted in ibid., p. 17.
88 For sympathetic approaches and enlightened proposals see, for example, ibid.; D.M. Cannings, 'Myths and stereotypes – obstacles to effective police intervention in domestic disputes involving a battered woman', *The Police Journal*, vol. 57, no. 1, 1984, pp. 43–56.
89 Metropolitan Police, *Domestic Violence – Policy and Practice*, Metropolitan Police, ND.
90 N. Knewstub, 'Guide for police on home violence', *Guardian*, 1 Aug., 1990, p. 7.
91 L. Smith, *Domestic Violence*, Home Office Research Study 107, London, HMSO, 1989.
92 D. Redding, 'Women at risk', *Guardian*, 4 July, 1990, p. 17.
93 S.S.M. Edwards, 'Police attitudes and dispositions in domestic disputes: The London study', *Police Journal*, July, 1986, pp. 230–41.
94 Bourlet, op. cit., pp. 92, 62.
95 S.R. Moody, *Diversion From the Criminal Justice Process: Report on the Diversion Scheme at Ayr*, Central Research Unit Papers, Edinburgh, Scottish Office, 1983.
96 For details of these cases and summaries of legislative efforts in the US contact the National Center on Women and Family Law, 799 Broadway, Room No. 402, New York, NY 10003.
97 The Women's Advocate, 'Battered woman awarded 2.3 million dollars by federal jury', *The Women's Advocate*, vol 6, no. 4, 1985, pp. 5–6, published by the National Center on Women and Family Law, New York, NY; S. Moore, 'Landmark court decision for battered women', *Response*, vol. 8, no. 5, 1985; A. Epplen, 'Battered women and the equal protection clause: Will the constitution help them when the police won't?', *Yale Law Journal*, vol. 95, 1986, pp. 788–809; S.M. Buel, 'Mandatory arrest for domestic violence', *Harvard Women's Law Journal*, vol. 11, pp. 213–26.
98 M.D. Fields, Municipal Liability for Police Failure to Arrest in Domestic Violence Cases, unpublished policy statement April, 1987; see also R. Gundle, 'Civil liability for police failure to arrest: Nearing v. Weaver', *Women's Rights Law Reporter*, vol. 9, no. 3/4, 1986, pp. 259–65.
99 S. Epstein, 'New Connecticut law on domestic violence', *The Women's Advocate, Newsletter of the National Center on Women and Family Law*, vol. 8, no. 1, 1987, pp. 1, 6–7; K. Triantafillou, 'Massachusetts: New legislation to help battered women', *The Judges' Journal*, Summer, 1988, pp. 20–3, 50–2.
100 Epstein, op. cit., p. 1.
101 S.W. Crane, personal correspondence, 15 Aug., 1985; see also S.W. Crane et al., *The Domestic Violence Act Evaluation Project*, Olympia, WA, Washington State Shelter Network, 1984; S.W. Crane, 'Washington's domestic violence prevention act: Mandatory arrest two years later', *The Women's Advocate*, vol. 8, no. 3, 1987, pp. 1, 4–5.
102 Epstein, op. cit.
103 Ibid., p. 6.
104 Crane, op. cit., 1987.
105 P. Jaffe, D.A. Wolfe, A. Telford and G. Austin, 'The impact of police

charges in incidents of wife abuse', *Journal of Family Violence*, vol. 1, no. 1, 1986, pp. 37–49.

106 Ibid., p. 43.

107 L.W. Sherman and R.A. Berk, 'The specific deterrent effects of arrest for domestic assault', *American Sociological Review*, vol. 49, no. 2, 1984, pp. 261–72; R.A. Berk and P.J. Newton, 'Does arrest really deter wife battery: An effort to replicate the findings of the Minneapolis spouse abuse experiment', *American Sociological Review*, vol. 50, 1985, pp. 253–62.

108 Ibid.

109 G.A. Goolkasian, *Confronting Domestic Violence: A Guide for Criminal Justice Agencies*, Washington DC, National Institute of Justice, 1986, p. 52, no. 16; for the full report see Berk and Newton, op. cit.

110 P.A. Langan and C.A. Innes, *Preventing Domestic Violence Against Women*, Bureau of Justice Statistics Special Report, Washington DC, US Department of Justice, 1986, p. 1.

111 R.A. Berk and L.W. Sherman, 'Data collection strategies in the Minneapolis domestic assault experiment', in L. Burstein, H.E. Freeman and P.H. Rossi, *Collecting Evaluation Data: Problems and Solutions*, Sage, London, 1985, pp. 35–48.

112 Jaffe et al., op. cit., p. 47.

113 Police Foundation, *Domestic Violence and the Police*, Studies in Detroit and Kansas City, vol. 9, 1977; for a slightly different approach to prevention see C. Petrie and J. Garner, 'Is violence preventable', in D.J. Besharov (ed.), *Family Violence: Research and Policy Issues*, Washington DC, AEI Press, pp. 164–84.

114 Buel, op. cit., p. 218.

115 A. Jolin, 'Domestic violence legislation: An impact assessment', *Journal of Police Science and Administration*, vol. 11, no. 4 1983, pp. 451–6.

116 F.W. Dunford, D. Huizinga and D.S. Elliott, 'The role of arrest in domestic assault: The Omaha police experiment', *Criminology*, vol. 28, no. 2, 1990, pp. 183–206.

117 T.D. Cook, 'Quasi-experimentation: Its ontology, epistemology and methodology', in G. Morgan (ed.), *Beyond Method: Strategies for Social Research*, Newbury Park, CA, Sage, 1986, pp. 74–94. As Cook points out quasi-experimental approaches are usually rigid and deterministic and thus restrict the use of background and contextual knowledge.

118 Berk and Sherman, op. cit.

119 Crane, op. cit., 1987.

120 Goolkasian, op. cit. The advisory panel involved in the preparation of this policy document included among its eight members Anne L. Ganley and Ellen Pence, both prominent feminists involved in programmes for violent men.

121 Probably the most persistent links have been established in Wales where a national conference brought police and representatives of the movement together to discuss continuing problems and future relationships. See The Welsh Office, *Dialogue for Change, Report of a Conference Between Women's Aid and Police Forces in Wales*, Cardiff, The Welsh Office.

122 For example, in 1987 a Dallas, Texas judicial judgment mandated changes in police and city policies and practices. The judgment also

specified the monitoring of compliance for two years. J.W. Vickery and
J.M. Alracht, 'Battered women win Dallas police suit', *The Women's
Advocate*, New York, National Center on Women and Family Law, p. 3.
123 D. Rose, 'Acts but no real faith', *Guardian*, 13 June, 1990, p. 25.
124 For example, N. Loving, *Responding to Spouse Abuse and Wife Beating.
A Guide for Police*, Washington DC, Police Executive Research Forum
1980, op. cit.; G.A. Goolkasin, *Confronting Domestic Violence: A
Guide for Criminal Justice Agency*, Washington DC, US Department of
Justice, 1986.
125 Women in Law, American Bar Association 'Fact Sheet', 1987; M.L.
Henry, E. Koslow, J. Soffer and J. Furey, *The Success of Women and
Minorities in Achieving Judicial Office, The Selection Process*, New
York, Fund for Modern Courts, 1985.
126 Solicitor, op. cit.
127 B. Richie, 'Battered black women: a challenge for the black community',
The Black Scholar, vol. 16, no. 2, 1985, pp. 40-4; A. Mama, *The
Hidden Struggle. Statutory and Voluntary Responses to Violence Against
Black Women in the Home*, London, London Race and Housing
Research Unit, 1990.
128 For early evidence of this pattern see W. LaFave, 'Noninvocation of the
criminal law by police', in D.R. Cressey and D. Ward (eds), *Delinquency,
Crime and Social Process*, New York: Harper and Row, 1967. For an
excellent analysis of this problem see V.D. Young, 'Gender expectations
and their impact on black female offenders and victims', *Justice Quarterly*, vol. 3, no. 3, 1986, pp. 305-27.
129 Young, ibid.
130 *SANEnews*, 'The police and wife battering', vol. 5, no. 1, Sept., 1987,
p. 4; Pence, op. cit., 1989.
131 L.W. Sherman and E.G. Cohn, 'The effects of research on legal policy in
the Minneapolis domestic violence experiment', in D.J. Besharov (ed.),
Family Violence, Washington DC, AEI Press, 1990, pp. 205-27, p. 211.
132 The following recent studies confirm patterns discovered in past research;
Metropolitan Police, op. cit., 1986; Bourlet, op. cit.; E.S. Buzawa, 'Police
officer response to domestic violence legislation in Michigan', *Journal of
Police Science and Administration*, vol. 10, no. 4, 1982, pp. 415-24;
D.N. Oppenlander, 'Coping or copping out', *Criminology*, vol. 20,
nos. 3/4, 1982, pp. 449-65; P.W. Davis, 'Structured rationales for non-
arrest: Police stereotypes of the domestic disturbance', *Criminal Justice
Review*, vol. 6, no. 2, 1982, pp. 8-15; A. Ford, 'Wife battery and
criminal justice: A study of victim decision-making', *Family Relations*,
vol. 32, 1983, pp. 463-75; L.H. Bowker, 'Police services to battered
women, bad or not so bad?', vol. 9, 1982, pp. 476-94; S.E. Brown,
'Police responses to wife beating: Neglect of a crime of violence', *Journal
of Criminal Justice*, vol. 12, 1982, pp. 227-88; D.J. Bell, 'The police
response to domestic violence: A multiyear study', *Police Studies*, vol. 8,
no. 1, 1985, pp. 58-64; D.J. Bell, 'A multiyear study of Ohio urban,
suburban, and rural police dispositions of domestic disputes',
Victimology, vol. 10, nos. 1-4, 1985, pp. 301-10; D. Quarm and M.D.
Schwartz, 'Domestic violence in criminal court: An examination of new
legislation in Ohio', *Women and Politics*, vol. 4, 1985, pp. 29-39; R.

Reiner, *The Politics of the Police,* Brighton, Wheatsheaf 1985; A. Sanders, 'Personal violence and public order: The prosecution of domestic violence in England and Wales', *International Journal of the Sociology of Law,* vol. 16, 1988, pp. 359–82; S.S.M. Edwards, 'Police attitudes and dispositions in domestic disputes: The London study', *Police Journal,* July, 1986, pp. 230–41; S.S.M. Edwards, *Policing 'Domestic' Violence,* Newbury Park, CA, Sage, 1989.

133 Metropolitan Police, op. cit.; Sanders, op. cit.; Ford, op. cit.; Davis, op. cit.

134 Sanders, op. cit.; Bourlet, op. cit.

135 For Britain see Edwards, op. cit., 1986, 1989 and Sanders, op. cit.; for the USA see Bowker, op. cit., pp. 485–6; Bell, op. cit., 1985; Buzawa, op. cit.; Oppenlander, op. cit.

136 Bourlet, op. cit., p. 78; Sanders, op. cit.

137 Sanders, op. cit., p. 381; see also Bell, op. cit.; Bourlet, op. cit.; Bowker, op. cit.

138 K.J. Ferraro, 'The legal response to woman battering in the United States,' in J. Hanmer, J. Radford and E. Stanko (eds), *Women, Policing and Male Violence,* London, Routledge, 1989, pp. 155–84 for a negative evaluation of LEAA intervention.

139 P.A. Morgan, 'Constructing images of deviance: A look at state intervention into the problem of wife-battery', in N. Johnson (ed.), *Marital Violence,* Sociological Review Monograph 31, London, Routledge, 1985, pp. 66–76.

140 Attorney General's Task Force, *Family Violence,* Washington DC, Attorney General, September, 1984.

141 Abolitionist thinking is perhaps strongest in Norway and the Netherlands, although it seems to be attracting adherents in North America. N. Christie, 'Conflicts as property', *British Journal of Criminology,* vol. 17, 1977, pp. 1–19; T. Mathiesen, *The Politics of Abolition,* London, Martin Robertson, 1974; J.R. Blad, H. van Mastrigt and N.A. Uildriks (eds), *The Criminal Justice System as a Social Problem: An Abolitionist Perspective,* Rotterdam, Erasmus University Press, 1987; H. Bianchi and R. van Swaaningen, *Abolitionism: Towards a Non-Repressive Approach to Crime,* Amsterdam, Free University Press, 1986. In Britain, some of the issues considered in this section have been debated by new 'left realists' and the old and new 'left idealists'. They are not included here because these debates are primarily academic and neither camp has been involved in specific social movements, although new 'left idealists' often identify with abolitionists.

142 H.E.H. Pepinksy, 'Better living through police discretion', *Law and Contemporary Problems,* vol. 47, no. 4, 1984, pp. 249–67.

143 L. Hulsman, 'Critical criminology and the concept of crime', in Bianchi and Swaaningen, op. cit.

144 L. Hulsman, 'The language of discourse on alternatives', paper presented at the International Criminology Conference, Hamburg, September, 1988.

145 Christie, op. cit.

146 Hulsman, op. cit., 1988; J.C. Hes, 'The patchwork of reality: Exploring non-criminal means of intervention', in Bianchi and Swaaningen, op. cit., pp. 219–27.

147 H. Davidson, 'Community control without state control', in Bianchi and Swaaningen, op. cit., pp. 133–43, p. 139.
148 For similar criticisms see L. van Outrive, Hulsman's abolitionism: The great reduction', in Blad, Mastrigt and Uildriks, op. cit., pp. 53–66; C. Debuyst, 'The negotiation of conflicts and the resistances which are revealed', in Blad, Mastrigt and Uildriks, op. cit., pp. 187–98.

7 THE THERAPEUTIC SOCIETY CONSTRUCTS BATTERED WOMEN AND VIOLENT MEN

1 *Response, '"Battered syndrome" now official'*, Response, vol. 3, no. 3, 1979, p. 5.
2 Ibid.
3 L.V. Davis, 'Battered women: The transformation of a social problem', *Social Work*, vol. 32, July–August, 1987, pp. 306–11; for an example of this wider approach see E.H. Bern, 'From violent incident to spouse abuse syndrome', *Social Casework*, vol. 63, no. 1, 1982, pp. 41–5. While we think Davis's analysis is generally correct, it should be stressed that the therapeutic literature stressed pathology from the beginning, although as she indicates when social work professionals first began to write about battering they were more likely to consider wider social factors.
4 J. Pfouts, H. Renz and C. Renz, 'The future of wife abuse programs', *Social Work*, vol. 26, November, 1981, pp. 451–5, p. 452.
5 Davis, op. cit., p. 310.
6 B. Bowder, 'The wives who ask for it' (interview with Gayford, McKeith and Pizzey) *Community Care*, 1 March, 1979.
7 E. Pizzey and J. Shapiro, *Prone to Violence*, London, Hamlyn, 1982.
8 Ibid., p. 170.
9 Ibid., p. 230.
10 Women's National Commission, *Violence Against Women*, London, Cabinet Office, 1985, p. 20.
11 H. Eisenstein, *Contemporary Feminist Thought*, London, George Allen and Unwin, 1984.
12 R. Castel, F. Castel and A. Lovell, *The Psychiatristic Society*, translated by A. Goldhammer, New York, Columbia University Press, 1982, B. Zilbergeld, *The Shrinking of America: Myths of Psychological Change*, Boston, Little Brown, 1983; R.N. Bellah, R. Madsen, W.M. Sullivan, A. Swidler and S.M. Tipton, *Habits of the Heart: Individualism and Commitment in American Life*, New York, Harper and Row, 1985.
13 Zilbergeld, op. cit., p. 32.
14 M. Straus and R. Gelles, 'Societal change and change in family violence from 1975 to 1985 as revealed by two national surveys', *Journal of Marriage and the Family*, 48, August, 1986, pp. 465–79, p. 477, n. 15.
15 Zilbergeld, op. cit., p. 33.
16 Ibid., p. 31.
17 Ibid.
18 Alexis de Tocqueville, *Democracy in America*, translated by G. Lawrence, J.P. Mayer (ed.), New York, Doubleday, Anchor Books, 1969.

19 Ibid., p. 37.
20 Ibid., p. 508.
21 Ibid., p. 506.
22 D.J. Rothman, *The Discovery of the Asylum*, Boston, Little Brown, 1971; M. Foucault, *Discipline and Punish*, translated by A. Sheridan, London, Allen Lane, 1977; M. Ignatieff, *A Just Measure of Pain*, London, Macmillan, 1978; N.H. Rafter, *Partial Justice: State Prisons and their Inmates, 1800–1935*, Boston, Northeastern University Press, 1985; R.P. Dobash, R. Dobash and S. Gutteridge, *The Imprisonment of Women*, Oxford, Basil Blackwell, 1986.
23 Dobash, Dobash and Gutteridge, op. cit., Rafter, op. cit., N.H. Rafter, 'Too dumb to know better: Cacogenci family studies and the criminology of women', *Criminology*, vol. 18, no. 1, 1980, pp. 3–25.
24 This development appears not to have occurred in Britain, possibly because of the under-development of clinical psychology in contrast to institutional medical psychiatry.
25 G.M. Beard, *American Nervousness*, New York, Arno Press and the *New York Times*, 1972 (1881), cited in Bellah et al., op. cit.
26 Quoted in Bellah et al., op. cit., p. 120.
27 C. Beers, *A Mind that Found Itself*, New York, Doubleday, 1908. See Castel, Castel and Lovell, op. cit., pp. 33–5.
28 Castel, Castel and Lovell, op. cit., pp. 39–48; M. Bush, *Families in Distress: Public, Private and Civic Responses*, Berkeley, CA, University of California Press, 1988.
29 Linda Gordon, *Heroes of Their Own Lives*, Boston, Viking, 1988, pp. 257, 278.
30 Bush, op. cit., p. 285.
31 Castel, Castel and Lovell, op. cit., pp. 276–95.
32 Ibid., Chapter five.
33 Ibid.
34 N. Shainess, *Sweet Suffering: Woman as Victim*, New York, Pocket Books, 1984; N. Shainess, 'Psychological aspects of wife-beating', in M. Roy (ed.), *Battered Women: A Psychological Study of Domestic Violence*, New York, Van Nostrand Reinhold, 1986. In places Norwood's style is particularly disturbing. She uses examples gleaned from media reports of women who had been seriously assaulted or murdered in order to speculate about how they might have avoided these incidents. This technique seems immoral since it may very well cause distress to these victims and, if they were murdered, to their surviving relatives and friends. In the end it is, of course, another form of victim blaming.
35 Ibid., p. 12.
36 Ibid., p. 125.
37 Ibid., p. 139.
38 Ibid., pp. 141–2.
39 R. Norwood, *Women Who Love Too Much*, New York, Pocket Books, 1985; R. Norwood, *Letters From Women Who Love Too Much. A Closer Look at Relationship Addiction and Recovery*, London, Arrow Books, 1988. See C. Jackson, 'Steps to heaven', *Trouble and Strife*, vol. 17, 1990, pp. 14–17, for an incisive critique of Norwood's ideas.

40 Norwood, op. cit., 1988, p. 98.
41 Norwood, op. cit., 1988, p. 93; Norwood, op. cit., 1985, p. 183.
42 Norwood, op. cit., 1988, p. 267.
43 Ibid., p. 205.
44 Ibid., p. 207.
45 B. Star, C.G. Clark, K.M. Goetz and L. O'Malia, 'Psychological aspects of wife battering', in S. Howell and M. Bayes (eds), *Women and Mental Health*, New York, Basic Books, 1981, pp. 426–38; E.W. Gondolf (with E.R. Fisher), *Battered Women as Survivors*, Lexington, MA, Lexington, 1988; L. Okun, *Women Abuse: Facts Replacing Myths*, Albany, NY, State University of New York Press, 1986. Even the most vehement supporter of 'learned helplessness' and the 'battered woman syndrome' failed to find significant and meaningful differences between a group of women who had experienced violence and a group who had not: L.E.A. Walker, *The Battered Woman Syndrome*, New York, Springer, 1984.
46 Star et al., op. cit., p. 432.
47 L.E.A. Walker, 'What counselors should know about the battered woman', in D.J. Sonkin, D. Martin and L.E.A. Walker, *The Male Batterer: A Treatment Approach*, New York, Springer, 1985, pp. 152–6.
48 A. Shupe, W.A. Stacey and L.R. Hazelwood, *Violent Men, Violent Couples. The Dynamics of Domestic Violence*, Lexington, MA, Lexington Books, 1987; R. Kuhl, 'Personality traits of abused women: Masochism myth refuted', *Victimology*, vol. 9, no. 4, 1984, pp. 450–63.
49 P.H. Neidig, 'Women's shelters, men's collectives and other issues in the field of wife abuse', *Victimology*, vol. 9, no. 34, 1984, pp. 464–76.
50 M. Hendricks-Matthews, 'The battered woman: Is she ready for help?', *Social Casework*, vol. 63, no. 3, 1982, pp. 131–46.
51 Ibid., p. 133.
52 H. Lantz, *A Community in Search of Itself*, Carbondale, IL, Southern Illinois University Press, 1972, cited in Gondolf, op. cit., p. 13.
53 L.E.A. Walker, 'Battered women and learned helplessness', *Victimology*, vol. 2, nos. 3–4, 1977–8, pp. 525–34.
54 Ibid., p. 525.
55 Ibid., p. 529.
56 L.E.A. Walker, R.K. Thyfault and A. Browne, 'Beyond the juror's ken: Battered women', *Vermont Law Review*, vol. 7, no. 1, Spring, 1982, pp. 2–14, p. 9; Walker, op. cit., 1985.
57 Walker, op. cit., 1977–8, L.E.A. Walker, *The Battered Woman*, New York, Harper and Row, 1979. Douglas is one of the few clinicians who clearly asserts, 'Not all women who are battered suffer from the BWS ...': M.A. Douglas, 'The battered woman syndrome', in D.J. Sonkin (ed.), *Domestic Violence on Trial. Psychological and Legal Dimensions of Family Violence*, New York, Springer, 1987, pp. 39–54, p. 39.
58 Walker, op. cit., 1977–8, p. 525.
59 Ibid., p. 530.
60 Walker, op. cit., 1979, p. xvi.
61 Walker, op. cit., 1985, p. 159.
62 Walker, 1977–8, p. 530.
63 Douglas, op. cit.
64 Walker, op. cit., 1977–8, p. 530.

65 Walker, op. cit., 1985, pp. 158–9.
66 Ibid., 1985, p. 158.
67 Walker, op. cit., 1977–8, p. 531.
68 Douglas, op. cit., p. 50.
69 Ibid.
70 E.M. Schneider, 'Women's self defense work and the problem of expert testimony on battering', *Women's Rights Law Reporter*, vol. 9, nos. 3/4 1986, pp. 191–5, p. 195; E.M. Schneider, 'Describing and changing: Women's self-defense work and the problem of expert testimony on battering', *Women's Rights Law Reporter*, vol. 9, nos. 3/4, 1986, pp. 196–222; V.M. Mather, 'The skeleton in the closet: The battered woman syndrome, self-defense, and expert testimony', *Mercer Law Review*, vol. 39, 1988, pp. 545–89.
71 Schneider, op. cit.; Mather, op. cit.
72 Schneider, op. cit., p. 198.
73 Ibid.
74 Schneider, op. cit.; Mather, op. cit.
75 Schneider, op. cit., p. 216.
76 R.E. Dobash and R.P. Dobash, *Violence Against Wives*, New York, Free Press, 1979, Chapter 6 and pp. 137–43; R.E. Dobash and R.P. Dobash, 'The nature and antecedents of violent events', *British Journal of Criminology*, vol. 24, no. 3, 1984, pp. 269–88; Okun, op. cit., pp. 76–7. These works present a much more dynamic view of the violent event and its impact on the lives of women. Ellen Pence made us aware of how women adamantly reject the use of the word 'honeymoon' to describe the events occurring immediately after the violent event.
77 J. Pahl, *A Refuge for Battered Women*, London, HMSO, 1978; Dobash and Dobash, op. cit., 1979; R.E. Dobash, R.P. Dobash and C. Cavanagh. 'The contact between battered women and social and medical agencies', in J. Pahl, 1985, pp. 142–65; M.D. Pagelow, *Women-Battering: Victims and Their Experiences*, Beverly Hills, Sage, 1981; V. Binney, G. Harkell and J. Nixon, *Leaving Violent Men: A Study of Refuges and Housing for Battered Women*, Leeds, Women's Aid Federation England, 1982; E. Evason, *Hidden Violence: A Study of Battered Women in Northern Ireland*, Belfast, Farset Press, 1982; L.H. Bowker, *Beating Wife Beating*, Lexington, MA, Lexington Books, 1983; M. Homer, A.E. Leonard and M.P. Taylor, *Private Violence: Public Shame*, Middlesbrough, Cleveland Women's Aid, 1984; J. Pahl, *Private Violence and Public Policy: The Needs of Battered Women and the Response of the Public Service*, London, Routledge, 1985; N. Johnson (ed.), *Marital Violence*, London, Routledge, 1985; S. Vaughn, *Breaking the Silence: Voices on Battered Women. An Oral History*, Radio History Series, KUOM radio, University of Minnesota, 1987, available from 728 Osceola Avenue, St Paul, MN 55105; Gondolf, op. cit.; L.A. Hoff, *Battered Women as Survivors*, London, Routledge, 1990.
78 E. Stark, A. Flitcraft and W. Frazier, 'Medicine and patriarchal violence: The construction of a "private" event', *International Journal of Health Services*, vol. 9, 1979, pp. 461–93; Okun, op. cit., B. Andrews and G.W. Brown, 'Marital violence in the community: A biographical approach', *British Journal of Psychiatry*, vol. 153, 1988, pp. 305–12.

79 Dobash and Dobash, op. cit., 1979; Dobash, Dobash and Cavanagh, op. cit.

80 Dobash and Dobash, 1979, op. cit.

81 Dobash, Dobash and Cavanagh, op. cit.

82 Dobash and Dobash, op. cit., 1979; Dobash, Dobash and Cavanagh, op. cit., Hoff, op. cit.

83 Dobash and Dobash, 1979, op. cit.

84 Dobash and Dobash, op. cit., 1979; Bowker, op. cit., Gondolf, op. cit.; Vaughn, op. cit.

85 Dobash and Dobash, op. cit., 1979; Bowker, op. cit.

86 We now have overwhelming evidence that the most important factors in a woman's efforts to leave a violent relationship are her economic and employment status. For a review of this evidence see: M.J. Strube, 'The decision to leave an abusive relationship: Empirical evidence and theoretical issues', *Psychological Bulletin*, vol. 104, no. 2, 1988, pp. 236–50; J.H. Pfouts, 'Violent families: Coping responses of abused wives', *Child Welfare*, vol. 57, 1978, pp. 101–11; M.J. Strube and L.S. Barbour, 'The decision to leave an abusive relationship: Economic dependence and psychological commitment', *Journal of Marriage and the Family*, vol. 45, 1983, pp. 785–93; M.J. Strube and L.S. Barbour, 'Factors related to the decision to leave an abusive relationship', *Journal of Marriage and the Family*, vol. 46, 1984, pp. 837–44; Pahl, op. cit., 1985.

87 M. Fine, 'Coping with rape: Critical perspectives on consciousness', *Imagination, Cognition and Personality*, vol. 3, no. 3, 1983–4, pp. 249–67, p. 252, 256; see also Michelle Fine, 'Contextualizing the study of social injustice', in M. Saks and L. Saxe (eds), *Advances in Applied Social Psychology*, New Jersey, Erlbaum, 1985, pp. 103–26.

88 See Strube, op. cit., for a discussion of entrapment theory, cost–benefit assessment and the reasoned action model, approaches which are more contextual and less reductionist than the learned helplessness approach; see also Fine, op. cit., 1985.

89 Eisenstein, op. cit., pp. 130–1; see K. Ferraro, 'Processing battered women', *Journal of Family Issues*, vol. 2, no. 4, 1981, pp. 415–38 for an example of the transformation of an activist shelter into one with a strong therapeutic orientation.

90 Eisenstein, op. cit., p. 131.

91 See Bush, op. cit.

92 See for example, Star et al., op. cit.; Bern, op. cit. It is interesting, however, that these arguments appear infrequently in the more recent therapeutic literature. When they do it is usually to emphasize the need to counsel women about their supposed economic and social opportunities and not to stress efforts to change these wider problems.

93 Walker's writing are exemplary. When she first put her arguments about learned helplessness she discussed wider social and economic factors, e.g. Walker, op. cit., 1977–8; in more recent work these discussions rarely appear, e.g. Walker, op. cit., 1985. See R. Emerson Dobash and R.P. Dobash, 'Research as social action: The struggle for battered women', in K. Yllo and M. Bograd (eds), *Feminist Perspectives on Wife Abuse*, Beverly Hills, Sage, pp. 51–74.

94 F. Power Cobbe, 'Wife torture in England', *Contemporary Review*, vol. 32, April, 1878, pp. 55–87.
95 L.G. Schultz 'The wife assaulter', *Journal of Social Therapy*, vol. 6, no. 2, 1960, pp. 103–12, p. 103.
96 Ibid.
97 J. E. Snell, R. Rosenwald and A. Robey, 'The wifebeater's wife: A study of family interaction', *Archives of General Psychiatry*, vol. 11, 1964, pp. 107–12, p. 111.
98 L. B. Schlesinger, M. Benson and M. Zornitzer, 'Classification of violent behavior for the purposes of treatment planning: A three-pronged approach', in M. Roy (ed.), *The Abusive Partner: An Analysis of Domestic Battering*, New York, Van Nostrand Reinhold, 1982, pp. 148–69, p. 148.
99 Ibid., p. 152.
100 A. Schauss, 'Effects of environmental and nutritional factors on potential and actual batterers', in Roy, op. cit., pp. 76–89, p. 78.
101 Cited in Schauss, ibid., p. 86.
102 Ibid., p. 87.
103 R.J. Powers and I.L. Kutash, 'Alcohol, drugs, and partner abuse', in Roy, op. cit., pp. 39–75, p. 44.
104 J.P. Deschner, *The Hitting Habit: Anger Control for Battering Couples*, New York, Free Press, 1984.
105 Schlesinger et al., op. cit., p. 163.
106 Deschner, op. cit., p. 51.
107 Ibid.
108 Shupe et al., op. cit., p. 36.
109 Ibid.
110 Ibid., p. 37.
111 M. Elbow, 'Theoretical considerations of violent marriages', *Social Casework*, vol. 58, 1977, pp. 515–26, p. 515.
112 Quoted in Shupe et al., op. cit., p. 60.
113 Ibid., p. 61.
114 F.G. Bolton and S.R. Bolton, *Working with Violent Families*, Newbury Park, CA, Sage, 1987, p. 31.
115 J. Weitzman and K. Dreen, 'Wife beating: A view of the marital dyad', *Social Casework*, vol. 63, no. 5, 1982, pp. 259–65, p. 261.
116 Ibid., p. 261.
117 Shupe et al., op. cit., p. 31.
118 R.J. Shapiro, 'Therapy with violent families', in S. Saunders, A.M. Anderson and C.A. Hart (eds), *Violent Individuals and Families*, Springfield, IL, Charles C. Thomas, 1984, pp. 112–36, p. 119.
119 P.H. Neidig, 'Women's shelters, men's collectives and other issues in the field of spouse abuse', *Victimology*, vol. 9, nos. 3/4, 1984, pp. 464–76, p. 475.
120 Shapiro, op. cit., p. 119.
121 J. Geller, 'Conjoint therapy: Staff training and treatment of the abuser and the abuse', in Roy, op. cit., p. 205.
122 Weitzman and Dreen, op. cit., p. 264.
123 Shapiro, op. cit., p. 119.
124 Geller, op. cit., p. 201.

125 For an excellent discussion of these limitations see J. Myers Avis, 'Deepening awareness: A private study guide to feminism and family therapy', *Journal of Psychotherapy and the Family*, vol. 3, no. 4, 1988, pp. 15–46.
126 J. Flanzer, 'Alcohol and family violence: Double trouble', in Roy, op. cit., pp. 136–42, p. 136.
127 Bolton and Bolton, op. cit., p. 31.
128 For interpretative approaches to explaining violence see H. Toch, *Violent Men: An Inquiry into the Psychology of Violence*, Chicago, Aldine, 1969; L. Athens; *Violent Criminal Acts and Actors*, New York: Routledge, 1980. For feminist approaches to violence see the Violence Against Women section in the next chapter.
129 Raging Words of Wisdom, unpublished paper presented at NCADV National Conference, Milwaukee, 1982.
130 Ibid.
131 M. Morrison, 'Yes, I am angry', *Aegis*.
132 B. Hart, 'Visions forum', Appendix A, *Safety for Women: Monitoring Batterers' Programs*, Harrisburg, PA, Pennsylvania Coalition Against Domestic Violence, 1988, pp. 135–40.
133 Ibid., p. 136.
134 Ibid.
135 Shupe et al., op. cit., p. 14.
136 Ibid.
137 Emerge, *Emerge: A Men's Counseling Service on Domestic Violence*, Boston, 1981; D. Adams, 'Treatment models of men who batter: A profeminist analysis', K. Yllo and M. Bograd, op. cit., pp. 176–97.
138 A.L. Ganley, *Court-Mandated Counseling for Men Who Batter: A Three Day Workshop for Mental Health Professionals*, Washington, DC, Available from the Center for Women's Policy Studies, 1981.
139 Emerge, op. cit., p. 49.
140 A.L. Ganley, 'Perpetrators of domestic violence: An overview of counseling the court-mandated client', in Sonkin, op. cit., 1987, pp. 155–73.
141 F. Purdy and N. Nickel, 'Practice principles for working with groups of men who batter', *Social Work with Groups*, vol. 4, 1981, pp. 111–12.
142 Ganley, op. cit., 1987, p. 157.
143 Adams, op. cit., p. 177.
144 J.L. Edelson, 'Working with men who batter', *Social Work*, vol. 29, no. 3, 1984, pp. 237–42; J. Ptacek 'Why do men batter their wives', in Yllo and Bograd, op. cit., pp. 133–57.
145 Edelson, op. cit.
146 Quoted in Z. Metger, 'Help for men who batter: An overview of issues and program', *Response*, vol. 5–6, November/December, 1981, pp. 1–2, p. 2.
147 E. Pence and M. Paymar, *Power and Control: Tactics of Men who Batter. An Educational Curriculum*, Minnesota Program Development, 206 West Fourth Street, Duluth, MN 55806, 1986 (revised 1990).
148 J.L. Bernard and M.L. Bernard, 'The abusive male seeking treatment: Jekyll and Hyde', *Family Relations*, vol. 33, no. 4, 1984, pp. 543–7. Bernard and Bernard point out that a woman can identify sex biases even when sensitive men miss them and the presence of a woman may illicit responses that can become part of the learning process.

149 P. Freire, *Pedagogy of the Oppressed*, Harmondsworth, England, Penguin, 1977; P. Freire, *A Pedagogy for Liberation*, Basingstoke, Macmillan, 1987; for another explicit educational programme see P.B. Frank and B.D. Hougton, *Confronting the Batterer: A Guide to Creating the Spouse Abuse Educational Workshop*, Domestic Violence Project, Volunteer Counseling Service, ND; P.B. Frank, *Volunteer Service: The Setting of the Domestic Violence Project*, 1988, both available from 151 S. Main Street, New York, NY 10956.

150 L. Cantoni, 'Clinical issues in domestic violence', *Social Casework*, vol. 62, 1981, pp. 3–12.

151 Clarification of these ideas was much aided by R.A. Duff, *Trials and Punishments*, London, Cambridge University Press, 1986.

152 Ptacek, op. cit.

153 Duff, op; cit., discusses the requirement that meaningful punishment must be both retributive and reformative.

154 Hart, op. cit., provides a detailed analysis of the processes and problems associated with monitoring programmes for men.

155 H. Sinclair, The MAWS *Men's Program and the Issue of Male-Role Violence Against Women, A Training Manual*, Marin, CA, Marin Abused Women Services, ND, p. 25.

156 Emerge, op. cit., p. 55.

157 For an excellent review of the evaluation research on programmes for violent men see Z.C. Eisikovits and J.L. Edelson, 'Intervening with men who batter: A critical review of the literature', *Social Service Review*, September, 1989, pp. 384–414; M.A. Pirog-Good and J. Stets, 'Programs for abusers: Who drops out and what can be done', *Response*, vol. 9, no. 2, 1986, pp. 17–20.

8 KNOWLEDGE AND SOCIAL CHANGE

1 The start of this new conception of the conduct of science was heralded by T. Kuhn, *The Structure of Scientific Revolutions*, Chicago, University of Chicago Press, 1962; see also I. Lakatos and A. Musgrave (eds), *Criticism and the Growth of Knowledge*, Cambridge, Cambridge University Press, 1970; P. Feyerabend, *Against Method: Outline of an Anarchistic Theory of Knowledge*, London, New Left Books, 1975; for important discussions of these issues within the interpretive tradition see P. Rabinow and W.M. Sullivan (eds), *Interpretive Social Science*, Berkeley, University of California Press, 1979; D. Callahan and B. Jennings, *Ethics, the Social Sciences and Policy Analysis*, New York, Plenum, 1983; for feminist discussions around these issues see S. Harding, *The Science Question in Feminism*, Ithaca, Cornell University Press, 1983; N. Tuana (ed.), *Feminism and Science*, Bloomingon, Indiana University Press, 1989.

2 B. Jennings, 'Interpretive social science and policy analysis', in Callahan and Jennings, op. cit., pp. 6–26.

3 For an excellent discussion of the impact of science on social thinking see S. Rose, L.J. Kamin and R.C. Lewontin, *Not in Our Genes: Biology, Ideology and Human Nature*, New York, Penguin, 1984.

4 For details of the discovery of this hoax see L. Kamin, *The Science and Politics of IQ*, Potomac, Md.: Erlbaum, 1974; Rose, Kamin and Lewontin, op. cit.

5 J. Pahl, *A Refuge for Battered Women: A Study of The Role of a Women's Centre*, London, HMSO, 1978; R. Emerson Dobash and R.P. Dobash, *Violence Against Wives*, New York, Free Press, 1979; S. Delamont and R. Ellis, *Statutory and Voluntary Responses to Domestic Violence in Wales*, DHSS/Welsh Office Domestic Violence Project, SRU Working Paper no. 6, University College, Wales, 1979; V. Binney, G. Harknell and J. Nixon, *Leaving Violent Men*, ,London, Women's Aid Federation England, 1981; M. Borkowski, M. Murch and V. Walker, *Marital Violence – The Community Response*, London, Tavistock, 1983; S.S.M. Edwards, *Policing 'Domestic' Violence*, London, Sage, 1989.

6 NIMH has been the main financial supporter of research on the characteristics of 'violent families' and the battered woman syndrome as well as learned helplessness.

7 The following projects were collaborative efforts of academic researchers and the movement with the members of the movement playing the major role in formulating and carrying out the research, Binney, Harkell and Nixon, op. cit.; M. Homer, A. Leonard and P. Taylor, *Private Violence: Public Shame*, Middlesbrough, Cleveland Refuge and Aid for Women and Children, 1984; J. Browne, *Not Worth the Paper ...?*, Bristol, England, Women's Aid Federation England, 1990.

8 Dobash and Dobash, op. cit.; L. Smith, *Domestic Violence: An Overview of the Literature*, London, HMSO, 1989; M.A. Straus and R.J. Gelles, 'Societal change and change in family violence from 1975 to 1985 as revealed by two national surveys', *Journal of Marriage and the Family*, vol. 48, 1986, pp. 465–79.

9 United States Commission on Civil Rights, *Battered Women: Issues of Public Policy*, Washington DC, US Commission on Civil Rights, p. 103.

10 Lisa Leghorn, ibid., p. 139.

11 Parliament (1974–75), *Report from the Select Committee on Violence in Marriage*, vol. 2, London, HMSO, p. 61.

12 Commission on Civil Rights, op. cit., p. 139; Select committee, p. 264.

13 See S. Schechter, *Women and Male Violence*, Boston, South End Press, 1982; pp. 41–42.

14 J. Hanmer and D. Leonard, 'Negotiating the problem: The DHSS and research on violence in marriage', in C. Bell and H. Roberts (eds), *Social Researching: Politics, Problems, and Practice*, London, Routledge, 1984, pp. 32–53.

15 L. Leghorn, 'Grassroots services for battered women: A model for long-term social change', 'Funding The Battered Husband Myth'. Commission on Civil Rights, op. cit., pp. 450–3, p. 451; see also Hilberman, USCCR, ibid., p. 528 on self-defence.

16 Civil Rights Commission, op. cit., p. 139.

17 M.P. Pagelow, 'The "battered husband syndrome": social problem or much ado about little?', in N. Johnson (ed.), *Marital Violence*, London, Routledge, 1985, pp. 172–94, p. 174.

18 D. Adams, J. Jackson and M. Lauby, 'Family violence research: Aid or

obstacle to the battered women's movement', *Response*, vol. 11, no. 3, 1988, pp. 14–16.
19 D. Kurz, 'Social science perspectives on wife abuse: Current debates and future directions', *Gender and Society*, vol. 3, no. 4, December, 1989, pp. 489–505. We use the same term as Kurz for defining the family violence approach, but differ in defining the other approach as violence against women.
20 R.J. Gelles, *The Violent Home*, Newbury Park, CA, Sage, 1974.
21 M.A. Straus and R.J. Gelles, 'Societal change and change in family violence from 1975 to 1985 as revealed in two national surveys', in M.A. Straus and R.J. Gelles, *Physical Violence in American Families*, New Brunswick, NJ, Transaction, 1990, pp. 113–32, p. 118.
22 Ibid.
23 Ibid.
24 M. Straus, 'Wife-beating: How common and why?', *Victimology*, vol. 2, nos. 3/4, 1977–8, pp. 443–58.
25 A. Shupe, W.A. Stacey and L.R. Hazelwood, *Violent Men, Violent Couples. The Dynamics of Domestic Violence*, Lexington, MA, Lexington Books, 1987; J.E. Stets and M.A. Straus, 'Gender differences in reporting martial violence and its medical and psychological consequences', in Straus and Gelles, op. cit., pp. 151–65.
26 R.L. McNeely and G. Robinson-Simpson, 'The truth about domestic violence: A falsely framed issue', *Social Work*, Nov–Dec, 1987, pp. 485–90, p. 486.
27 Shupe, Stacey and Hazelwood, op. cit., p. 56.
28 S.K. Steinmetz, 'The battered husband syndrome', *Victimology*, vol. 2, nos. 3/4, 1977–8, pp. 499–509.
29 Steinmetz, quoted in A. Jones,, *Women Who Kill*, New York, Fawcett Columbine, 1980, p. 301, from 'Battered husbands', *Time*, 20 March, 1978, p. 69.
30 M. McLeod, 'Women against men: An examination of domestic violence based on an analysis of official data and national victimization data', *Justice Quarterly*, vol. 1, 1984, pp. 171–93, p. 191.
31 McNeely and Robinson-Simpson, op. cit., p. 486.
32 Straus, op. cit., p. 488.
33 M.A. Straus, 'Measuring intrafamily conflict and violence: The conflict tactics (CT) scales', *Journal of Marriage and the Family*, vol. 41, 1979, pp. 75–88; M.A. Straus, 'The Conflict Tactics Scales and its critics: An evaluation and new data on validity and reliability', in Straus and Gelles, op. cit., 1990.
34 McNeely and Robinson-Simpson, op. cit.
35 Ibid.
36 Steinmetz, op. cit., S.K. Steinmetz, 'Family violence. Past, present and future', in M.B. Sussman and S.K. Steinmetz (eds), *Handbook of Marriage and the Family*, New York, Plenum 1987, pp. 725–65; S.K. Steinmetz and J.S. Lucca, 'Husband battering', in V.B. Van Hasselt, R.L. Morrison, A.S. Bellack and M. Hersen, *Handbook of Family Violence*, New York, Plenum, 1988, pp. 233–46.
37 Steinmetz, op. cit.,1987, p. 727.
38 Straus and Gelles, op. cit., 1986, p. 471.

39 Steinmetz, op. cit., 1987, p. 727.
40 For a further discussion of this tactic see R.E. Dobash and R.P. Dobash, 'Research as social action: The struggle for battered women', in K. Yllo and M. Bograd (eds), *Feminist Perspectives on Wife Abuse*, Newbury Park, CA, Sage, 1988, pp. 51–74.
41 L. Wardell, D.L. Gillespie and A. Leffler, 'Science and violence against wives', in D. Finkelhor et al. (eds), *The Dark Side of Families*, Newbury Park, CA, Sage, 1983, pp. 69–84, p. 79.
42 Shupe, et al., op. cit., p. 46.
43 Steinmetz, op. cit., 1977–8, p. 507. Comments such as this seem to reflect an ignorance or lack of appreciation of the totally different economic circumstances of divorced men and women. Research on the financial consequences of divorce from several countries shows that a large percentage of men never pay any support and that women are much worse off than men after a divorce. See, for instance, L.J. Weitzman, *The Divorce Revolution*, New York, Free Press, 1985; J. Ekelaar and M. Maclean, *Maintenance After Divorce*, Oxford, Oxford University Press, 1986; R.E. Dobash and F. Wasoff, 'Moving the family: Changing housing circumstances after divorce', in P. Symon, *Housing and Divorce*, Studies in Housing No. 4, Glasgow, Centre for Housing Research, 1990.
44 Steinmetz, op. cit., 1977–8, p. 507.
45 Ibid.
46 Ibid., p. 506.
47 Straus and Gelles, op. cit., 1990, p. xvi; see Jones, op. cit., pp. 203–5 for additional evidence of the public activity of the FV researchers.
48 R.J. Gelles, 'Domestic criminal violence', in M.E. Wolfgang and N. A. Weiner (eds), *Criminal Violence*, Beverly Hills, CA, Sage, 1982, pp. 201–35. Pahl, op. cit.
49 Straus and Gelles, op. cit., 1986, p. 472.
50 Steinmetz, op. cit., 1987.
51 Ibid., p. 727.
52 Shupe, et al., op. cit., p. 45.
53 Ibid., p. 52.
54 McNeely and Robinson-Simpson, op. cit., p. 487.
55 Ibid., p. 488.
56 Ibid., p. 487.
57 M.A. Straus, 'The national family violence surveys', in Straus and Gelles, op. cit., 1990, pp. 3–16, p. 11.
58 Ibid.
59 It must be pointed out that not all researchers who accept the asymmetry of violence in the family have adopted these methods. This is especially true for those researchers who have attempted to establish the supposedly distinct psychological attributes of women who have been abused.
60 M. Daly and M. Wilson, *Homicide*, New York, Aldine de Gruyter, 1988.
61 M.H. Lystad, 'Violence at home: A review of the literature', *American Journal of Orthopsychiatry*, vol. 45, no. 5, 1975, pp. 328–45; Dobash and Dobash, op. cit., 1979; R. Emerson Dobash and R.P. Dobash, 'Wives: The "appropriate" victims of marital violence', *Victimology*, vol. 2, 1977–8, pp. 426–42; D. Martin, *Battered Wives*, San Francisco CA, Glide.

62 Lystad, op. cit., p. 332.
63 Dobash and Dobash, op. cit., 1977–8; 1979.
64 C. R. Watkins, *Victims, Aggressors and the Family Secret: An Exploration into Family Violence*, St Paul, Minnesota, Department of Public Welfare, 1982; J.A. Byles, 'Family violence: Some facts and gaps: A statistical overview', in D'Oyley, *Domestic Violence: Issues and Dynamics*, Toronto, The Ontario Institute for Studies in Education, 1978; P.J. Kincaid, *The Omitted Reality: Husband–Wife Violence in Ontario and Policy Implications for Education*, Maple, Ontario, Learners Press, 1982; D. Quarm and M.D. Schwartz, 'Domestic violence in criminal court', in C. Schweber and C. Feinman (eds), *Criminal Justice, Politics and Women*, New York, Haworth, 1985, pp. 29–46; San Diego, San Diego Association of Governments, 1981; McLeod, op. cit.; D.J. Bell, 'Domestic violence in rural areas', unpublished paper presented at the annual meeting of the Academy of Criminal Justice Sciences, 1985; B.E. Vanfossen, 'Intersexual violence in Monroe County, New York', *Victimology*, vol. 4, 1979, pp. 299–305.
65 Dobash and Dobash, op. cit., 1977–8. German research revealed that over 90 per cent of the victims of violence in the family are females. The researcher concluded 'The rare cases in which male victims do occur mostly refer to disputes between parents and children ...'. W. Steffen, 'Help seeking women and the police: An empirical study on the settling of family disputes', paper presented at the XII World Congress of Sociology, Madrid, July, 1990.
66 D.A. Gaquin, 'Spouse abuse: Data from the National Crime Survey', *Victimology*, vol. 2, 1977–8, pp. 634–5.
67 McLeod, op. cit.
68 M.D. Schwartz, 'Gender and injury in spousal assault', *Sociological Focus*, vol. 20, no. 1, 1987, pp. 61–75.
69 H. Johnson, 'Wife assault in Canada', paper presented at the annual conference of the American Society of Criminology, November, 1989.
70 A. Worral and K. Pease, 'Personal crime against women: Evidence from the British Crime Survey', *The Howard Journal*, vol. 25, 1986, pp. 118–24.
71 R.A. Berk, S.F. Berk, D.R. Loseke and D. Rauma, 'Mutual combat and other family violence myths', in Finkelhor et al., op. cit., pp. 197–212, p. 207.
72 Schwartz, op. cit., p. 67.
73 Dobash and Dobash, op. cit., 1979.
74 L.P. Rouse, R. Breen and M. Howell, 'Abuse in intimate relationships. A comparison of married and dating college students', *Journal of Interpersonal Violence*, vol. 3, pp. 414–29.
75 Kincaid, op. cit., p. 91.
76 Kincaid, op. cit.
77 Dobash and Dobash, op. cit., 1979; J. O'Faolain and L. Martines (eds), *Not in God's Image: Women in History*, London, Virago, 1979; E. Pleck, *Domestic Tyranny*, Oxford, Oxford University Press, 1987; L. Gordon, *Heroes of Their Own Lives*, New York, Viking, 1988. Although we know that women have always been the predominant victims of violence in the home, this does not mean that there was no variation over

time in the violence and the responses to it. There is some evidence to suggest that English communities in the late eighteenth century were likely to conduct shaming rituals to protect women and it may always have been considered more of an offence among patrician and bourgeois families. Indeed, this is an area which needs additional investigation.

78 R.P. Dobash and R. Emerson Dobash, 'Community response to violence against wives: Charivari, abstract justice and patriarchy', *Social Problems*, vol. 28, no. 5, 1978, pp. 563–81.

79 Jones, op. cit.; Pleck, op. cit.; Gordon, op. cit.; Daly and Wilson, op. cit.

80 Daly and Wilson, op. cit., p. 69; Jones, op. cit., p. 59 reaches similar conclusions, 'Women in desperate circumstances turned to infanticide'.

81 Daly and Wilson, op. cit., Chapter 3.

82 Jones, op. cit.; Daly and Wilson, op. cit.

83 N. Zemon Davis, 'The reasons of misrule: Youth groups and Charivaris in sixteenth century France', *Past and Present*, vol. 51, 1971, pp. 51–77; E.P. Thompson 'Rough music: "*le charivari anglais*"', translated for the authors by M. Malkowski, *Annales (Economie, Societies, Civilization)*, vol. 27, no. 2, 1972, pp. 285–312; Dobash and Dobash, op. cit., 1981; R.P. Dobash, R. Emerson Dobash and S. Gutteridge, *The Imprisonment of Women*, Oxford: Basil Blackwell, 1986.

84 Dobash, Dobash and Gutteridge, ibid.

85 E. Shorter, *The Making of the Modern Family*, New York, Basic Books, 1975. In her efforts to confirm the existence of battered husbands, Steinmetz persistently misinterprets the evidence regarding these rituals. For example, she erroneously claims that men who beat their wives were forced to 'kiss a large set of ribboned horns', whereas this 'punishment' was reserved for the cuckold. Steinmetz, op. cit., 1977–8; Steinmetz and Lucca, op. cit.

86 S. Schama, *The Embarrassment of Riches*, London, Fontana, 1988, p. 445.

87 Ibid., pp. 443–58.

88 Shorter, op. cit., p. 200.

89 See, for example, Dobash and Dobash, op. cit., 1979; E.A. Stanko, 'Typical violence, normal precaution: Men, women and interpersonal violence in the US, England, Wales and Scotland', in J. Hanmer and M. Maynard (eds), *Women, Violence and Social Control*, London, Macmillan, 1987; L. Kelly, *Surviving Sexual Violence*, Oxford, Polity Press, 1988.

90 Dobash and Dobash, op. cit., 1979; R.E. Dobash and R.P. Dobash, 'The nature and antecedents of violent events', *British Journal of Criminology*, vol. 24, no. 3, 1984, pp. 269–88.

91 Dobash and Dobash, op. cit., 1979, 1984; Kincaid, op. cit.; S. Eisenberg and P. Micklow, 'The assaulted wife: "Catch-22" revisited', unpublished paper, University of Michigan Law School, 1974 (edited and reprinted in *Women's Rights Law Reporter*, Spring/Summer, 1977); M. Pagelow, *Woman-Battering*, Newbury Park, CA, Sage, 1981; E. Evason, *Hidden Violence. A Study of Battered Women in Northern Ireland*, Belfast, Farset Press, 1982; D. Russell, *Rape in Marriage*, New York, Collier, 1982; L. Bowker, *Beating Wife Beating*, Lexington, MA, Lexington Books, 1983; L.E. Walker, 'Psychological impact of the criminalization

of domestic violence on victims', *Victimology*, vol. 10, 1985, pp. 281–300; J. Pahl, *Private Violence and Public Policy*, London, Routledge, 1985; T. Jones, B. Maclean and J. Young, *The Islington Crime Survey*, Aldershot, Gower, 1986 (one of the few surveys to investigate the nature of assaults and resulting injuries).

92 Russell, op. cit.; I.H. Frieze, 'Investigating the causes and consequences of marital rape', *Signs*, vol. 8, no. 3, 1983, pp. 532–53.

93 Frieze, ibid.

94 L. Kelly, *Surviving Sexual Violence*, Oxford, Polity Press, 1988.

95 See Note 91 for references.

96 Dobash and Dobash, op. cit., 1979, 1984; Pagelow, op. cit.; Bowker, op. cit.; D.G. Saunders, 'When battered women use violence: Husband-abuse or self-defense?', *Violence and Victims*, vol. 1, 1986, pp. 47–60; D.G. Saunders, 'Wife abuse, husband abuse, or mutual combat?', in K. Yllo and M. Bograd (eds), *Feminist Perspectives on Wife Abuse*, Newbury Park, CA, Sage, 1988; R.P. Dobash, R. Emerson Dobash, M. Wilson and M. Daly, 'The asymmetrical nature of domestic violence: The myth of battered husbands', *Social Problems*, 1992.

97 Dobash and Dobash, op. cit., 1979; pp. 108–9.

98 Dobash and Dobash, op. cit., 1979; Eisenberg and Micklow, op. cit.

99 Saunders, op. cit.

100 Steinmetz, op. cit., 1987; Shupe, Stacey and Hazelwood, op. cit.

101 Shupe, Stacey and Hazelwood, op. cit.

102 Ibid., p. 62.

103 For a comprehensive review of the literature on sexual differences in killing see Daly and Wilson, op. cit.

104 Dobash, Dobash, Wilson and Daly, op. cit., forthcoming; Daly and Wilson, op. cit.

105 S.S.M. Edwards, *Policing 'Domestic' Violence*, London, Sage, p. 124.

106 Ibid.

107 Daly and Wilson, op. cit.; Jones, op. cit.; A. Browne, *When Battered Women Kill*, New York, Free Press, 1987.

108 Daly and Wilson, op. cit.; Jones, op. cit.; J. Boudouris, 'Homicide and the family', *Journal of Marriage and the Family*, vol. 33, no. 4, 1971, pp. 667–76, p. 671; W. Wilbanks, 'The female homicide offender in Dade County, Florida', *Criminal Justice Review*, vol. 8, no. 2, 1983, pp. 9–14, p. 13; B. Davidson, C. del Rio and P. Jenkins, 'Women's view of homicide: The battered woman offender', paper presented at the Family Violence Research Conference, Durham, New Hampshire, July 1987; M. Daly and M. Wilson, 'Evolutionary social psychology and family homicide', *Science*, vol. 242, pp. 519–24.

109 Straus, op. cit., 1990, p. 14.

110 K.A. Yllo and M.A. Straus, 'Patriarchy and violence against wives: The impact of structural and normative factors', in Straus and Gelles, op. cit., 1990, pp. 383–99, p. 386. In making this point FV researchers often invoke our own work in which we discuss the limitations of quantitative and positivist methods. It seems that FV commentators have confused the rejection of certain forms of positivisim and empiricism with the rejection of quantification since we have actually used and endorsed quantitative methods for certain tasks.

111 M.A. Straus, 'Injury and frequency of assault and the "representative sample fallacy" in measuring wife beating and child abuse', in Straus and Gelles, op. cit., 1990, pp. 75–91.

112 D. Willer and J. Willer, *Systematic Empiricism: A Pseudoscience*, Englewood Cliffs, NJ, Prentice-Hall, 1973; Callahan and Jennings, op. cit.; C.G.A. Bryant, *Positivism in Social Theory and Research*, Basingstoke, England, Macmillan, 1985.

113 Willer and Willer, op. cit.

114 E. Pleck, J.H. Pleck, M. Grossman and P.B. Bart, 'The battered data syndrome: A comment on Steinmetz' article', *Victimology*, vol. 2, 1977–8, pp. 680–3; Dobash and Dobash, op. cit., 1979; R.E. Dobash and R.P. Dobash, 'Research as social action: The struggle for battered women', in K. Yllo and M. Bograde, Feminist Perspectives on Wife Abuse, Newbury Park, CA, Sage, 1988, pp. 51–74; R.P. Dobash and R.E. Dobash, 'How research makes a difference to policy and practice', in D.J. Besharov (ed.), *Family Violence: Research and Public Policy Issues*, Washington DC, AEI Press, 1990; R.P. Dobash, R. Emerson Dobash, M. Wilson and M. Daly, op. cit., forthcoming; W. Breines and L. Gordon, 'Review essay: The new scholarship in family violence', *Signs*, vol. 8, 1983, pp. 490–531; M. Pagelow, 'The "battered husband syndrome": social problem or much ado about little?', in N. Johnson (ed.), *Marital Violence*, London, Routledge, 1985; Saunders, op. cit., 1986, 1988; Kurz, op. cit., 1989.

115 Straus, op. cit., 1990, p. 76.

116 Dobash and Dobash, op. cit., 1979, Kelly, op. cit.

117 G. Margolin, 'The multiple forms of aggressiveness between marital partners; How we identify them', *Journal of Marital and Family Therapy*, vol. 13, 1987, pp. 77–84.

118 M. Szinovacz, 'Using couple data as a methodological tool: The case of marital violence', *Journal of Marriage and the Family*, vol. 45, 1983, pp. 633–44; E.N. Jouriles and K.D. O'Leary, 'Interpersonal reliability of reports of marital violence', *Journal of Consulting and Counseling Psychology*, vol. 53, 1985, pp. 419–21; J.L. Edelson and M.P. Brygger, 'Gender differences in reporting of battering incidences', *Family Relations*, vol. 35, 1986, pp. 377–82.

119 Dobash et al., op. cit., forthcoming.

120 Straus, op. cit., 1990, p. 69.

121 J.E. Stets and M.A. Straus, 'Gender differences in reporting marital violence and its medical and psychological consequences', in Straus and Gelles, op. cit., pp. 151–65, p. 153.

122 M.A. Straus, 'The Conflict Tactics Scales', in Straus and Gelles, op. cit., 1990, pp. 49–73, p. 71.

123 Ibid., p. 53.

124 Ibid., p. 56.

125 Ibid., p. 58.

126 M.A. Straus, 'Injury and frequency of assault and the "representative sample fallacy" in measuring wife beating and child abuse', in Straus and Gelles, op. cit., 1990, pp. 75–91, p. 88.

127 Straus, 'The Conflict Tactics Scale', op. cit., p. 59.

128 Straus, 'Injury and frequency of assault', op. cit., p. 71.

129 Ibid., p. 88.
130 Straus, 'The Conflict Tactics Scale', op. cit., p. 52.
131 F. Suppe, *Structure of Scientific Theories*, Urbana, University of Illinois Press, 1977.
132 Rabinow and Sullivan, op. cit.; Callahan and Jennings, op. cit.; G. Morgan (ed.), *Beyond Method: Strategies for Social Research*, Newbury Park, CA: Sage, 1986; R. Bellah et al., *Habits of the Heart*, Appendix: Social Science as Public Philosophy, New York, Harper and Row, 1985.
133 See for example Steinmetz, op. cit., 1987; R.J. Gelles and M.A. Straus, 'Determinants of violence in the family: Toward a Theoretical integration', in W.R. Burr et al. (eds), *Contemporary Theories of the Family*, Vol. 1, New York, Free Press, 1979.
134 For an excellent review of this tendency in American family sociology see D.L. Thomas and J.E. Wilcox, 'The rise of family theory', in Sussman and Steinmetz, op. cit., pp. 81–102; for additional criticisms of American sociology of the family see M.W. Osmond 'Radical-critical theories', in Sussman and Steinmetz, op. cit., pp. 104–24.
135 W.R. Burr, *Theory Construction and the Sociology of the Family*, New York, Wiley, 1973, p. 1.
136 H.T. Christensen, 'Development of the field of study', in H.T. Christensen (ed.), *Handbook of Marriage and the Family*, Chicago, Rand McNally, 1964.
137 R.P. Dobash and R. Emerson Dobash,; Kuhn, op. cit.; Feyerabend, op. cit.; D. Shapere, 'Notes toward a post-positivistic interpretation of science', in P. Achinstein and S.F. Barker (eds), *The Legacy of Logical Positivism*, Baltimore, Johns Hopkins University Press, 1969.
138 Thomas and Wilcox, op. cit.
139 Thomas and Wilcox, op. cit., p. 96.
140 H.L. Dreyfus and P. Rabinow, *Michel Foucault: Beyond Structuralism and Hermeneutics*, Chicago, University of Chicago Press, 1982.
141 T.D. Cook, 'Quasi-experimentation: Its ontology, epistemology and methodology', in Morgan, op. cit., pp. 74–94.
142 Dobash and Dobash, op. cit., 'Research as social action', 1988.
143 R.N. Bellah, 'Social science as practical reasoning', in Callahan and Jennings, op. cit., Dobash and Dobash 'The context specific approach to researching violence against wives', in D. Finkelhor, R. Gelles, G. Hoteling and M.A. Straus (eds) *The Dark Side of Families*, 1983, pp. 261–76.

9 INNOVATION AND SOCIAL CHANGE

1 Conservative MP Nicolas Fairbairn, 'MP attacks aid for battered wives', *Glasgow Herald*, 22 September, 1975.
2 E. Pleck, *Domestic Tyranny*, New York, Cambridge University Press, 1988, p. 197 makes a similar point.
3 See K.J. Ferraro, 'Processing battered women', *Journal of Family Issues*, vol. 2, no. 4, 1981, p. 435 for a discussion of just such a transformation within a refuge in the USA.
4 S. Vaughan, 'The last refuge: Shelter for battered women', *Victimology*, vol. 2, 1977, pp. 113–15, p. 118.

5   National Center on Women and Family Law, 'State laws exempting battered women from mediation', *The Women's Advocate, Newsletter of the National Center on Women and Family Law,* New York, NCOWFL, vol. 11, no. 5, 1990, p. 2.

6   In 1990 a rise in the number of assaults reported to the London Metropolitan police was primarily associated with a 13 per cent increase in the number of arrests for domestic violence. D. Campbell, 'Victims readier to report rape attacks, police say', *Guardian,* 16 November, 1990.

7   K. Arnot, 'Leaving the pain behind – Women's Aid in Scotland', in S. Henderson and A. Mackay (eds), *Grit and Diamonds: Women in Scotland Making History, 1980–1990,* Edinburgh, Stramullion Ltd, 1990, pp. 78–80.

8   CHANGE began in 1989 and was followed by the creation of a second experimental programme, the Lothian Probation Project, created in 1990. The Lothian project emerged from within social work and probation, but Women's Aid is involved in an advisory capacity.

9   For a useful model, see B. Hart, *Safety for Women: Monitoring Batterers' Programs,* Harrisburg, PA, Pennsylvania Coalition Against Domestic Violence, 1988.

Selected references

Anderson, Bonnie S. and Zinsser, Judith P. (1990) (first pub. 1988), *A History of Their Own: Women in Europe from Prehistory to the Present*, Vol. II, London, Penguin.

Attorney General's Task Force (1984), *Family Violence*, Washington DC, Attorney General, September.

Banks, Olive (1981), *Faces of Feminism: A Study of Feminism as a Social Movement*, Oxford, Martin Robertson.

Barrett, Michele and McIntosh, Mary (1982), *The Anti-Social Family*, London, Verso.

Barron, Jackie (1990), *Not Worth the Paper ...?*, Bristol, England, Women's Aid Federation England.

Berk, Richard A., Rauma, D., Loseke, D.R. and Berk, S.F. (1982), 'Throwing the cops back out: The decline of a local program to make the criminal justice system more responsive to incidents of domestic violence', *Social Science Research*, vol. 11, pp. 245 79.

Besharov, Douglas A. (1990), *Family Violence: Research and Policy Issues*, Washington, DC, AEI Press.

Binney, Val, Harkell, Gina and Nixon, Judy (1981), *Leaving Violent Men: A Study of Reguges and Housing for Battered Women*, Leeds, England, Women's Aid Federation England.

Bowker, L. (1983), *Beating Wife Beating*, Lexington, MA, Lexington Books.

Breines, W. and Gordon, L. (1983), 'Review essay: The new scholarship in family violence', *Signs*, vol. 8, pp. 490–531.

Brophy, Julia and Smart, Carol (eds) (1985), *Women-in-Law*, London, Routledge, 1985.

Browne, Angela (1987), *When Battered Women Kill*, New York, The Free Press.

Bush, Malcolm (1988), *Families in Distress. Public, Private and Civic Responses*, Berkeley, University of California Press.

Castel, Robert, Castel, Francoise and Lovell Anne (1982), *The Psychiatric Society*, trans. by A. Lovell, New York, Columbia University Press.

Coote, Anna and Campbell, Beatrix (1987), 2nd edition, *Sweet Freedom: The Struggle for Women's Liberation*, Oxford, Basil Blackwell.

Dahl, Tove Stang (1987), *Women's Law, An Introduction to Feminist Jurisprudence*, Oxford, Oxford University Press.

Dahlerup, Drude (ed.) (1986), *The New Women's Movement: Feminism and*

352   *Women, violence and social change*

Polical Power in Europe and the USA, London, Sage.

Dale, Jennifer and Foster, Peggy (1986), *Feminist and State Welfare*, London, Routledge.

Daly, Kathleen (1989), 'Criminal justice ideologies and practices in different voices: Some feminist questions about justice', *International Journal of Sociology of Law*, vol. 17, no. 1, pp. 1–18.

Daly, Martin and Wilson, Margo (1988), *Homicide*, New York, Aldine De Gruyter.

Delamont, Sara and Rhian Ellis (1979), *Statutory and Voluntary Responses to Domestic Violence in Wales: A pilot project*, DHSS/Welsh Office, Domestic Violence Project, SRU Working Paper no. 6.

Dobash, R. Emerson (1988), 'Violence against women – A worldwide view', *Report of the International Women's Aid Conference, Cardiff, Wales 1988*, Welsh Women's Aid 38/42 Crwys Road, Cardiff, Wales, UK, pp. 21–6.

Dobash, R. Emerson and Dobash, Russell P. (1977–8), 'Wives: The "appropriate" victims of marital violence', *Victimology*, vol. 2, nos. 3–4, pp. 426–42.

Dobash, R. Emerson and Dobash, Russell P. (1970), *Violence Against Wives*, New York, The Free Press, and Macmillan Distributing, Brunel Road, Houndmills, Basingstoke, England.

Dobash, R. Emerson and Dobash, Russell P. (1984), 'The nature and antecedents of violent events', *The British Journal of Criminology*, vol. 24, no. 3, July, pp. 269–88.

Dobash, R. Emerson and Dobash, Russell P. (1987), 'The response of the British and American women's movements to violence against women', in J. Hanmer and M. Maynard (eds), *Women, Violence and Social Control*, London, Macmillan Press, pp. 169–79.

Dobash, R.E. and Dobash, R.P. (1988), 'Research as social action: the struggle for battered women', in K. Yllo and M. Bograd, *Feminist Perspectives on Wife Abuse*, Newbury Park CA, Sage, 1988, pp. 51–74.

Dobash, Russell P. and Dobash, R. Emerson (1981), 'Community response to violence against wives: Charivari, abstract justice and patriarchy', *Social Problems*, vol. 28, no. 5, pp. 563–81.

Dobash, R.P. and Dobash, R. Emerson (1990), 'How research makes a difference to policy and practice', in D.J. Besharov (ed.), *Family Violence: Research and Public Policy Issues*, Washington DC, AEI Press.

Dobash, R. Emerson, Dobash, Russell P. and Cavanagh, Katherine (1985), 'The contact between battered women and social and medical agencies', in Jan Pahl (ed.), *Private Violence and Public Policy*, London, Routledge, pp. 142–65.

Dobash, R.E., Dobash, R.P., Cavanagh, K. and Wilson, M. (1977–78), 'Wifebeating: The victims speak', *Victimology*, vol. 2 (3–4), pp. 608–22.

Dobash, R.P., Dobash, R. Emerson and Gutteridge, S. (1986), *The Imprisonment of Women*, Oxford, Basil Blackwell.

Dobash, R.P., Dobash, R. Emerson, Wilson, M. and Daly, M. 'The myth of the asymmetrical nature of domestic violence', *Social Problems*, 1992.

Edelson, Jeffrey L. and Eisikovits, Zvi (1985), 'Men who batter women: A critical review of the evidence', *Journal of Family Issues*, vol. 6, no. 2, June, pp. 229–47.

Edwards, Susan S.M. (1981), *Female Sexuality and the Law*, Oxford, Martin Robertson.

Edwards, Susan S.M. (1986), 'Police attitudes and dispositions in domestic disputes: The London study', *Police Journal*, July, pp. 230–41.

Edwards, Susan S.M. (ed.), (1989), *Policing 'Domestic' Violence*, London, Sage.

Eisenstein, H. (1984), *Contemporary Feminist Thought*, London, George Allen and Unwin.

Eisikovits, Zvi C. and Edelson, Jeffrey L. (1989), 'Intervening with men who batter: A critical review of the literature', *Social Service Review*, September, pp. 384–14.

Elshtain, Jean Bethke (1981), *Public Man, Private Woman: Women in Social and Political Thought*, Oxford, Martin Robertson.

Emerge (1981), *Emerge: A Men's Counseling Service on Domestic Violence*, Boston.

Epplen, A. (1986), 'Battered women and the equal protection clause: Will the constitution help them when the police won't?', *Yale Law Journal*, vol. 95, pp. 788–809.

Evason, Eileen (1982), *Hidden Violence: A Study of Battered Women in Northern Ireland*, Belfast, Farset Press.

Ferraro, Kathleen, J. (1989), 'The legal response in the United States', in J. Hanmer, J. Radford and E. Stanko (eds), (1989), *Women, Policing and Male Violence*, London, Routledge.

Fields, Marjorie (1978), 'Wife beating: Government intervention, policies and practices', in US Commission on Civil Rights, *Battered Women*, Washington DC, USCCR, pp. 228–87.

Fine, Michelle (1983–4), 'Coping with rape: Critical perspectives on consciousness', *Imagination, Cognition and Personality*, vol. 3, no. 3, pp. 249–67.

Finn, P. and Colson, S. (1990), *Civil Protection Orders: Legislation, Current Court Practice, and Enforcement*, Washington DC, National Institute of Justice, US Department of Justice.

Freeman, Jo (1975), *The Politics of Women's Liberation*, New York, Longman.

Ganley, Anne L. (1981), *Court-Mandated Counseling for Men Who Batter: A Three Day Workshop for Mental Health Professionals*, Washington DC., Available from the Center for Women's Policy Studies.

Gilligan, Carol (1982), *In A Different Voice*, Cambridge, Harvard University Press.

Gondolf, E.W. (with E.R. Fisher) (1988), *Battered Women as Survivors*, Lexington, MA, Lexington Books.

Goolkasin, Gail A. (1986), *Confronting Domestic Violence: A Guide for Criminal Justice Agencies*, Washington DC, US Department of Justice, National Institute of Justice.

Gordon, Linda (1988), *Heroes of Their Own Lives: The Politics and History of Family Violence, Boston 1880–1960*, New York, Viking.

Grau, J. Fagan, Jeffrey and Wexler, Susan (1984), 'Restraining orders for battered women: Issues of access and efficacy', *Women and Politics*, vol. 4, no. 3, pp. 13–28.

Hall, Stuart (1984), 'The state in question', in G. McLennan, D. Held and S.

Hall (eds), *The Idea of the Modern State*, Milton Keynes, Open University Press.

Hanmer, Jalna (1977), 'Community action, women's aid and the women's liberation movement', in Marjorie Mayo (ed.), *Women in the Community*, London, Routledge, pp. 91–108.

Hanmer, Jalna, Radford, Jill and Stanko, Elizabeth A. (1989), *Women, Policing and Male Violence*, London, Routledge.

Hart, Barbara (1988), *Safety for Women: Monitoring Batterers' Programs*, Harrisburg, PA, Pennsylvania Coalition Against Domestic Violence.

Hartmann, Heidi (1976), 'Capitalism, patriarchy, and job segregation by sex', *Signs: Journal of Women in Culture and Society*, vol. 1, no. 3, pp. 137–69.

Held, David (1984), 'Central perspectives on the modern state', in G. McLennan, D. Held and S. Hall (eds), *The Idea of the Modern State*, Milton Keynes, Open University Press, pp. 29–79.

Held, David (1984), 'Beyond liberalism and Marxism?', in G. McLennan, D. Held and S. Hall (eds), *The Idea of the Modern State*, Milton Keynes, Open University Press, pp. 223–40.

Hoff, Lee A. (1990), *Battered Women as Survivors*, London, Routledge.

Homer, Marjorie, Leonard, Anne and Taylor, Pat (1984), *Private Violence: Public Shame, A Report on the Circumstances of Women Leaving Domestic Violence in Cleveland*, England, Cleveland Refuge and Aid for Women and Children (CRAWC).

Jones, Ann (1980), *Women who Kill*, New York, Fawcett Columbine.

Kelly, Liz (1988), *Surviving Sexual Violence*, Cambridge, Polity Press.

Kincaid, P.J. (1982), *The Omitted Reality: Husband–Wife Violence in Ontario and Policy Implications for Education*, Maple, Ontario, Learners Press.

Kurz, D. (1989), 'Social science perspectives on wife abuse: Current debates and future directions', *Gender and Society*, vol. 3, no. 4, pp. 489–505.

Langan, Patrick and Innes, Christopher (1986), 'Preventing domestic violence against women', US Dept. of Justice, Bureau of Justice Statistics, Special Report, Washington DC 20531, August.

Leghorn, Lisa and Warrior, Betsy (1974), *Houseworker's Handbook*, 1st Ed., c/o Woman's Center, 46 Pleasant St., Cambridge, MA.

Lerman, Liza A. (1984), 'A Model State Act, remedies for domestic abuse', *Harvard Journal on Legislation*, vol. 21, no. 1, pp. 61–143.

Lerman, Liza A. (1984), 'Mediation of wife abuse cases: The adverse impact of informal dispute resolution on women', *Harvard Women's Law Journal*, vol. 7, no. 1, pp. 57–113.

MacKinnon, Catharine A. (1989), *Toward a Feminist Theory of the State*, Cambridge, MA, Harvard University Press.

MacLeod, Linda (1980) *Wife Battering in Canada: The Vicious Circle*, Hull, Quebec, Canadian Government Publishing Centre.

Mama, Amina (1989), *The Hidden Struggle : Statutory and Voluntary Sector Responses to Violence Against Black Women in the Home*, London, London Race and Housing Research Unit.

Martin, D. (1976), *Battered Wives*, San Francisco, CA, Glide.

Mathiesen, Thomas (1974), *The Politics of Abolition*, London, Martin Robertson.

Metropolitan Police, (1986), *Report of the Metropolitan Police Working Party into Domestic Violence*, London, January.

Okun, L. (1986), *Woman Abuse: Facts Replacing Myths*, Albany, NY, State University of New York Press.

Pagelow, M A. (1981), *Woman-Battering*, Newbury Park, CA, Sage.

Pahl, Jan (1978), *A Refuge for Battered Women: A Study of the Role of a Women's Centre*, London, Her Majesty's Stationery Office.

Pahl, Jan (ed.) (1985), *Private Violence and Public Policy: The Needs of Battered Women and the Response of the Public Service*, London, Routledge.

Parliament (1974–75), *Report from the Select Committee on Violence in Marriage, Together with the Proceedings of the Committee, Vol. 1. Report*, London, HMSO, H.C.553-I.

Parliament (1974–75), *Report from the Select Committee on Violence in Marriage, Together with the Proceedings of the Committee, Vol. 2, Report, Minutes of Evidence and Appendices*, London, HMSO, H.C.553-II.

Pence, Ellen (1983), 'The Duluth Domestic Abuse Intervention Project', *Hamline Law Review*, vol. 6, no. 2, pp. 247–75.

Pence, Ellen (with M. Duprey, M. Paymar and C. McDonnell) (1989), *Criminal Justice Response to Domestic Assault Cases: A Guide for Policy Development* (revised), Duluth, MN, Domestic Abuse Intervention Project.

Pence, E. and Paymar, M. (1986), *Power and Control: Tactics of Men Who Batter. An Educational Curriculum* (revised 1990), Duluth, MN, Minnesota Program Development.

Pierson, Christopher (1991), *A New Political Economy of the Welfare State*, Cambridge, Polity.

Pleck, Elizabeth (1987), *Domestic Tyranny*, Oxford, Oxford University Press.

Pleck, E. Pleck, J.H. Grossman, M. and Bart, P.B. (1977–8), 'The battered data syndrome: A comment on Steinmetz' article', *Victimology*, vol. 2, 1977–8, pp. 680–3.

Rendall, Jane (1985), *The Origins of Modern Feminism: Women in Britain, France and the United States 1780–1860*, London, Macmillan.

Rose, Hilary (1978), 'Women's refuges: Creating new forms of welfare?' (1985), in Clare Ungerson (ed.), *Women and Social Policy*, London, Macmillan, pp. 243–59.

Rowbotham, Sheila (1989), *The Past is Before Us: Feminism in Action Since the 1960s*, London, Penguin.

Russell, Diana (1982), *Rape in Marriage*, New York, Collier.

Sachs, Abie and Wilson, J. Hoff (1978), *Sexism and the Law. A Study of Male Beliefs and Judicial Bias*, Oxford, Martin Robertson.

San Francisco Family Violence Project (1982), *Domestic Violence is a Crime*, San Francisco, Family Violence Project (revised in 1985).

Schechter, Susan (1982), *Women and Male Violence: The Visions and Struggles of the Battered Women's Movement*, Boston, South End Press.

Schneider, E.M. (1986), 'Describing and changing: Women's self-defense work and the problem of expert testimony on battering', *Women's Rights Law Reporter*, vol. 9, nos. 3–4, pp. 196–222.

Sherman, Lawrence W. and Berk, Richard A. (1984), 'The specific deterrent effects of arrest for domestic assault', *American Sociological Review*, vol. 49, pp. 261–72.

Sinclair, H. (No Date), *The MAWS Mens Program and the Issue of Male-Role*

Violence Against Women, A Training Manual, Marin, CA, Marin Abused Women Services.

Smart, Carol (1989), *Feminism and the Power of Law*, London, Routledge.

Smith, L. (1989), *Domestic Violence: An Overview of the Literature*, London, HMSO.

Soler, Ester (1987), 'Domestic violence is a crime: A case study – San Francisco Family Violence Project' in D.J. Sonkin (ed.), *Domestic Violence on Trial*, New York, Springer.

Solicitor, A. (1983), 'The Matrimonial Homes Act – working at last', *SCOLAG: The Bulletin of the Scottish Legal Action Group*, October, no. 85, pp. 152–7.

Stark, Evan, Flitcraft, Ann and Frazier, W. (1979), 'Medicine and patriarchal violence: The construction of a "private" event', *International Journal of Health Services*, vol. 9, pp. 461–93.

Straus, M.A. and Gelles, R.J. (1990), *Physical Violence in American Families*, New Brunswick, NJ, Transaction.

Strube, M.J. and Barbour, L.S. (1984), 'Factors related to the decision to leave an abusive relationship', *Journal of Marriage and the Family*, vol. 46, pp. 837–44.

Sutton, Jo (1978), 'The growth of the British movement for battered women', *Victimology*, vol. 2, nos. 3–4, pp. 576–84.

SWA, Scottish Women's Aid (1988), *The Herstory of Women's Aid in Scotland*, 11 St Colme St., Edinburgh, Scotland.

Touraine, Alain (1981), *The Voice and the Eye: An Analysis of Social Movements*, trans. by Maison des Sciences de l'Homme and Cambridge University Press, Cambridge, Cambridge University Press.

United States Attorney General's Task Force on Family Violence (1984), *Final Report*, Washington, DC, US Department of Justice.

United States Commission on Civil Rights (1978), *Battered Women: Issues of Public Policy*, Washington DC, US Commission on Civil Rights.

United States Commission on Civil Rights (1982), *The Federal Response to Domestic Violence*, Washington DC, US Commission on Civil Rights.

Vaughan, Sharon (1987), Breaking the Silence: Voices on Battered Women. An Oral History, Radio History Series, KUOM radio, University of Minnesota, 1987, available from 728 Osceola Avenue, St Paul, MN 55105.

Walker, L.E.A. (1984), *The Battered Woman Syndrome*, New York, Springer.

Warrior, Betsy (1976), *Working on Wife Abuse*, 1st Ed., subsequent editions published annually, c/o Betsy Warrior, 46 Pleasant St., Cambridge, MA.

Wilson, Elizabeth (1983), *What is to be Done About Violence Against Women?*, Harmondsworth, Middlesex, Penguin.

Zilbergeld, B. (1983), *The Shrinking of America; Myths of Psychological Change*, Boston, Little Brown.

Name index

Subject index

229, 234, 285, 287, 289, 293, 298
diversion 152, 159, 165, 166, 167, 176, 179, 184, 197, 206, 296
Duluth/Domestic Abuse Intervention Project (DAIP) 180–6, 205, 208, 247

economic change 25, 27, 71, 75
education 25, 29
employment 68, 135
equal rights 23, 24, 74, 75, 110, 130
experts 32, 48, 144

feminism 14, 16, 17, 23, 24, 70, 72, 234, 288, 289
  liberal 23, 24, 71, 72, 74, 75
  radical 23, 24, 73, 75
  socialist 23, 24, 72, 75

health care 27, 120, 135, 143, 294
homicide 5, 6, 7, 8, 9, 202, 273–4
housing 29, 93–98, 118, 119–24, 128, 135, 142–3, 286, 294

individualism 74, 216, 221, 234
innovations 13, 28–9, 58, 110, 121, 167, 174, 212, 285

justice system 27–9, 38, 99, 206, 295–6
  criticisms of 132–3, 146, 150

Labour and left politics 23–4, 74–5
law 24–5, 27, 128, 149, 155, 295
  arrest 119, 150, 152, 163, 168–9, 180, 186–7, 198, 203, 207, 297
  civil 168, 171, 186
  compensation 168
  equal protection 132, 150–1, 198
  exclusion orders 168, 172, 186–8
  housing 93–6
  injunctions 119, 149, 151, 156, 167–8, 171, 186, 189, 191–2, 194
  interdicts 171, 186
  peace bond 154, 156, 160
  protection orders 152, 167, 168, 186

spouse abuse statutes 168
Women's Self-Defense Law Project, 228
law enforcement (*see also* police, battered-women's movement) 176, 295
laws, Britain: (1857) (1878) Matrimonial Causes Acts 156, (1976) The Domestic Violence and Matrimonial Proceedings Act 124, 170, 172, 186, 192, 193, (1978) The Domestic Proceedings and Magistrates' Court Act 124, 170, 172, (1981) The Matrimonial Homes (Family Protection) (Scotland) Act 124, 170, 188, 189, (1983) The Matrimonial Homes Act, [England and Wales] 125, 170, 172; USA: (1946) National Mental Health Act 219, (1978) The Child Abuse Prevention and Treatment Act 138, 140, 141, (1984) The Family Violence Prevention and Services Act 141, (1984) Victims of Crime Act (VOCA) 141, (1976) Pennsylvania Protection from Abuse Act 167, The Domestic Violence Prevention and Services Act [bill] 138, The Domestic Violence Prevention and Treatment Act [bill] 136, The Family Violence Prevention and Treatment Act [bill] 137
LEAA 161–2, 167, 174–6, 184–5, 205, 254
  Family Violence Program 176, 180
legal
  aid 135
  protection 136, 142–3
legal change 25, 71, 75, 112, 120, 122, 136, 142, 143, 149, 151, 153, 154, 165, 167, 189, 190, 200, 202, 204, 206, 211, 295

male violence 1, 2, 28, 29, 43, 88, 116, 119, 155, 267, 271, 273, 290

and the state 111, 136
definition of 23, 32–3, 48, 121,
    142, 159, 160, 161, 211, 221,
    225, 255, 257, 283, 293
definition of problem 115, 197,
    204, 215, 229–30, 234
nature of 2, 3, 4, 269
recognition of 15, 27, 112, 156,
    190, 255, 285, 298
sexual 270
social problem 27, 48, 120, 131
solutions 14, 23, 112, 116, 117,
    118, 119, 131, 132, 143, 149,
    150, 151, 153, 156, 159, 160,
    195, 197, 199, 211, 221, 223,
    227, 233, 234, 253, 293

victim blaming 4, 116, 120, 214,
    222, 224, 235, 237, 239, 241
worldwide 9–11

women
    changing status 21, 23–4, 28–9,
        38, 88, 120, 288, 290, 298
    subordination of 27, 38, 126,
        132, 155, 292
    violence of 259–63, 266, 267–9,
        271, 272, 274
Women's Aid (*see* battered-
    women's movement, refuge/
    shelter)
women's movement 15–17, 21–5,
    30, 57–8, 73, 139, 287, 289